Cerebral Arterial Disease

Cerebral Arterial Disease

Edited by
R. W. Ross Russell
Physician to the Department of Neurology, St Thomas' Hospital;
The National Hospital for Nervous Diseases, Queen Square; and
Moorfields Eye Hospital, City Road. London

CHURCHILL LIVINGSTONE
Edinburgh London and New York 1976

CHURCHILL LIVINGSTONE
Medical Division of Longman Group Limited

Distributed in the United States of America by Longman Inc., 19 West 44th Street, New York, N.Y. 10036 and by associated companies, branches and representatives throughout the world.

ISBN 0 443 01414 0

Library of Congress Cataloging in Publication Data
Main entry under title:

Cerebral arterial disease.

   1.   Cerebrovascular disease. I. Ross Russell, R. W.
[DNLM: 1. Cerebral artery diseases. WL355 C353]
RC388.5.C37   616.8'1   76-6504

Printed in Great Britain

Preface

There is little that the physician of today can add to the classical descriptions of the clinical and pathological effects of cerebral infarction and haemorrhage. Recent years have, however, seen advances in certain related fields which have stimulated a fresh approach to an old subject. The first of these has been the discovery of methods for the measurement of cerebral blood flow and metabolism and the large amount of subsequent research on the regulation of the cerebral circulation in health and on the disturbance which may occur in disease. Second have been the carefully planned epidemiological studies which have indicated the various genetic and environmental influences underlying vascular disease. Physicians concerned with arterial disease and with hypertension have again turned their attention to the brain where so many of the most significant lesions occur in terms of morbidity and mortality. The results of these researches are already apparent in the field of prevention.

This leads on directly to the third advance, which concerns the pathogenesis of arterial degeneration or atherosclerosis. Although many questions are still unanswered there is now a clearer understanding of the dual factors of the arterial wall and the circulating blood, and of how these relate to rupture, thrombosis and embolism.

The fourth advance is the gradual improvement in diagnostic techniques mainly in the field of angiography and more recently in the introduction of computerised axial tomography. The differentiation in life between cerebral haemorrhage and infarction, which has so long been a stumbling block in clinical management and in epidemiological studies, has been removed, leaving the way open to further progress in related conditions such as cerebral oedema and microvascular disease.

It must be admitted that these advances, although valuable as indicators of how cerebral vascular disease may be prevented, have not been matched by similar spectacular changes in the field of therapy in established stroke. In the acute stages of stroke there is a need for a critical evaluation of intensive therapy and for careful clinical studies to indicate which patients are capable of useful recovery. Once the prognosis of a severely brain damaged patient can be accurately forecast then the available resources can be applied most usefully. That intensive therapy and early intervention can have a place in cerebral vascular disease there can be no doubt, and this point is illustrated by Dr Hutchinson and Mr Richardson in acute cerebellar infarction and haemorrhage, but it is bad medicine as well as bad economics to apply intensive therapy indiscriminately.

Once the acute phase of the stroke has passed, far too often the patient survives with the quality of life severely impaired by permanent physical or mental disability, to succumb eventually to the effect of vascular disease in the brain or elsewhere. For the less severely affected patient, often in middle age, the techniques and advances in rehabilitation have attracted scant attention in the past from medical authors, and for this reason Dr Langton Hewer's chapter is given special emphasis.

Finally there is a growing awareness that cerebral arterial disease is not seen only in the setting of senescence and degenerative disease but is a frequent complicating factor in a wide variety of systemic disorders at all ages. Earlier recognition and better management of these patients can be achieved only by bringing neurology back into closer relationship with other medical disciplines.

1976   R. W. Ross Russell

Acknowledgements

Acknowledgement is gratefully made to the following for permission to reproduce material previously published elsewhere:

To Dr Shurtleff and the Department of Health, Education and Welfare for Figures 1.1 to 1.10, 1.12 to 1.14 and Tables 1.1 to 1.10, and to the U.S. Government Printing Office for Figure 1.11; to Munksgaard, Copenhagen, Publishers of *The Natural History of Acute Cerebrovascular Disease* (1969) for Figures 2.1 to 2.3; to Dr R. F. Dodson and to the Editor and Publishers of the *Journal of Neuropathology and Experimental Neurology* for Figures 4.1 and 4.2.; to Dr W. S. Fields, and to C. C. Thomas, Publishers of *Pathogenesis and Treatment of Cerebrovascular Disease* (1961) for Figure 4.3; to the Editor and Publishers of *Neurology* (Minneapolis) for Figures 4.4 to 4.6 and 5.3; to Dr E. Stoica and colleagues for Figure 4.6; to Dr N. A. Lassen for Figure 5.1; to Drs M. E. Raichle and H. L. Stone and the Editor and Publishers of *European Neurology* for Figure 5.2; to Dr J. Gawler for Figure 6.5; to Dr M. Gross and the Editor and Publishers of *Traité de Radio Diagnostic* for Figure 6.6.; to Dr G. D. Friedman and colleagues and the Editor and Publishers of the *Journal of the American Medical Association* for Table 7.1; to Dr J. W. D. Bull for Figure 7.1D; to Dr G. Frank for Table 7.3; to Dr M. J. G. Harrison, Professor J. Marshall and the Editor and Publishers of the *British Medical Journal* for Table 7.2; to Dr W. K. Hass and colleagues and to the Editor and Publishers of the *Journal of the American Medical Association* for Figure 7.2; to Dr F. B. Byrom and to Wm. Heinemann Limited, Publishers, for Figure 10.4; to Dr C. M. Fisher, and to the Editor and Publishers of *Acta Neuropathologica* (Berlin) for Figures 10.9 and 10.14; to Dr H. B. Locksley, and to the Editor and Publishers of the *Journal of Neurosurgery* for Figures 12.1, 12.2 and 12.5; to Dr E. C. Alvord and the Editor and Publishers of *Archives of Neurology* (Chicago) for Figure 12.2, and Tables 12.3 and 12.4; to Professor V. Logue for Figure 12.6; to Dr W. E. Hunt and Dr. R. M. Hess for Table 12.2; to Dr C. H. Millikan and the Publishers of *Stroke* for Figures 13.5 and 7.3.; to Dr G. H. duBoulay for Figures 14.1, 14.4 and 14.6; to Dr Athasit Vejjejiva for Figure 14.3; to Dr M. Lea Thomas for Figure 14.2; to Dr B. E. Kendall for Figure 14.7; to Dr L. Jorgensen and Dr A. Torvik and the Editor and Publishers of the *Journal of Neurological Sciences* for Table 14.1.

My especial thanks are also due to Professor G. H. duBoulay for his valuable advice on Chapter 14 and in the selection of radiographs, and to Mrs Marion Greenwood and Miss Beryl Łaatz for unstinted secretarial help.

Contributors

M. Rufus Crompton
St. George's Hospital, London SW1X7EZ

Vinod D. Deshmukh
Baylor College of Medicine, Houston, Texas 77025, U.S.A.

Cesare Fieschi
Department of Neurology, University of Siena, Italy

J. C. Gautier
Hôpital de a Salpêtrière, 47 Bd. d l'hôpital, 75364 Paris, France

M. J. G. Harrison
The Middlesex Hospital, London W1P7PN

R. Langton Hewer
Frenchay Hospital, Bristol BS1 61LE

E. C. Hutchinson
North Staffordshire Royal Infirmary, Stoke-on-Trent ST47LM

William B. Kannel
National Heart and Lung Institute, National Institutes of Health, Bethesda, Md., U.S.A.

Jørgen Marquardsen
Fredriksberg Hospital, Copenhagen, Denmark

John Marshall
Institute of Neurology, The National Hospital for Nervous Diseases, Queen Square, London WC1N3BG

John Stirling Meyer
Baylor College of Medicine, Houston, Texas 77025, U.S.A.

Alan Richardson
Atkinson Morley's Hospital (St. George's Hospital) London SW20ONE

Michel Des Rosiers
National Institute of Mental Health, Bethesda, Md., U.S.A.

R. W. Ross Russell
The National Hospital for Nervous Diseases, Queen Square, London WC1N3BG
St. Thomas' Hospital, London SE17EH

Lindsay Symon
The National Hospital for Nervous Diseases, Queen Square, London WC1N3BG

K. M. A. Welch
Baylor College of Medicine, Houston, Texas 77025, U.S.A.

Contents

1. Epidemiology of Cerebrovascular Disease

William B. Kannel

There is general agreement that atherosclerotic cardiovascular disease is foremost among the health problems in affluent countries. Atherothrombotic brain infarction (ABI), although not as lethal as coronary heart disease, is nevertheless the most devastating manifestation of atherosclerosis, for it may rob its victims of their dignity, physical prowess, ability to communicate, and independence.

A review of the epidemiology of cerebrovascular disease, relying heavily on Framingham Study data, reveals that it is a sizeable but predictable force of cardiovascular morbidity. Uncertain diagnosis, vagaries in case finding, reliance on retrospective data and on indirect evidence have led to some confusion and contradictory reports. Nevertheless, numbers of major factors contributing to the incidence of strokes, particularly to atherothrombotic brain infarction, the most common variety, have been identified. Prospective epidemiological investigations have established the major precursors as: hypertension, cardiac impairment, impaired glucose tolerance, a high normal blood haemoglobin, the cigarette habit (in men), lipid abnormalities (under age 55), and other clinical evidence of atherosclerosis such as coronary heart disease or transient cerebral ischaemic attacks (Council on Cerebrovascular Disease, 1971). Using some of these to formulate a stroke risk profile it is possible to identify, while still asymptomatic, a tenth of the general population, from which about half the ABIs will emerge, thus providing a basis for prevention.

From data provided by Framingham and other prospective studies information has been gleaned on the incidence of stroke in the general population, the way it evolves, hallmarks of vulnerability, clues to pathogenesis, a profile of the potential candidate, and the disability and mortality following the stroke. Each of these features of the epidemiology of ABI will be explored.

Over the past two decades at Framingham, a cohort of 5209 men and women aged 30 to 62 at entry to the study in 1949 were classified at entry and biennially thereafter according to a variety of personal attributes and living habits. These were then examined in relation to the subsequent rate of development of clinical manifestations of atherosclerosis, including ABI. Criteria, methods of examination, and sampling procedures have been described in detail elsewhere (Shurtleff, 1970; Gordon, Sorlie, and Kannel, 1971). Follow-up of this representative population sample has been reasonably complete over the 18 years of follow-up herein reported, with about 85 per cent receiving every possible biennial examination; the rest have been seen at less frequent intervals. Admissions to the only hospital in town have been monitored daily. Only 2 per cent of the population have been completely lost to follow-up. Hospitalised cases and those examined in the clinic suspected of a stroke have in recent years been examined by a neurologist assigned to the study (Shurtleff, 1974).

EPIDEMIOLOGIC ASSESSMENT OF THE STROKE ENTITY

There is reason to believe that not all strokes have the same epidemiologic features, and the four major stroke entities must be distinguished: atherothrombotic brain infarction, intracerebral haemorrhage, subarachnoid haemorrhage, and cerebral embolism. Also, to gain a better understanding of atherothrombotic strokes and their natural history it is desirable to identify those due to extracranial vascular disease, those due to lesions in the small penetrating branches in the brain substances (lacunar strokes), and those due to major intracerebral arterial lesions (Fisher, 1968). These are often difficult to distinguish on clinical grounds alone. Since transient ischaemic cerebral attacks and permanent brain infarction may occur without vascular occlusion, may be caused by emboli from proximal atherothrombotic lesions, or may result from ill-defined lesions in the smaller penetrating branches, the term 'cerebral thrombosis' seems inappropriate. It should fall into disuse as has the term 'coronary thrombosis'.

Although now accorded an important role in the development of strokes, the contribution of atherosclerosis of extracranial arteries is difficult to evaluate because it so often co-exists with intracranial arterial disease, because it requires invasive procedures to demonstrate it accurately, and because it is commonly found in asymptomatic persons. Consequently, the risk of an ABI in persons with asymptomatic stenosis of extracranial cerebral arterial stenosis is unknown, as are its precursors. In such persons with transient cerebral ischaemic attacks the incidence of ABI has been estimated to be about 5 per cent (Martin, Whisnant, and Sayre, 1960; Acheson and Hutchinson, 1964; Fields *et al.*, 1970), but this is based only on selected clinical cases and not general population surveys.

The lacunar stroke described by Fisher is not to be confused with the 'lacunar state' often incorrectly used to describe progressive intellectual impairment in the elderly in the absence of discrete episodes of focal neurologic deficit. Fisher (1968) has described focal neurological deficits, abrupt in onset, which he has demonstrated to be associated with lacunes deep within the brain. These are manifested clinically as a pure motor hemiparesis, a pure sensory stroke, crural paresis with homolateral ataxia, or dysarthria with clumsiness of one hand. In Framingham, careful neurological evaluation revealed that 13 per cent of ABIs in men and 23 per cent in women could, by these criteria, be attributed to lacunar pathology.

Epidemiological investigation of cerebral embolism is also a somewhat speculative enterprise. The condition is most accurately diagnosed in younger persons with a clear source for emboli from the heart and accompanying evidence of extracerebral emboli. It is probably overdiagnosed in older persons with established atrial fibrillation due to hypertensive or ischaemic heart disease. In other circumstances it is very likely to be underdiagnosed, for post-mortem dissections have recently suggested that as many as half of ostensibly thrombotic strokes may be embolic, derived from proximal atherothrombotic lesions (Jorgensen and Torvik, 1966). From an epidemiologic point of view this is not a serious drawback since atherosclerosis in the vessels of the neck probably has the same precursors as that occurring within the cranium.

Intracerebral haemorrhage is usually clinically distinguishable from subarachnoid haemorrhage and from ABI, but since it is relatively infrequent, prospective epidemiological data concerning intracranial haemorrhage are sparse.

Frequency of strokes by type

Difficulties in diagnosis constitute a major obstacle to obtaining a consistent picture of the epidemiologic features of stroke, particularly from mortality data. Review of death certificate data gives undue prominence to intracerebral haemorrhage because of its high case fatality rate and grossly underestimates the occurrence of subarachnoid haemorrhage and 'cerebral thrombosis' (Kurtze, 1968). Because they contain all the cases, living as well as dead, hospitalised or not, prospective population data such as that from Framingham provide less distorted information on the relative frequency of each variety of stroke. These data reveal that the preponderance of strokes in the general population are ABIs—almost 60 per cent (Table 1.1). This is true even in those occurring under age 55. Subarachnoid haemorrhages seem to be more common in men. In the Framingham cohort, strokes resulting from emboli arising in the heart were about as frequent in men as in women, particularly before age 55. Intracranial bleeding resulted twice as frequently from subarachnoid haemorrhage (about 10 per cent) as from intracerebral haemorrhage (about 5 per cent). Only 10 per cent of cerebrovascular disease in men

Table 1.1 Relative frequency of various types of cerebrovascular disease, men and women, 30 to 60. (Framingham Study: 18 year follow-up).

Type of stroke	30–54 Men No.	30–54 Men %	30–54 Women No.	30–54 Women %	55–62 Men No.	55–62 Men %	55–62 Women No.	55–62 Women %
Atherothrombotic brain infarction[a]	38	53	14	53	32	55	27	69
Transient ischaemic attack[a]	6	8	2	8	3	5	–	–
Lacunar stroke[a]	2	3	1	4	2	3	4	10
Cerebral embolus	9	12	4	15	12	20	5	13
Subarachroid haemorrhage	10	14	2	8	9	15	3	8
Intracerebral haemorrhage	4	6	2	8	2	3	2	5
Other	5	7	2	8	1	2	2	5

[a]Number of initial strokes with TIA, ABI, and lacunar strokes may overlap and are not mutually exclusive.

and 8 per cent in women manifested itself as transient cerebral ischaemic attacks. In Framingham 14 per cent of ABIs in men and 12 per cent in women were preceded by definite transient cerebral ischaemic attacks. If less definite attacks are included, the proportion rises to 24 and 20 per cent, respectively. The 13 per cent of ABIs in men and 23 per cent in women which were designated as lacunar strokes constituted too small a number to allow a determination of their epidemiologic features, and they are included with the ABIs.

Similar prospective epidemiologic data are needed from other, less affluent areas of the world where intracerebral haemorrhage is said to predominate. Because of diagnostic difficulties and lack of sufficient information, this report will focus on the antecedents and evolution of ABI.

Incidence

It is estimated that there are about half a million new strokes and 200 000 deaths annually from atherosclerotic brain infarction in the U.S.A., comprising 11 per cent of the total mortality (National Heart and Lung Institute, 1971). However, death certificate data classified by underlying cause are likely to underestimate cerebrovascular disease as a contributor to mortality by about half. Of all the deaths in the Framingham cohort, stroke was listed as the cause by the attending physician in 5 per cent of men and 8 per cent of women, whereas a stroke occurred in 15 per cent. Based on Framingham data the chances of an ABI before age 70 are 1 in 20. Although strokes primarily afflict the elderly, one-fifth occur in persons under 65. There was no striking difference in the average age of occurrence of ABI com-

Table 1.2 Average age at occurrence of different types of stroke. Men and women aged 30 to 62 at entry, followed for two decades.

Type of stroke	Men No.	Men Mean age	Men s.d.	Women No.	Women Mean age	Women s.d.
Atherothrombotic brain infarction	83	64.6	8.4	91	66.4	8.8
Transient ischaemic attack	14	63.2	8.3	12	67.1	8.9
Cerebral embolus	21	62.5	9.2	22	66.8	8.6
Subarachnoid haemorrhage	13	59.4	10.1	18	62.5	10.1
Intracerebral haemorrhage	9	63.1	10.1	5	67.5	10.6
Other	4	61.3	4.8	4	58.8	14.4

Note: Age composition of the two sexes in the cohort is roughly equivalent, consisting largely of married couples.

pared to other types of stroke. In this cohort, originally aged 30 to 62 and followed for two decades, the average age of each major type of stroke was slightly greater in women than men, and this cannot be accounted for by differences in age distribution in the two sexes in the sample (Table 1.2).

The incidence of ABI, as expected, increases sharply with age in both sexes but without the anticipated male predominance (Fig. 1.1). Curiously, ABI is the only one of the major clinical manifestations of atherosclerosis which fails to afflict men in preference to women. In women the incidence of brain and myocardial infarctions is at all ages virtually identical. In men, on the other hand, there is a distinct prediliction for myocardial infarction at all ages (Fig. 1.1). The

PREMORBID FACTORS

Coronary heart disease frequently occurs in persons who appear to be well. This is not the case in ABI, where about 70 per cent had established hypertension and 20 per cent had advanced to the point where there was ECG evidence of left ventricular hypertrophy (ECG–LVH). About 30 per cent had co-existing coronary heart disease, 15 per cent congestive heart failure, 30 per cent occlusive peripheral arterial disease, and 15 per cent were under treatment for diabetes. About 13 per cent of the strokes were preceded by transient ischaemic attacks.

Before overt disease processes appear, a number of features presaging stroke can be discerned. Chief among these are the blood pres-

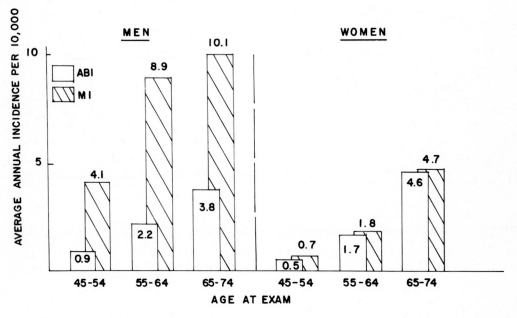

Fig. 1.1   Incidence of atherothrombotic brain infarction vs. myocardial infarction in each sex. Men and women, 45 to 74. (Framingham Study: 18 year follow-up).

greater immunity of women to coronary than to cerebral atherosclerosis may stem from the later onset and slower progress of atherosclerosis in the cerebral than in the coronary vessels. It apparently does not reach major proportions in the cerebral vessels until women have already lost their premenopausal immunity.

sure, the blood lipids, and impaired carbohydrate tolerance.

BLOOD PRESSURE
Evaluation of the various personal attributes and environmental factors which are known to contribute to the occurrence of strokes in general

and ABIs in particular leads to the inescapable conclusion that hypertension plays a dominant role (Table 1.3). Judging from the size of its multivariate regression coefficient (taking into account the effect of other co-existing major contributors to ABI) and after standardisation to allow for different units of measurement it is clear that blood pressure is the most powerful precursor of ABI (Table 1.4). Not only is hypertension the most potent contributor to ABI incidence but it is also a highly prevalent one afflicting 20 per cent of the adult U.S. population (National Center for Health Statistics, 1974). Since it is readily detected and in most instances easily controlled, the practising physician can in

Table 1.3 Logistic regression of two year ABI incidence on various risk characteristics. Men and women, 45 to 74. (Framingham Study: 18 year follow-up).

	Average standardised univariate regression coefficient	
Characteristics	Men	Women
Systolic blood pressure	0.694	0.688
Serum cholesterol	0.274	0.127[a]
Phospholipid	0.267	−0.057[a]
Blood sugar	0.200	0.223
Relative weight	0.162[a]	0.436
Vital capacity height	−0.258[a]	−0.215[a]
Cigarettes	0.308	−0.016[a]
Cardiac enlargement (X-ray)	0.242	0.555
ECG–LVH	0.513	0.480
Non-specific ECG abnormality	0.270	0.317

[a]Coefficient not statistically significant at a 0.05 level.

Table 1.4 Standardised multivariate regression coefficients of six specified contributors to incidence of atherothrombotic brain infarction. (Framingham Study: 18-year follow-up).

	Coefficient		T-value	
	Men	Women	Men	Women
Systolic blood pressure	0.619	0.501	5.57	4.62
Age	0.545	0.537	3.65	3.67
Serum cholesterol	0.210	0.109	1.62	0.85
Cigarettes	0.441	−0.011	3.01	−0.07
LVH by ECG	0.108	0.221	1.30	3.63
Glucose intolerance	0.052	0.150	0.45	1.81

Note: Persons at risk of developing atherothrombotic brain infarction are those persons aged 45 to 74 years and free of cerebrovascular accident at exam.

theory make a substantial impact on stroke incidence. There is evidence from controlled clinical trials that early, vigorous, and sustained control of hypertension with antihypertensive agents does indeed prevent strokes (Veterans Administration Cooperative Study Group,1967, 1970). This warrants a detailed examination of the role of blood pressure in the development of ABI, in order to clarify the indications for therapy. Categorically speaking 'hypertensives' develop about seven times as many strokes as do 'normotensives' (Shurtleff, 1970; Gordon *et al.*, 1971). Such arbitrary designations of 'hypertension' (usually greater than 160/95 mmHg) by and large identify persons at high risk, but the risk of ABI is related to the height of the blood pressure not only among hypertensives but throughout the range of blood pressure (Fig. 1.2). No discernible critical value of either systolic or diastolic blood pressure demarcates the stroke candidate from the general population (Table 1.5). Risk is simply proportional to blood pressure, at any age in either sex (Fig. 1.3).

There is no evidence to support the clinical teaching that the risk of stroke derives chiefly from the diastolic component of the blood pressure. Examination of the gradients of risk of ABI over 18 years in the Framingham cohort classified at each biennial examination by their systolic and by their diastolic pressure reveals nothing to suggest a closer association with diastolic than with systolic pressure. This is also evident from multivariate analysis taking into account other components of the pressure. This multivariate analysis, considering net and joint effects, reveals that risk of ABI is most closely linked to the systolic or mean arterial pressure. Neither pulse pressure, lability of pressure, nor tension–time index (systolic pressure × heart rate) adds appreciably to risk calculated from systolic pressure alone (Table 1.5). Thus, the simple casual systolic blood pressure appears as good a predictor of ABI incidence in populations as does any other component or derivative of blood pressure.

There is no direct evidence from Framingham which bears on the importance of *isolated* systolic hypertension in elderly persons. Indirect

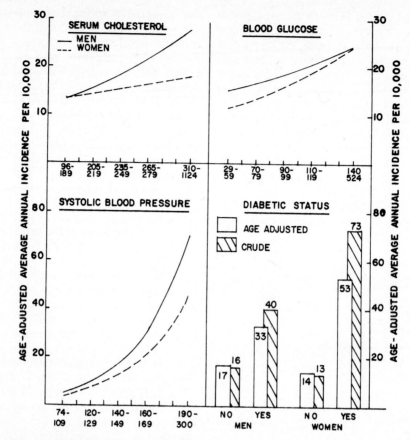

Fig. 1.2   Risk of atherothrombotic brain infarction according to atherogenic traits at biennial exam. Men and women, 45 to 74. (Framingham Study: 18 year follow-up).

evidence, however, does not support the contention that the disproportionate rise in systolic pressure which accompanies ageing (and is attributed to inelastic vasculature) is innocuous. There is no decrease in the influence of systolic pressure with advancing age (Fig. 1.3).

A recent prospective study of isolated systolic hypertension in the elderly provides more direct evidence that this predisposes to strokes (Colandrea et al., 1970). However, only a clinical trial

Table 1.5   Risk of ABI according to various components of blood pressure. Likelihood ratio statistic for logistic function. Bivariate analysis, men and women, 45 to 74. (Framingham Study: 18 year follow-up).

| | Chi-squares −2 degrees of freedom | | | | | |
| | Men | | | Women | | |
	45–54	55–64	65–74	45–54	55–64	65–74
Systolic blood pressure (SBP) and pulse pressure	10.06	24.46	5.63	10.68	13.68	12.55
SBP^1 and SBP^2 and liability SBP	10.41	28.19	5.00	10.34	14.66	10.73
Systolic blood pressure and tension time index	10.06	23.68	5.24	10.63	13.24	7.71
Systolic blood pressure alone	9.96	22.56	4.80	10.05	13.11	7.62
Population (P-Y)/cases	4708/8	3431/12	1500/11	5858/6	4559/18	2092/22

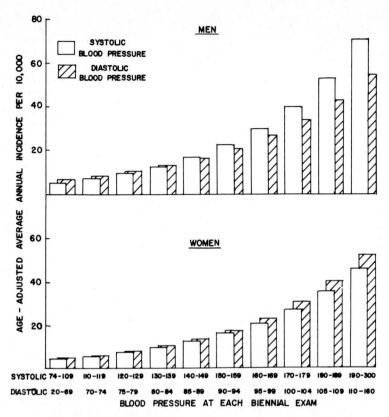

Fig. 1.3   Incidence of atherothrombotic brain infarction according to systolic vs. diastolic blood pressure at biennial exam. Men and women, 45 to 74 (Framingham Study: 18 year follow-up).

of antihypertensive therapy in such persons can settle whether the fault lies in the systolic pressure or the rigidity of the vessel.

It is apparent that blood pressure makes an independent contribution to risk, and substantial risk gradients proportional to blood pressure level are present in otherwise high- and low-risk subjects (Fig. 1.3). Blood pressure is the strongest independent contributor to ABI risk (Table 1.4) as judged from multivariate regression coefficients, and those with moderate hypertension who are in jeopardy from a stroke may be distinguished from those in need of surveillance only by taking into account associated risk characteristics (Fig. 1.4).

It is a common belief that women, particularly in the postmenopausal state, tolerate hypertension better than men. As regards risk of ABI, there is no evidence that either the relative or absolute risk is substantially different in the sexes (Fig. 1.3). Despite lack of controlled trials in women, it seems unwise to withhold antihypertensive treatment from them, even after the menopause.

BLOOD LIPIDS

A considerable body of evidence has accumulated linking blood lipids with accelerated atherogenesis. Evidence implicating blood lipids and particularly cholesterol in the development of coronary heart disease is substantial and quite consistent. Evidence incriminating lipids in the development of cerebrovascular disease is more fragmentary and inconclusive (Meyer *et al.*, 1959; Paterson, Dyer, and Armstrong, 1960; Robinson, Higano, and Cohen, 1963;

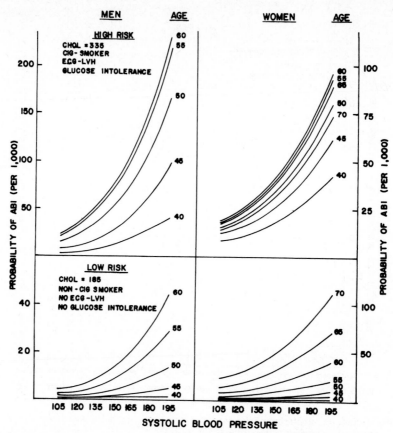

Fig. 1.4   Risk of atherothrombotic brain infarction in 8 years according to systolic blood pressure in each sex. (Framingham Study: 18 year follow-up).

Cumings *et al.*, 1967). Prospective data in particular are quite sparse.

The association of blood lipids with ABI incidence in the Framingham cohort is considerably weaker than for coronary heart disease (Shurtleff, 1970; Gordon *et al.*, 1971). A relationship can be demonstrated only in persons having premature strokes whose lipids are examined before the age of 55. Below this age, but not above it, risk of ABI is related to the concentration both of the cholesterol-rich beta lipoprotein and the triglyceride-rich pre-beta lipoprotein in the blood (Fig. 1.5). Even here, the relationship is statistically significant only for men. The same is true for serum cholesterol where a statistically significant gradient of risk proportional to the level of the lipid can be demonstrated only

for men in the age range of 45 to 54 years (Fig. 1.6).

Accurate methods for measuring triglyceride were developed too recently to allow direct assessment of its role in the development of ABI in the Framingham cohort. However, its effect may be inferred from the S_f 20-400 pre-beta lipoprotein data, since endogenous triglyceride is carried chiefly in this lipoprotein fraction. Despite the fact that these were non-fasting values, it can be seen that there is indeed an association of this lipid with premature ABI incidence (Fig. 1.5). However, from multivariate analysis to determine the net effect of each lipid (taking other risk factors into account as well) only cholesterol appears to make an independent contribution to risk (Fig. 1.7).

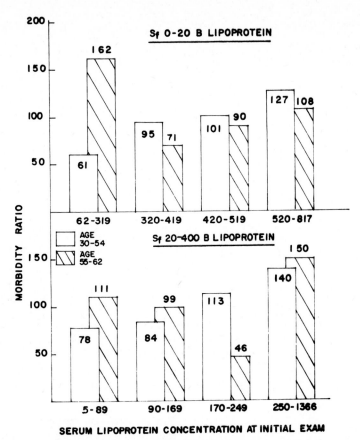

Fig. 1.5 Risk of atherothrombotic brain infarction according to lipoprotein concentration. Men and women, 30 to 62, at entry. (Framingham Study: 18 year follow-up).

More prospective data from other sources are required to determine if these findings, which are based on rather sparse data in this age group, hold up. However, the findings are consistent with those for coronary heart disease, where more adequate data are available. The lack of a relationship of serum cholesterol to ABI incidence beyond age 55 seems reasonable since it has been found that in coronary heart disease the risk associated with cholesterol wanes with advancing age (Shurtleff, 1970; Gordon *et al.*, 1971). Failure to demonstrate a statistically significant association between ABI incidence and cholesterol level in women is very likely a consequence of the small number of premature strokes in this cohort.

However, even in men aged 50, the computed probability of a stroke in relation to serum cholesterol is relatively slight in the absence of other contributors to ABI incidence, particularly hypertension. At any level of blood lipid risk varies profoundly depending on the level of other stroke precursors (Fig. 1.8).

IMPAIRED CARBOHYDRATE TOLERANCE

Although considerably less potent than blood pressure in its impact on ABI incidence, impaired glucose tolerance is a significant contri-

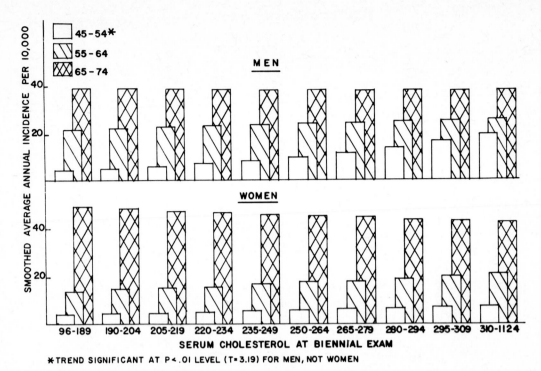

Fig. 1.6   Incidence of atherothrombotic brain infarction according to serum cholesterol at specified ages in each sex. Men and women, 45 to 74. (Framingham Study: 18 year follow-up).

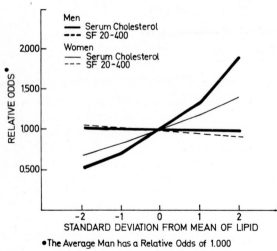

Fig. 1.7   Relative odds of ABI according to lipids (multivariate). (Framingham Study: 18 year follow-up).

butor (Table 1.3). The gradient of risk is more pronounced in women than men and is proportional to the blood glucose value (Fig. 1.2), and there may be some unique effect (Fig. 1.9). Either as a consequence of a greater impairment of carbohydrate tolerance, a different type of metabolic aberration, or as the result of treatment, the insulin-treated diabetics were at greatest risk (Garcia *et al.*, 1973).

CARDIAC PRECURSORS

In addition to reflecting sustained hypertension and its damaging effects on the vascular system, it seems that poor cardiac function directly precipitates strokes. Not only does overt congestive failure and coronary heart disease contribute to stroke incidence, but more subtle evidences of cardiac impairment do as well (Fig. 1.10). Cardiac enlargement on X-ray, and ECG abnormalities such as left ventricular enlargement, intraventricular conduction disturbances, and even non-specific S-T and T-wave abnormalities are all associated with a substantially increased risk (Fig. 1.10). These cardiac impairments exert an influence independent of the hypertension with which they are

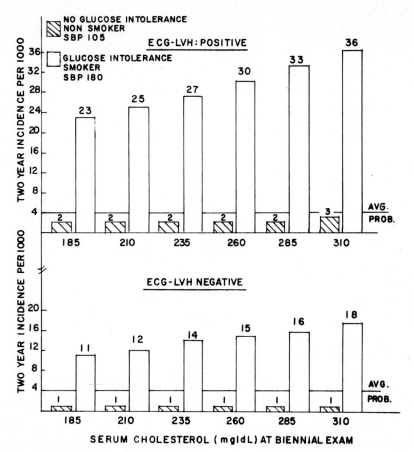

Fig. 1.8   Two-year probability of atherothrombotic brain infarction according to serum cholesterol and other risk factors. Men, aged 60. (Framingham Study: 18 year follow-up).

often associated (Wolf *et al.*, 1973). Three of every four stroke victims have one or more of these cardiac impairments, and it is cardiac disease, particularly coronary disease, which is chiefly responsible for mortality following a stroke (Table 1.6).

Other cardiac disorders, such as chronic rheumatic valvular disease, subacute bacterial endocarditis, acute myocardial infarction, congenital heart defects, and dysrhythmias such as atrial fibrillation and complete heart block, are also reported to be associated with an increased risk of stroke, including ABI. Stroke is also an important complication of prosthetic heart valves. Data from Framingham are too sparse to provide accurate estimates of the risk from

these cardiac causes. Strokes of this type are more likely to be embolic in origin than to be caused by occlusions *in situ*; they do not account for a sizeable proportion of ABIs.

Table 1.6   Survival after initial ABI. Men and women 30 to 62 on entry.

Years after diagnosis	Proportion Surviving			
	Men		Women	
	All ABI	Excluding CHD & CHF	All ABI	Excluding CHD & CHF
0	78.8	95.2	86.8	95.8
2	66.7	83.3	81.2	91.0
4	58.3	74.1	75.5	78.9

CHD = Coronary heart disease.
CHF = Congestive heart failure.

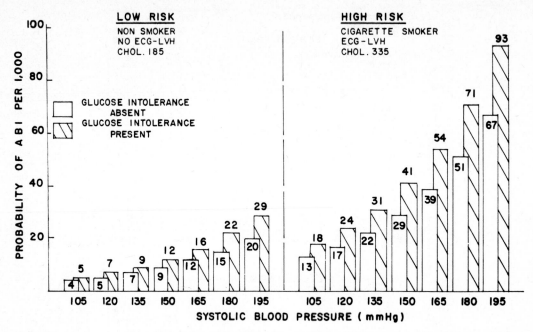

Fig. 1.9   Risk of atherothrombotic brain infarction in eight years according to diabetic status and level of other risk factors; 55-year-old women. (Framingham Study: 18 year follow-up).

Systemic disease

Strokes occurring under age 45 are decidedly infrequent in the general population, and unusual causes such as polycythemia vera, leukemia, macroglobulinemia, hypertensive encephalopathy, severe diabetes, and subacute bacterial endocarditis must be sought. These were rare in the Framingham cohort precluding reliable estimates of the risk entailed.

An increased propensity to strokes has been noted to occur in persons with polycythemia vera. It is interesting to note that in the Framingham cohort risk of an ABI was proportional to the blood haemoglobin value *within the normal range* of values (Kannel *et al.*, 1972). Those in the upper end of the distribution developed about twice as many strokes as did those with lower haemoglobin values (Fig. 1.11). The mechanism is obscure but it is interesting to note that there is a modest correlation between blood haemoglobin and blood pressure, and when allowance is made for the associated hypertension only a small residual independent

effect of haemoglobin is discernible (Kannel *et al.*, 1972).

Young women taking oral contraceptives sometimes exhibit an alarming rise in atherogenic traits such as blood lipids, blood glucose, and blood pressure (Weir, Briggs, and Mack, 1974) as well as enhanced blood coagulation (Medical Letter on Drugs & Therapeutics, 1974; Inman and Vessey, 1968; Vessey and Doll, 1968). There is some evidence to suggest that their risk of strokes is increased (Heyman *et al.*, 1969; Collaborative Group for the Study of Stroke in Young Women, 1973). However, while the relative risk may be high (4- to 11-fold) the absolute risk is small (Heyman *et al.*, 1969; Collaborative Group for the Study of Stroke in Young Women, 1973; Sartwell *et al.*, 1969; Boston Collaborative Surveillance Program, 1973). The tendency to thrombosis appears to be related to the dose of estrogen in the oral contraceptive, and those which contain only progestin, while slightly less effective contraceptives, provide a safer alternative. Progestin therapy or a differ-

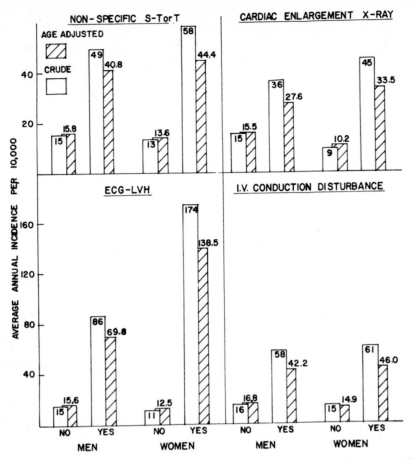

Fig. 1.10   Risk of atherothrombotic brain infarction according to X-ray and ECG cardiac impairments. Men and women, 45 to 74. (Framingham Study: 18 year follow-up).

ent method of contraception would seem prudent in women who develop atherogenic traits while on estrogen-containing oral contraceptives. Women with a history of thromboembolic disease, migraine, hypertension, diabetes, or hyperlipidemia should also be encouraged to use other methods of contraception.

It has been alleged that premature surgical menopause may predispose to stroke in women (Robinson et al., 1959). Although definitive studies have not been completed, about 26 per cent of menopauses in women who developed a stroke in Framingham were surgical, compared to 30 per cent in the general population, providing little support for this claim.

Environmental factors

Few potent environmental contributors to stroke incidence have been found despite the reported sizeable geographic differences in stroke mortality (Stallones, 1965; Goldberg and Kurland, 1962; Baker et al., 1967; Gifford, 1966; Williams, Resch, and Loewenson, 1969; World Health Organization, 1969) and the seasonal (McDonnell, Louis, and Manohan, 1970) and secular trends (Kuller et al., 1968) in stroke incidence. The cigarette habit (Jorgensen et al., 1966; Kurtze, 1968) and living habits which promote obesity (Gordon and Kannel, 1973) appear to have some influence. Diet, salt intake,

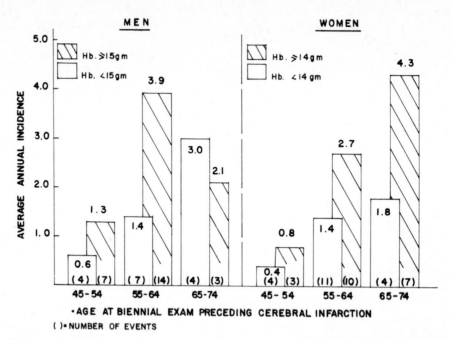

Fig. 1.11   Average annual incidence of cerebral infarction according to antecedent haemoglobin. Men and women, 45 to 74. (Framingham Study: 16 year follow-up).

hardness of water (Schroeder, 1960; Crawford, Gardner, and Morris, 1968), alcohol, psychosocial factors (Paffenbarger and Wing, 1967) and physical activity (Paffenbarger *et al.*, 1970) have yet to be convincingly connected with stroke incidence.

The role of *cigarettes* in the development of ABI and the mechanism involved require further evaluation. In the Framingham cohort men who smoked heavily developed almost three times as many strokes as did non-smokers (Table 1.7). In women no relationship was noted. Among men the impact was strongest in the youngest group (Schroeder, 1960; Crawford, Gardner, and Morris, 1968; Paffenbarger and Wing, 1967; Paffenbarger *et al.*, 1970; Klassen, Lowenson, and Resch, 1974; Dawber, Kannel, and Gordon, 1974; Foder, Pfeiffer, and Papezik, 1971; Katsuki and Hirota, 1966; McGee, 1973; Gresham *et al.*, 1973), waned with advancing age, and increased with the number of cigarettes smoked per day (Shurtleff, 1970; Gordon *et al.*, 1971), and in multivariate analysis had a significant independent effect taking

other factors into account (Table 1.4). In young men, heavy smokers (>20 cigarettes/day) had a doubled risk of ABI at any level of blood pressure. The mechanism by which smoking enhances risk of stroke in men is uncertain. Rather than promoting atherogenesis, it more probably precipitates strokes in susceptible subjects who have a compromised cerebral circulation by enhancing platelet aggregation, raising carboxyhaemoglobin values, or increasing myocardial irritability (National Heart and Lung Institute, 1971).

Even in coronary heart disease where the effect of cigarettes is more pronounced, it also wanes with advancing age and applies more strongly to men (Shurtleff, 1970; Gordon *et al.*, 1971). Studies of male college graduates (Paffenbarger *et al.*, 1967) and U.S. Veterans (Kahn, 1966) have also shown an increased mortality from ABI in cigarette smokers but have failed to demonstrate a clear relationship to the intensity of the habit.

An association between obesity and ABI has not been firmly established (Klassen *et al.*, 1974).

Table 1.7   Average annual incidence of ABI according to cigarette habit. Men and women, 45 to 74. (Framingham Study: 18 year follow-up).

Cigarettes per day	Person–years at risk	No. of ABI events	Crude Rate/10 000 Actual	Crude Rate/10 000 Smoothed	Age-adjusted rate/10 000[a]
Men					
None	12544	18	14	13.9	11.3
<20	4336	6	14	16.7	15.6
20	5710	12	21	20.0	21.4
>20	5398	13	24	24.0	29.3
Women					
None	23716	46	19	17.7	16.2
<20	7162	2	3	13.0	14.7
20	3808	6	16	9.5	13.4
>20	1636	2	12	7.0	12.1

Trend in:
  [a]Univariate:
        Men: $T = 2.62$
        Women: $T = -0.50$
    [b]Multivariate: (Takes into account age, systolic blood pressure, cholesterol, glucose, ECG–LVH)
        Men: $T = 3.01$
        Women: $T = -0.07$

In the Framingham cohort obesity is weakly related to ABI incidence, but the effect is significant and sizeable only in women (Fig. 1.12). The effect appears to derive from the fact that obesity generates atherosclerotic traits, notably hypertension. Multivariate coefficients are substantially lower than univariate indicating that most of its effect is mediated through other risk factors (Table 1.8). However, to the extent that obesity promotes these atherogenic traits it is a contributor to ABI incidence. Autopsy studies have shown findings consistent with this statement (Kahn, 1966).

Despite adverse effects on serum lipids and on the myocardium reported in alcoholics the usual range of alcohol consumed in the Framingham cohort was unrelated to ABI incidence (Fig. 1.13). Although a modest trend was noted in men, it was not statistically significant. In women, no trend was observed. Likewise, coffee intake was unrelated to ABI incidence in either sex (Dawber et al, in press).

Table 1.8   Regression of atherothrombotic brain infarction incidence on relative weight. Men and women, 45 to 74. (Framingham Study: 18 year follow-up).

	Men			Women		
	Regression coefficient	s.e.	T-value	Regression coefficient	s.e.	T-value
45–54	0.006	0.018	0.32	0.031	0.008	3.87
55–64	0.022	0.013	1.73	0.017	0.007	2.41
65–74	−0.007	0.017	−0.41	0.011	0.008	1.26
Average all ages	0.010	0.009	1.14	0.020	0.004	4.36
Univariate	0.008	0.009	0.91	0.019	0.004	4.46
Bivariate[a]	0.010	0.009	1.13	0.018	0.005	3.94
Multivariate[b]	0.003	0.009	0.35	0.009	0.005	1.76

[a]Bivariate = Metropolitan relative weight and age.
[b]Multivariate = Relative weight, age, systolic blood pressure, serum cholesterol, glucose tolerance, cigarette habit, and ECG–LVH.

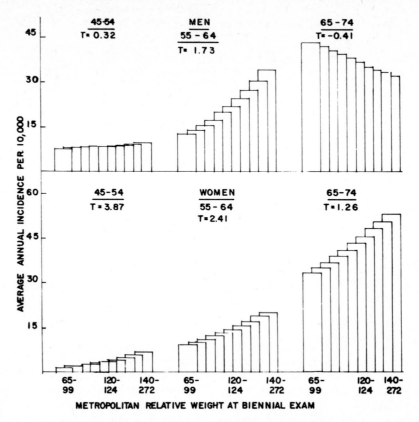

Fig. 1.12   Risk of atherothrombotic brain infarction according to relative weight. Men and women, 45 to 74. (Framingham Study: 18 year follow-up).

A role of personality, life style, and work pattern has been suggested (Paffenbarger and Wing, 1967). The reported lower incidence of strokes in the summer months may be a clue to factors which precipitate strokes in susceptible persons (McDonnell *et al.*, 1970). More rigorously designed studies are needed to evaluate the relation of the quality of drinking water to stroke incidence. A belt of high stroke mortality has been noted along the eastern coast of the U.S.A., an area characterised by soft drinking water (Foder *et al.*, 1971).

The incidence of strokes due to intracranial haemorrhage and infarction seems to be distinctly higher in some populations than others (Katsuki *et al.*, 1966), and within the U.S.A. in some areas than others. The reason for this is obscure, and differences in diagnostic sophistica-

tion, hospital admission practices, genetics, and death certification practices, as well as the prevalence of hypertension, all seem to be involved. Accepted at face value mortality from intracerebral haemorrhage has been declining while that from cerebral infarction has been rising (Katsuki *et al.*, 1966). The secular and geographic differences suggest powerful environmental influences at work. They have not yet been identified.

THE STROKE RISK PROFILE

Although it is clear that hypertension is the chief contributor to ABI incidence it is also apparent that there is no logical basis for determining the need for treatment of hypertension to

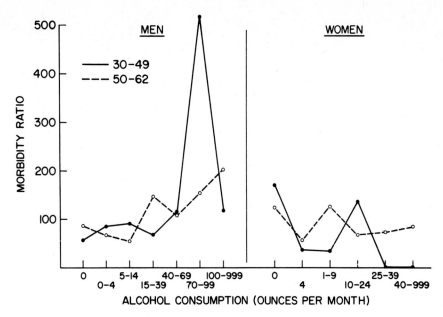

Fig. 1.13 Risk of atherothrombotic brain infarction according to alcohol intake. Men and women, 30 to 62 at entry. (Framingham Study: 18 year follow-up).

prevent strokes unless other contributing factors are taken into account. Since among hypertensives the risk of ABI is proportional to the height of the blood pressure, it would seem essential to take into account the actual blood pressure value. Also, at any blood pressure level risk varies over more than a five-fold range depending on the associated risk factors (Fig. 1.14). Thus risk factors, including blood pressure, are most efficiently dealt with as ingredients of a stroke risk profile.

Risk factor information can be efficiently synthesised into a composite risk estimate using multiple logistic equations, which describe the conditional probability of a cerebrovascular event for any given set of risk variables from their known coefficients of regression on incidence and constants for the intercept (Gordon *et al.*, 1971). This allows a more logical selection of patients for preventive management and avoids underestimating the risk of persons with multiple marginal 'abnormalities' according to categorical assessments of 'risk factors'. It also avoids over-reacting to those with only a single 'abnormality'.

Using such formulations risk estimates can be obtained over a wide range depending on the combined strength of the ingredients. Using an efficient set of ingredients (systolic blood pressure, serum cholesterol, glucose tolerance, cigarette habit, and ECG–LVH) one-tenth of the asymptomatic population can be identified from which about half the ABIs will emerge. This segment of the population has a 40 to 47 per cent chance of an ABI in eight years (Table 1.9).

Such an approach is feasible for computerised health agencies screening the normal population. Since such multiple logistic formulations can seldom be applied in medical office practice, handbooks have been computed which display the risk for a wide range of combinations of relevant risk factors (McGee, 1973). This makes it feasible to estimate the risk of an ABI for any combination of factors at any given age in either sex (Table 1.10). For example, a 60-year-old man who does not smoke cigarettes, has no glucose intolerance or ECG–LVH, but has a systolic blood pressure of 165 mmHg and a serum cholesterol of 285 mg/100 ml will have a 2.4 per

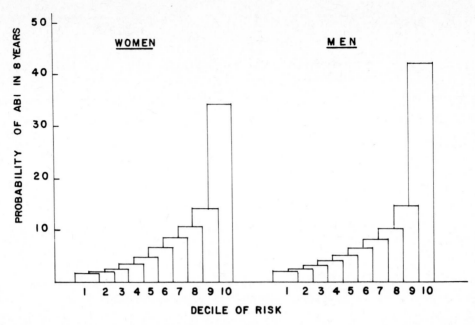

Fig. 1.14   Risk of atherothrombotic brain infarction according to decile of risk function profile. Men and women, 45 to 74. (Framingham Study: 18 year follow-up).

Table 1.9   Risk of specified cardiovascular events according to decile of risk score. Men and women, 35 to 74.

| Decile of risk | Average probability (in thousands) | | | | |
	Coronary disease	Brain infarction	Intermittent claudication	Hypertensive heart failure	Total C–V disease
Men					
1	16.4	0.2	1.4	0.4	18.9
2	31.1	0.6	3.2	1.0	36.5
3	44.6	1.3	5.3	1.6	53.9
4	59.0	2.3	7.6	2.4	72.8
5	73.6	3.6	10.2	3.3	92.7
6	88.9	5.5	13.2	4.7	115.1
7	105.3	7.9	17.7	6.5	140.1
8	124.0	11.2	24.3	8.8	170.7
9	150.3	17.1	34.9	13.6	215.0
10	225.6	47.4	68.5	44.4	343.6
Women					
1	3.2	0.2	0.9	0.4	6.5
2	6.7	0.5	1.6	0.7	12.2
3	10.7	1.1	2.4	1.2	18.3
4	16.1	1.9	3.2	1.8	26.2
5	23.9	3.4	4.3	2.6	37.4
6	34.5	5.4	6.0	3.7	52.1
7	46.6	8.0	7.9	5.5	70.2
8	62.8	11.5	10.6	8.0	95.0
9	82.2	16.8	14.8	12.9	127.5
10	140.9	39.8	37.0	37.9	224.4

cent probability of developing an ABI in eight years (Table 1.9). A man of the same age with a similar blood pressure and serum cholesterol but who smokes, has glucose intolerance and ECG–LVH has a risk of 10.3 per cent, about four times as great. These compare with an average risk of 1.6 per cent for men this age.

The variables selected are an efficient set of independent contributors to risk. They also have the virtue of being objective, obtainable from an unprepared, non-fasting patient, without trauma or undue expense, and, most important, they apply to other cardiovascular outcomes as well (McGee, 1973).

The tables are based on a population free of all major cardiovascular diseases such as coronary and rheumatic heart disease, intermittent claudication, congestive heart failure, and previous strokes. Persons with such diseases have a markedly enhanced risk of strokes by virtue of these alone. The variables chosen are not the only set which could be selected, but it is an efficient set for the reasons given above. Other information which should be taken into account in evaluating risk includes: other ECG abnormalities, cardiac dysrhythmias, cardiac enlargement on X-ray (Fig. 1.10), congestive heart failure, overweight (Fig. 1.12), and elevated haemoglobin values (Fig. 1.11).

Family history

Atherosclerosis and brain infarction in particular appear to evolve under the influence of multiple contributors. While hypertension is the most powerful contributor, it is an oversimplification to focus on it to the exclusion of all else. In fact, the concept of a single essential cause for most chronic disease has fallen into justified disrepute. To date, no essential factor, without which ABI fails to occur, has been implicated.

Genetic factors undoubtedly may affect individual susceptibility to non-genetic promoters of stroke. Also, with improved hygiene and nutrition, control of infectious disease, and artificial control of family size we may be exerting a sizeable influence on our evolution, formerly left to natural selection. It is possible we may

be breeding a population more susceptible to atherosclerotic disease as well as an ecology which promotes the disease.

Atherosclerosis appears to be ubiquitous in man beyond 20 years of age and can be looked upon as a concomitant of ageing or regarded as a function of the type of vasculature inherited. As for most chronic disease of the nervous system it is difficult to say to what extent ABIs are exogenous or genetic in origin. There is much to suggest a strong genetic component in hypertension, and since hypertension is such a dominant component of the stroke profile, it seems we must accept a strong familial influence. Direct evidence ȯn the issue is hard to obtain, for family studies of stroke have had too many shortcomings to allow ready acceptance of the findings. Aggregations of stroke in families are very difficult to demonstrate convincingly in one-time, cross-sectional prevalence studies, and index case-control approaches can be misleading since they are seldom representative of the population from which they originate. Prospective rather than cross-sectional studies are required to obtain a true assessment and these are sparse indeed.

While the general tendency to deposit lipid in the arterial intima may be largely a consequence of the level of blood lipids and the blood pressure, dynamics of flow and the integrity of the vascular intima determine where the atheromata will form. However, to contend that the architecture of the vasculature is the chief determinant of atheroma formation appears to be as faulty in logic as to invoke cholesterol or blood pressure as the only cause.

Host susceptibility and resistance to any noxious influence including blood pressure varies over a wide range; hence it would seem wise to single out those families with a strong family history of premature atherosclerotic cardiovascular catastrophies for earlier, more sustained, and more vigorous management of any abnormalities of blood pressure, blood lipids, or carbohydrate intolerance. An unfavourable cardiovascular risk profile should be even more ominous in such persons.

Atherosclerosis is very much a family affair. Not only do families appear to share an in-

Table 1.10 Probability (per 1000) of developing atherothrombotic brain infarction in eight years according to specified characteristics.(FraminghamStudy:18yearfollow-up).

60-year-old man: does not smoke cigarettes   **60-year-old man: smokes cigarettes**

LVH–ECG Negative

Glucose intolerance absent

	Chol.	SBP 105	120	135	150	165	180	195		Chol.	SBP 105	120	135	150	165	180	195
	185	4	6	8	13	20	30	44		185	7	11	16	25	37	56	83
	210	4	6	9	14	21	31	47		210	7	11	17	26	39	59	87
	235	4	6	9	14	22	33	48		235	8	12	18	27	41	62	91
	260	4	6	10	15	23	34	51		260	8	12	19	29	43	65	95
	265	4	7	10	16	24	36	54		285	9	13	20	30	45	68	100
	310	5	7	11	16	25	38	56		310	9	14	21	32	47	71	104
	335	5	7	11	17	26	39	59		335	10	14	22	33	50	74	109

Glucose intolerance present

	Chol.	SBP 105	120	135	150	165	180	195		Chol.	SBP 105	120	135	150	165	180	195
	185	7	11	17	26	39	59	87		185	14	22	33	49	74	108	157
	210	8	12	18	27	41	61	91		210	15	23	35	52	77	113	163
	235	8	12	19	29	43	64	95		235	16	24	36	54	81	118	170
	260	9	13	20	30	45	67	99		260	17	25	38	57	84	124	177
	285	9	14	21	31	47	70	104		285	17	26	40	60	88	129	185
	310	9	14	22	33	49	74	108		310	18	28	42	62	92	135	192
	335	10	15	23	35	52	77	113		335	19	29	44	65	97	140	200

LVH–ECG Positive

Glucose intolerance absent

	Chol.	SBP 105	120	135	150	165	180	195		Chol.	SBP 105	120	135	150	165	180	195
	185	4	7	10	15	23	35	52		185	8	13	19	29	44	66	97
	210	5	7	11	16	24	37	55		210	9	13	20	31	46	69	102
	235	5	7	11	17	25	38	57		235	9	14	21	32	49	72	106
	260	5	8	12	18	27	40	60		260	10	15	22	34	51	76	111
	285	5	8	12	19	28	42	63		285	10	16	24	36	53	79	116
	310	6	8	13	19	29	44	66		310	11	16	25	37	56	83	121
	335	6	9	13	20	31	46	69		335	11	17	26	39	58	87	127

Glucose intolerance present

	Chol.	SBP 105	120	135	150	165	180	195		Chol.	SBP 105	120	135	150	165	180	195
	185	9	13	20	31	46	69	101		185	17	26	39	58	86	126	181
	210	9	14	21	32	48	72	106		210	18	27	41	61	90	132	188
	235	10	15	22	34	51	75	111		235	19	28	43	64	94	137	196
	260	10	15	23	35	53	79	116		260	20	30	45	67	99	143	204
	285	11	16	25	37	56	82	121		285	21	31	47	70	103	149	212
	310	11	17	26	39	58	86	126		310	22	33	49	73	108	156	220
	335	12	18	27	41	61	90	132		335	23	34	52	77	113	162	229

Note: Framingham men aged 60 years have an average SBP of 140/mmHg and an average serum cholesterol of 234 mg%. Fifty per cent smoke cigarettes, 1.3 per cent have definite LVH by ECG, and 7.1 per cent have glucose intolerance. At these average values the probability of developing atherothrombotic brain infarction in 8 years is 16/1000.

creased propensity to disease, but they tend to share all of the atherogenic traits which predispose, including blood pressure, hyperlipidemia, impaired glucose tolerance, overweight, and hyperuricemia. Since spouses as well as siblings and offspring tend to share these liabilities, environment as well as genes must be at work. Intervention against risk factors should involve the entire family, particularly the younger members. The faulty life style which promotes atherosclerosis is conditioned in youth, and these habits and the lesions they provoke are more reversible then than later.

Although direct prospective evidence that a family history of stroke is of itself associated with an increased vulnerability to ABI is sparse, it would seem reasonable that because families tend to share atherogenic traits and may be more vulnerable to them, to regard a family history of premature strokes as a predisposing factor.

Residual disability

Following recovery from a stroke about 30 per cent are dependent on others for assistance and supervision of their daily activities. This compares with less than 10 per cent for persons the same age without strokes. About 10 per cent require nursing home, rest home, or chronic hospital care versus 3 per cent in the general population of this age. About 70 per cent will no longer be able to lead an active social life outside the house (compared to 4.6 per cent). Some 70 per cent have enough functional disability to interfere with either mobility, employment, socialisation, or daily living. Of those surviving a stroke in Framingham 23 per cent had some persistent residual sensory deficit, 14 per cent hemianopia, 34 per cent dysarthric or dysphasic speech disturbance, and 46 per cent some degree of hemiparesis (Gresham et al., 1973). If we are to keep people living to advanced age, the medical profession should have an obligation to ensure that the quality of life at this age is not impaired unduly by the effects of cerebral vascular disease.

Potential for reducing risk

A review of the epidemiology of ABI reveals that although there are gaps in our knowledge, we are now in a position to make prophylactic recommendations. This is not to say that the search for stroke precursors is completed, for there are still differences in vulnerability between and within populations which are not entirely explained by the identified factors. Many findings remain to be clarified, including the role of vascular anatomy, the epidemiologic features of lacunar strokes and intracerebral haemorrhage, the role of cigarettes and obesity, the impact of isolated systolic hypertension, and the equal sex ratio in ABI. The contribution of chronic atrial fibrillation and of TIAs in relation to ABI is still incompletely assessed as is the rate of recurrence in ABI victims and the factors which affect this.

However, from the data presented the conclusion seems inescapable that the occurrence of an ABI in a hypertensive patient constitutes a failure of medical preventative treatment. Conditions such as asymptomatic hypertension, when accompanied by ECG–LVH, impaired glucose tolerance, the cigarette habit, or hypercholesterolemia are not medical trivia. Such abnormalities are in fact responsible for the bulk of cerebrovascular catastrophies in the general population.

Since therapy is of only limited value in stroke we must learn to assess vulnerability to atherosclerotic disease and to correct the impairments which predispose long in advance of the first symptom. We are now able to identify stroke candidates employing nothing more than ordinary office procedures and simple laboratory tests. These risk factors can be synthesised into a composite risk estimate providing a logical basis for intervention. However, unless effective intervention can be mounted there is little point in seeking out stroke candidates. Coping with risk factors is no simple enterprise. The key to prevention of ABI would appear to be the early detection and vigorous and sustained treatment of hypertension and impaired cardiac function. The risk of precipitating strokes in persons with stenotic cerebral vessels by antihypertensive treatment have been exaggerated, for it has been shown that control of hypertension may actually *improve* cerebral blood flow and, on the whole, treated hypertensives develop fewer strokes and live longer (Veterans Administration Cooperative Study Group, 1970). However, it is no simple matter to convince asymptomatic hypertensives to take costly, symptom-producing medicines for long periods or their physicians to prescribe them.

There is no convincing evidence that lowering lipids, reducing overweight, taking physical exercise, treating diabetes, or giving up cigarettes will lessen the chances of a stroke. However, it seems prudent to include such measures in a comprehensive program to reduce atherosclerotic cardiovascular disease in hypertensives. Persons with coronary heart disease and congestive heart failure are at high risk of ABI and warrant careful control of hypertension and measures to support the failing myocardium. There is no evidence that the solution to the problem of ABI lies in more expert management of the completed brain infarction. The main hope appears to lie in an aggressive approach to prevention in the presymptomatic stage, and at present the most effective measure is early, vigorous, and sustained control of hypertension before organ damage has occurred.

REFERENCES

Acheson, J. & Hutchinson, E. C. (1964) Observations on the natural history of transient cerebral ischaemia. *Lancet*, ii, 871.
Baker, A. B., Flora, C. C., Resch, J. A. & Loewenson, R. (1967) The geographic pathology of atherosclerosis: a review of the literature with some personal observations on cerebral atherosclerosis. *Journal of Chronic Diseases*, **20**, 685.
Boston Collaborative Surveillance Program (1973) *Lancet*, i, 1399.
Colandrea, M. A., Friedman, G. D., Nichaman, M. Z. & Lynd, C. N. (1970) Systolic hypertension in the elderly. An epidemiologic assessment. *Circulation*, **41**, 239.
Collaborative Group for the Study of Stroke in Young Women (1973) Oral contraception and increased risk of cerebral ischaemia or thrombosis. *New England Journal of Medicine*, **288**, 871.
Council on Cerebrovascular Disease (1971) Risk factors in stroke due to cerebral infarction. *Stroke*, **2**, 423.
Crawford, M. D., Gardner, M. J. & Morris, J. N. (1968) Mortality and water hardness of local water supplies. *Lancet*, i, 827.
Cumings, J. N., Grundt, I. K., Holland, J. T. & Marshall, J. (1967) Serum lipids and cerebrovascular disease. *Lancet*, ii, 194.
Dawber, T. R., Kannel, W. B. & Gordon, T. (1974) Observations from the Framingham Study. *New England Journal of Medicine*, **291**, 871.
Fields, W. S., Maslenikov, V., Meyer, J. S., Hass, W. K., Remington, R. D. & MacDonald, M. (1970) Joint study of extracranial arterial occlusion. (V). Progress report of prognosis following surgery or nonsurgical treatment for transient cerebral ischaemic attacks and cervical carotid artery lesions. *Journal of the American Medical Association*, **211**, 1993.
Fisher, C. M. (1968) The arterial lesions underlying lacunes. *Acta Neuropathologica*, **12**, 1.
Fodor, J. G., Pfeiffer, L. J. & Papezik, V. S. (1973) Relationship of drinking water quality to cardiovascular mortality in Newfoundland. *Canadian Medical Association Journal*, **108**, 1369.
Garcia, M. McNamara, P. M., Gordon, T. & Kannel, W. B. (1973) Cardiovascular complications in diabetes. In *Early Diabetes: Advances in Metabolic Disorders*. Suppl. 2, 493.
Gifford, A. J. (1966) An epidemiological study of cerebrovascular disease. *American Journal of Public Health*, **56**, 452.
Goldberg, I. D. & Kurland, L. T. (1962) Mortality in 33 countries from diseases of the nervous system. *World Neurology*, **3**, 444.
Gordon, T., Sorlie, P., Kannel, W. B. (1971) An epidemiological investigation of cardiovascular disease. Coronary heart disease, atherothrombotic brain infarction, intermittent claudication. A multivariate analysis of some factors related to their incidence. *The Framingham Study. 16 Year Follow-up*. Washington, D.C.: United States Government Printing Office.
Gordon, T. & Kannel, W. B. (1973) The effects of overweight on cardiovascular diseases. *Geriatrics*, **28**, 80.
Gresham, G. E., Fitzpatrick, T. Wolf, P. A., McNamara, P. M., Kannel, W. B. & Dawber, T. R. (1973) The disability status of survivors of completed stroke in the Framingham Study (abstract). *Circulation*, **48**, Suppl. 4, 49.
Heyman, A., Arons, M. Quinn, M. & Camplong, L. (1969) The role of oral contraceptive agents in cerebral arterial occlusion. *Neurology* (Minneapolis), **19**, 519.
Inman, W. H. W. & Vessey, M. P. (1968) Investigation of deaths from pulmonary, coronary, and cerebral thromboses and embolism in women of child bearing age. *British Medical Journal*, ii, 193.
Jorgensen, L. & Torvik, J. (1966) Ischaemic cerebrovascular diseases in an autopsy series I. Prevalence, location and predisposing factors in verified thrombo-embolic occlusions and their significance in the pathogenesis of cerebral infarction. *Journal of the Neurological Sciences*, **3**, 490.
Kahn, H. A. (1966) The Dorn study of smoking and mortality among U.S. veterans. Report on $8\frac{1}{2}$ years of observation. In *National Cancer Institute Monogram No. 19*, 1.
Kannel, W. B., Gordon, T., Wolf, P. A. & McNamara, P. M. (1972) Haemoglobin and the risk of cerebral infarction: the Framingham Study. *Stroke*, **3**, 409.
Katsuki, S. & Hirota, Y. (1966) Recent trends in incidence of cerebrovascular haemorrhage and infarction in Japan. *Japanese Heart Journal*, **7**, 26

Klassen, A. C., Loewenson, R. L. B. & Resch, J. A. (1974) Body weight, cerebral atherosclerosis and cerebral vascular disease. An autopsy study. *Stroke*, **5**, 312.

Kuller, L., Seltser, R., Paffenbarger, R. S., Jr. & Kruger, D. E. (1968) Trends in cerebrovascular disease mortality based on multiple cause tabulation of death certificates 1930–1960. A comparison of trends in Memphis and Baltimore. *American Journal of Epidemiology*, **88**, 307.

Kurtze, J. F. (1968) Epidemiology of cerebrovascular disease –geographic distribution. *Transactions of the American Neurological Association*, **93**, 229.

McDonnell, F. W., Louis, I. & Manohan, K. (1970) Seasonal variation of non-embolic cerebral infarction. *Journal of Chronic Diseases*, **23**, 29.

McGee, D. (1973) The probability of developing certain cardiovascular diseases in 8 years at specified values of some characteristics. In *An Epidemiological Investigation of C–V Disease*, ed. Kannel, W. B. & Gordon, T. Washington, D.C.: Department of Health Education and Welfare.

Martin, M. J., Whisnant, J. P. & Sayre, G. P. (1960) Occlusive vascular disease in the extracranial cerebral circulation. *Archives of Neurology*, **3**, 530.

Medical Letter on Drugs & Therapeutics (1974) Topical and systemic contraceptive agents, **16**, 37.

Meyer, J. S., Waltz, A. G., Hess, J. W. & Zak, B. (1959) Serum lipid and cholesterol levels in cerebrovascular disease. *Archives of Neurology*, **1**, 303.

National Center for Health Statistics (1974) Vital and health statistics (Series II, No. 4). In *Blood Pressure of Adults by Age and Sex 1960–1962*. Washington, D.C.: United States Government Printing Office.

National Heart & Lung Institute Task force on Arteriosclerosis. (1971) *Arteriosclerosis*. Washington, D.C.: Department of Health Education and Welfare.

Paffenbarger, R. S., Jr. & Wing, A. L. (1967) Characteristics in youth predisposing to fatal stroke in later years. *Lancet*, i, 753.

Paffenbarger, R. S., Jr. Laughlin, M. E., Gima, A. S. & Black, R. A. (1970) Work activity of longshoremen as related to death from coronary heart disease and stroke. *New England Journal of Medicine*, **282**, 1109.

Paterson, J. C., Dyer, L. & Armstrong, E. C. (1960) Serum cholesterol level in human atherosclerosis. *Canadian Medical Association Journal*, **82**, 6.

Robinson, R. W., Cohen, W. D., Higano, N., Meyer, R., Lowkowsky, G. H., McLaughlin, B. & MacGilpin, H. H. (1959) Life-table analysis of survival after cerebral thrombosis; ten-year experience. *Journal of the American Medical Association*, **169**, 1149.

Robinson, R. W., Higano, N. & Cohen, W. D. (1963) Comparison of serum lipid levels in patients with cerebral thrombosis and in normal subjects. *Annals of Internal Medicine*, **59**, 180.

Sartwell, P. E., Masi, A. T., Arthes, F. G., Green, G. R. & Smith H. E. (1969) Thromboembolism and oral contraceptives: an epidemiologic case-control study. *American Journal of Epidemiology*, **90**, 365.

Schroeder, H. A. (1960) Relations between mortality from cardiovascular disease and treated water supplies. *Journal of the American Medical Association*, **172**, 1902.

Shurtleff, D. (1970) An epidemiological investigation of cardiovascular disease. Some characteristics related to the incidence of cardiovascular disease and death. *The Framingham Study. 16 Year Follow-up*. Section 26. Washington, D.C.: United States Government Printing Office.

Shurtleff, D. (1974) Some characteristics related to the incidence of cardiovascular disease and death. *The Framingham Study. 18 Year Follow-up*. Washington, D.C.: Department of Health Education and Welfare.

Stallones, R. A. (1965) Epidemiology of cerebrovascular disease. A review. *Journal of Chronic Diseases*, **18**, 859.

Vessey, M. P. & Doll, R. (1968) Investigation of relation between use of oral contraceptives and thromboembolic disease. *British Medical Journal*, ii, 199.

Veterans Administration Cooperative Study Group on Antihypertensive Agents (1970) Effects of treatment on morbidity in hypertension. *Journal of the American Medical Administration*, **202**, 1028.

Weir, R. J. Briggs, E. & Mack, A. (1974) Blood pressure in women taking oral contraceptives. *British Medical Journal*, i, 533.

Williams, A. O., Resch, J. A. & Loewenson, R. B. (1969) Cerebral atherosclerosis –a comparative autopsy study between Nigerian Negroes and American Negroes and Caucasians. *Neurology* (Minneapolis), **19**, 205.

Wolf, P. A., Kannel, W. B., McNamara, P. M. & Gordon, T. (1973) The role of impaired cardiac function in atherothrombotic brain infarction: The Framingham Study. *American Journal of Public Health*, **63**, 52.

World Health Organization (1969) *World Health Statistics*, Report 22, No. 9.

2. Natural History and Prognosis of Cerebrovascular Disease

Jørgen Marquardsen

Acute cerebrovascular disease, being a frequent cause of death and disability, is now a major public health problem in most parts of the world. An accurate knowledge of the natural history of cerebrovascular disorders is therefore necessary not only for the reliable prediction of the outcome in individual cases, but also for the evaluation of new methods of prevention and treatment and for the planning of comprehensive health services aimed at the control of vascular diseases in the community. Many reports on the subject have been published over the past 15 years; the present chapter, dealing exclusively with *acute* cerebrovascular disorders, is based on these reports and on the author's personal experience.

The term 'acute cerebrovascular disease', synonymous with 'cerebrovascular accident' or 'stroke', is here used according to the definition adopted by the World Health Organization (WHO), i.e. 'rapidly developed clinical signs of a focal disturbance of cerebral function of presumed vascular origin and of more than 24 hours' duration'. This purely clinical definition includes most cases of intracerebral haemorrhage, subarachnoid haemorrhage, and cerebral infarction (with or without demonstrable arterial occlusion), but *not* cases of transient cerebral ischaemia or diffuse cerebrovascular disease of insidious onset. The prognosis of subarachnoid haemorrhage, being dealt with in another chapter of the book, will be commented on very briefly here.

IMMEDIATE PROGNOSIS FOR LIFE

In spite of modern advances in the management of cerebrovascular diseases a stroke is still a serious and immediate threat to life. Of patients admitted to general hospitals about 30 to 60 per cent have been reported to die within three or four weeks of the stroke (Boyle and Reid, 1965; Marquardsen, 1969; Acheson and Fairbairn, 1970; Whisnant *et al.*, 1971). The widely varying fatality rates clearly reflect the fact that very few, if any, hospital series are representative of the general run of cerebrovascular accidents. In the few hitherto published community studies of cerebrovascular disease – based on experience both in hospitals and in general practice and thus including also very mild cases – about one-fourth to one-third of the strokes were fatal (Eisenberg, 1964; Acheson *et al.*, 1968). Fatality rates of the same magnitude have very recently been observed in an international WHO stroke project, based on the prospective registration of cerebrovascular accidents in selected communities in different parts of the world (Hatano, 1974).

In individual cases the immediate outlook for life depends on several factors, such as the age of the patient and the type, size, and anatomical site of the cerebrovascular lesion. Very high fatality rates, ranging from 60 to 90 per cent, have been observed in series of patients with a diagnosis of intracerebral haemorrhage (Kelly, 1958; Eisenberg, 1964; Acheson and Fairbairn, 1970). Even for such patients who are considered as possible candidates for surgery the chances of surviving the haemorrhage do not exceed 50 per cent, irrespective of treatment (McKissock *et al.*, 1961). Haemorrhages rupturing into the ventricular system and those primarily affecting the brain stem or the cerebellum are almost invariably fatal. This is true also of cerebellar haemorrhages, unless surgical evacuation of the clot can be undertaken immediately (McKissock *et al.*, 1960).

Ischaemic lesions carry a better prognosis

24

than do haemorrhagic ones. About one-quarter to one-third of patients admitted to hospital with a diagnosis of atheromatous cerebral infarction die from the original stroke (Carter, 1964). Most of the fatal ischaemic lesions are either extensive hemispheric infarcts with brain oedema or primary brain stem lesions. By contrast, the immediate prognosis is very favourable in cases of so-called 'lacunar strokes'; this term refers to various well-defined vascular syndromes caused by very small softenings in the basal ganglia or the pons (Fisher, 1967).

Attempts have been made to relate the immediate mortality of ischaemic strokes to the presence of arterial occlusion as demonstrated by angiography. Strokes due to occlusion of the middle cerebral artery appear to be fatal more often than those associated with occlusion of the internal carotid artery, or those without angiographically demonstrable occlusion (Thygesen et al., 1964; Rompel and Wiedermann, 1970).

A special type of ischaemic stroke is that caused by embolism as a manifestation of certain heart diseases, e.g., rheumatic endocarditis. One-fifth to one-fourth of patients in this category have been reported to die from the cerebral episode (Carter, 1965). What characterises these patients as a separate prognostic group is that they are comparatively young people, who, because of previously intact cerebral vessels, are more likely to establish a collateral blood supply than are patients with atheromatous cerebral infarction. According to some authors, however, atheromatous softenings are also often caused by embolism, the source of which may be the heart or the large arteries in the neck (Blackwood et al., 1969).

The type of cerebral lesion influences not only the ultimate outcome but also the length of the survival time. More than half of the patients who succumb to cerebral haemorrhage die within two days of the onset of symptoms, and about 80 per cent die within one week. In contrast, less than one-third of deaths due to cerebral infarction occur within a week of the stroke (Brown and Glassenberg, 1973). The difference clearly reflects the fact that in most cases of cerebral haemorrhage the cerebral lesion

itself is the immediate cause of death, whereas many patients with cerebral infarction, after having actually survived the cerebral catastrophe per se, are left in a precarious condition that makes them easy victims of incidental causes of death, such as pneumonia or heart failure. In a personal series of 340 fatal cases of stroke (haemorrhages as well as infarcts) the causes of death were analysed. In little over half of these cases the cerebral lesion was thought to be the immediate or direct cause of death; nearly all such fatalities occurred within a few days of the stroke. The remaining cases were either severely paralysed patients who eventually succumbed to extracerebral complications or patients who were apparently recovering from the immediate effects of the stroke but died from acute cardiopulmonary disease, e.g., unexpected pulmonary embolism. It is of practical interest to note that the last-mentioned category of potentially preventable deaths accounted for one-fifth of all the fatal cases.

A short comment on the relation between cerebrovascular disease and 'sudden death' seems appropriate. Although large intracranial haemorrhages can be very rapidly fatal, death will only rarely occur earlier than one or two hours after onset. In cases of instantaneous, unexpected death the cause 'cerebral apoplexy' is sometimes given by the certifying physician, but in actual fact such instances are nearly always caused by sudden cardiopulmonary failure.

In every case of fatal cerebral lesion, irrespective of its type and primary site, the direct cause of death is irreversible failure of vital functions of the brain stem. Primary subtentorial haemorrhages or infarcts are therefore often rapidly fatal, as they affect the brain stem directly, producing either disruption, necrosis, or compression of the tissue. In supratentorial lesions, on the other hand, any brain stem damage is a secondary phenomenon, resulting either from caudal expansion of the pathological process itself, or from transtentorial herniation of the brain. The latter term implies a downward displacement of the brain through the tentorial notch, accompanied by vasoparalysis and oedema proceeding caudally to diencephalic, midbrain, pontine, and finally medullary structures, thereby producing serial functional transections (Plum and Posner, 1972). In most supratentorial lesions the question of death or survival depends therefore mainly on whether or not a transtentorial herniation will follow; when herniation has actually started, the speed of the process is the main factor deciding the length of survival. The propagation usually takes some time, except in cases of intraventricular haemorrhage, where the sudden extravasation of blood probably creates a pressure wave that immediately propagates downwards to the fourth ventricle, causing compression of the surrounding brain stem tissue. This explains the usually very short survival after rupture of a haemorrhage into the ventricular system. In contrast, a hemisphere infarct, however large, becomes fatal only if a secondary oedematous swelling of the brain causes transtentorial herniation. Such swelling, reaching a maximum in three to five days, seems to occur only when an infarct involves the entire territory of the middle cerebral artery (Ng and Nimmannitya, 1970).

Clinical signs of prognostic value

A clinician who wants to assess his patient's chances of surviving a recent stroke must focus his attention on such neurological signs that are known to be suggestive of impending brain stem damage. Most important, and easily recognisable, is impairment of consciousness. Figure 2.1 clearly illustrates the prognostic significance of the level of consciousness, as observed in a large series of hospitalised stroke patients. Nearly all the patients who were deeply comatose at the time of admission died, most of them within 24 hours of the stroke. Those who were semi-comatose – i.e., inaccessible to questioning but responsive to painful stimuli – also fared badly, whereas the vast majority of the initially alert patients survived the acute phase.

Although the immediate outlook for life can be estimated with fair reliability on the basis of the conscious level alone, more detailed information can be gained by observing certain ocular, respiratory, and motor signs. Thus the caudal propagation of a supratentorial lesion is accompanied by pupillary constriction, which may be replaced by unilateral or bilateral mydriasis, with loss of the reaction to light. Patients in whom this sequence of pupillary changes is observed are unlikely to survive for more than a few hours. An enlarged pupil on the side of the cerebral lesion indicates herniation of the homolateral temporal lobe through the tentorial notch, often caused by a rapidly expanding hemispheric haemorrhage. In the personal series referred to above this sign was observed in 23

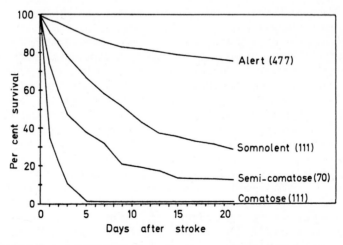

Fig. 2.1   Immediate survival after stroke by level of consciousness on admission (Marquardsen, 1969). (The figures in parentheses indicate the number of patients.)

patients, 19 of whom died within 24 hours of the stroke.

The pupillary changes may be accompanied by abnormal respiratory patterns such as Cheyne-Stokes respiration, central hyperventilation, ataxic breathing, etc., all of which are of ominous prognostic significance. This has been demonstrated also by means of analyses of the respiratory gases and acid-base balance in the blood: out of 11 stroke patients with a P_{CO_2} of less than 35 mmHg and a pH of more than 7.46 in the arterial blood, only one survived (Rout *et al.*, 1971).

In the motor system, as a result of the downward progression of the lesion, the originally unilateral defect becomes bilateral: decorticate and later decerebrate rigidity may develop, indicating irreversible brain stem damage.

The signs enumerated above are only some of the several clinical manifestations that occur in various combinations, each of which reflects a particular stage in the process of transtentorial herniation. For a full account of these clinical syndromes the reader is referred to the monograph of Plum and Posner (1972).

Finally, in patients who are fully alert and who are therefore unlikely to die from the cerebral lesion itself, the prognosis for life depends on the presence or absence of complicating extra-cerebral disease, in particular, cardiac, pulmonary, and renal disorders.

PROGNOSIS FOR FUNCTIONAL RECOVERY

When a patient has survived the acute phase of stroke, the next step in the prognostic evaluation is to assess the chances of recovery of function. Such an assessment meets with certain difficulties, mainly concerned with the definition and measurement of 'recovery'. In theory, the natural history of cerebrovascular accidents could be recorded in terms of the more or less complete restoration of normal anatomical and physiological conditions in the brain. In practice, however, the current state of cerebral dysfunction, being inaccessible to direct observation, can only be measured indirectly, usually by means of the resulting neurological deficit.

This type of prognostic evaluation, based on repeated neurological examinations, is very useful in the individual case, but has serious drawbacks as a basis for the statistical analysis of large series of patients. In particular, the method requires for each patient a detailed, quantitative registration of numerous neurological modalities, subsequently to be fitted into a scoring system. Many elaborate systems for stroke patients have in fact been devised, but none of them has gained universal acceptance.

The simplest yardstick by which to measure the recovery after stroke is the overall functional capacity of the patient, as illustrated by his ability to perform the ordinary activities of daily living. This method of evaluation, which has been used in most reports on the functional prognosis, only requires a rating scale for the grouping of the patients. A simple and practical scale is that of Rankin (1957) using five grades of disability:

Grade I. No disability: able to carry out all usual activities.

Grade II. Slight disability: unable to carry out some previous activities, but able to look after own affairs without assistance.

Grade III. Moderate disability: able to walk unaided, but needing some help with dressing.

Grade IV. Moderately severe disability: requiring help with both walking and self-care.

Grade V. Severe disability: bedfast or chairfast, usually incontinent; requiring constant nursing care and attention.

In the author's series of 404 immediate survivors from stroke the final functional levels achieved by the patients were as shown in Table 2.1. About 15 per cent of the patients made apparently complete recoveries (Grade I); 37 per cent remained slightly disabled (Grade II); 16 per cent moderately disabled; whereas the remaining 32 per cent either became more severely disabled or died within a couple of months. These results are in good accordance with those of other follow-up examinations of hospitalised stroke patients (Rankin, 1957; Adams and Merrett, 1961; Katz *et al.*, 1966; Shafer *et al.*, 1973). Briefly summarised, these studies show that 50 to 75 per cent of stroke survivors become able to walk unaided; 20 to 30

Table 2.1 Maximum functional capacity achieved by 404 immediate survivors[a] by age and sex.

| Age (years) | Males Disability grade | | | | | | | Females Disability grade | | | | | | |
	I	II	III	IV	V	Died within 2 months	Total	I	II	III	IV	V	Died within 2 months	Total
−59	10	25	7	4	2	–	48	9	24	3	10	4	–	50
60–69	12	22	8	5	2	2	51	13	34	10	8	9	3	77
70–79	5	12	13	9	3	–	42	10	28	17	19	16	10	100
80–	1	1	2	–	2	1	7	1	3	3	7	9	6	29
Total	28	60	30	18	9	3	148	33	89	33	44	38	19	256
%	18.9	40.5	20.3	12.2	6.1	2.0	100.0	12.9	34.8	12.9	17.2	14.8	7.4	100.0

[a]In three cases the disability grade was unascertainable.

per cent become permanently and severely handicapped.

Recovery rates far better than those given above have been reported from rehabilitation centres, particularly in the U.S.A. This is hardly surprising, since most of the patients admitted to such centres are relatively young persons who have been specially selected as suitable candidates for rehabilitation. Indeed, the study of Feldman et al. (1962) has shown that the majority of hemiparetic stroke victims can be adequately rehabilitated in ordinary medical or neurological wards without formal rehabilitation services, if proper attention is given to ambulation and self-care.

Factors influencing the functional recovery

Type of stroke. Since haemorrhagic strokes are less frequent but much more lethal than ischaemic ones, all representative series of survivors from stroke consist mainly of cases of cerebral infarction. Little is actually known about the functional prognosis after cerebral haemorrhage, but there is no reason to believe that recovery should be less complete after intracerebral haemorrhage than after cerebral infarction. In the category of primary subarachnoid haemorrhages the prospect for physical recovery is generally excellent, obviously because most of the survivors are youngish people with mild, if any, motor deficits. Patients with cerebral infarction caused by occlusion of major intracranial arteries have been reported

to fare worse than those without angiographically demonstrable occlusion (Thygesen et al., 1964), but the explanation may be that neurological signs are usually more severe in the former group than in the latter. It seems therefore fair to conclude that once the acute phase of a stroke is over, the anatomical type of the cerebral lesion is in itself no longer a prognostic factor of primary importance.

Extent and site of the lesion. The single most important factor governing the recovery from stroke is the extent of permanent cerebral damage. The larger a lesion is, the higher is the risk not only of interruption of motor pathways but, still more important, of widespread cortical or subcortical damage with loss of a variety of higher cerebral functions, all of which are involved in the process of recovery.

In addition to the size, the *site* of the lesion is prognostically relevant. Patients with ischaemic lesions in the brain stem, if they survive at all, are more likely to overcome a severe hemiparesis than are those with supratentorial lesions, the reason being that the cortical functions are intact in the former category, but often damaged in the latter. A typical example of small, strategically placed lesions are the 'lacunar strokes' which – whether situated in the pons or in the basal ganglia, almost invariably carry a favourable prognosis for recovery (Fisher, 1967).

The question of the prognostic significance of the *laterality* of supratentorial lesions has been a subject of some controversy. It was originally assumed that lesions of the dominant hemisphere, because of the accompanying disorders of language, might be more disabling than those affecting the other half of the brain. However, more recent reports suggest that the defects in visuomotor, temporal, and spatial concepts that often accompany lesions of the non-dominant hemisphere are more ominous prognostic signs than loss of speech. Thus, 21 per cent of the author's female patients with left-sided paresis became severely disabled, as compared with only 9 per cent of those with right-sided deficit.

Clinical predictors of functional outcome

Already at the initial neurological examination of the stroke patient the chances of recovery can be roughly estimated on the basis of the neurological deficit, which reflects the size of the cerebral lesion. At this very early stage, however, it is difficult to distinguish between permanent damage caused by neuronal loss and temporary dysfunction caused by remediable cerebral oedema. The clinical prognostication is therefore more reliable when based on a neurological examination performed one or two weeks after the stroke, or even later. Referring particularly to old and more handicapped survivors, Adams (1974) stated that confident predictions about their prospects can seldom be given in less than 12 to 16 weeks, nor can the ultimate grade of recovery be assessed in under 24 to 30 weeks.

In the following paragraphs a short account is given of some clinical signs which, separately or in combination, have significant prognostic implications.

Motor deficit. It is almost self-evident that the risk of becoming permanently disabled by a hemiplegia is directly proportional to the grade of paresis. However, there is some indication that the time that elapses before recovery begins is still more significant as a prognostic indicator than the initial severity of the motor deficit. This was first mentioned by Gowers (1888), who stated that patients in whom improvement begins within three days of onset will almost certainly become able to walk unaided, whereas a paralysis that is still complete after three months is likely to remain severe. Later reports suggest that even one month without improve-

ment indicates a bad prognosis. In the present author's series, for example, the ability to walk alone was regained by only 15 per cent of the patients who had not improved at the end of four weeks. In the upper limb progress is likely to be poor if there is no voluntary movement within three weeks.

A special type of motor deficit is paralysis of conjugate ocular movements. This sign, which is often co-existent with severe hemiplegia, indicates that the patient's chances of regaining independence are less than 50 per cent.

Sensory deficit. The importance of sensory regulation of movement patterns has often been stressed, and it is generally assumed that recovery from hemiplegia is severely impeded by loss of sensation in the paralysed limbs. Although this is probably true, a significant correlation between sensory loss and persistent motor handicap has not yet been satisfactorily established in stroke patients. In the author's series, independence in self-care was regained by 46 per cent of the patients with initial sensory deficit, and by 54 per cent of those with normal sensation; the difference is not significant. Similarly, in the series of severely disabled stroke patients reported by Isaacs and Marks (1973), the presence of heminaesthesia or proprioceptive loss did not apparently influence the ultimate outcome. On the other hand, Moskowitz, *et al.* (1972) found that stroke patients with hemisensory loss, despite significant motor recovery in many cases, did not attain the same ambulatory levels as those without such sensory disorders. It seems, therefore, that definite conclusions regarding the prognostic value of sensory deficit must await the results of further studies.

Visual disturbances, when present in surviving stroke patients, will obviously add to the difficulties of rehabilitation. It is particularly noteworthy that the presence of homonymous hemianopia, in spite of preserved central vision, is associated with poor recovery from hemiplegia (Haerer, 1973). The explanation may be that the hemianopia simply implies a larger lesion and therefore a poorer rehabilitative potential, or that the visual field defect is often accompanied by other more subtle perceptual defects, which are more serious handicaps than the hemianopia itself.

Disorders of higher nervous function. It is a common experience that some stroke patients fail to regain independence, although motor function improves and adverse prognostic factors are apparently absent. Many of these therapeutic failures–traditionally often ascribed to dementia or 'lack of motivation'–are the result of disorders of highly specialised mental functions, caused by focal lesions of cortical or subcortical structures. Adams and Hurwitz (1963) were able to demonstrate such 'mental barriers to the recovery from stroke' in one-half of a series of chronic hemiplegic invalids; among the disorders were: defect in comprehension, neglect of the hemiparetic limbs, denial of disease, disturbance of body-image, apraxia, motor perseveration, memory loss of recent events.

Of the above disorders, those characterised by unrealistic attitudes towards illness have attracted particular attention. In severe cases such defects cause striking and bizarre clinical pictures, dominated by the patient's complete denial of ownership of the paralysed limbs or by his unawareness of the motor deficit. Such patients, whose vascular lesions affect the parietal lobe of the non-dominant hemisphere, are usually inaccessible to rehabilitative treatment. In contrast to these dramatic manifestations, the milder forms of parietal lobe dysfunction, causing only partial neglect of the hemiplegia, may easily escape notice; suspicion should arise whenever an acute neurological deficit fails to evoke an adequate emotional response in the patient. Other signs of parietal lobe dysfunction of prognostic importance are the defects in the patient's concept of space, speed, and time; again, such signs may remain unnoticed, if not particularly looked for at the neurological examination.

Dysphasia, which is present in about one-third of immediate survivors from stroke, is another disorder that may impede recovery. This is true particularly when the dysphasia is of the receptive type, thus preventing the patient from understanding instructions; in addition, the loss of communication often results in severe frustra-tion, which further adds to the patient's difficulties. Nevertheless, the presence of dysphasia does not preclude a satisfactory functional recovery, as observed in the author's series of survivors with right hemiplegia: independence in walking was attained by 61 per cent of those who were dysphasic, as compared with 71 per cent of those without this defect. Generally speaking, the perceptual defects caused by lesions of the non-dominant hemisphere are more ominous as prognostic indicators than are disorders of language.

Dementia, indicating diffuse cerebral damage, is undoubtedly the most severe 'mental barrier' to recovery. Stroke patients with marked mental deterioration, particularly those presenting urinary incontinence and/or episodes of confusion, will almost certainly remain disabled and helpless.

Combinations of prognostic factors. It follows from the preceding paragraphs that, even in the acute phase of stroke, the chances of functional recovery can be assessed by paying due attention to the following adverse prognostic factors: old age, severe motor deficit, impairment of consciousness, disorders of higher nervous function, and conjugate ocular deviation. These signs, which are indicators of the extent of cerebral dysfunction, may occur in many combinations, each of which has a more or less distinct prognostic significance. As an example, for a patient under the age of 70 who has a complete or severe hemiplegia but without other signs of extensive lesion, the chances are two to one that he will regain independence in both walking and self-care. On the other hand, if more signs of extensive lesion are present, and particularly if any type of subsequent complication occurs, the patient is likely to remain incapacitated.

Social readaptation after stroke

An important part of the prognostic evaluation is the estimation of the patient's chances of ultimately returning home and of resuming his usual activities. Because of the high average age of patients with cerebrovascular disease, *vocational* rehabilitation after stroke is the exception rather than the rule: of the patients who were in employment at the time of the stroke no more than one-third can be expected to go back to work. In most cases, therefore, the realistic goal of rehabilitation is not re-employment but self-care and return home. According to reports from European and American hospitals, 60 to 80 per cent of survivors from stroke can finally be discharged home, whereas the remaining patients have to be transferred to nursing institutions.

In the individual case the chances of returning home, although primarily depending on the degree of functional recovery, are strongly influenced by such factors as the sex of the patient, the domestic structure, and the socio-economic status. This is illustrated by Table 2.2, which shows the discharge placement of the survivors in the author's series. Female patients living with a spouse were much more likely to return home than were those who were living with other relatives or alone. For males, on the other hand, the chances of being discharged home were apparently independent of the domestic structure.

closely knit units, virtually all surviving stroke patients, no matter how disabled, are discharged home and subsequently cared for by their children or other relatives. It is a sobering thought that even in such countries, now referred to as 'developing', social re-integration of handicapped patients may become more difficult with increasing industrialisation and prosperity.

LATE SURVIVAL

Until recently little was known about the late prognosis of patients who had recovered from stroke. Over the past 15 years, however, a number of follow-up studies have filled the gaps in our knowledge (Robinson et al., 1959; Marshall and Shaw, 1959; Adams and Merrett, 1961; Carter, 1964; Droller, 1965; Marquardsen, 1969; Whisnant et al., 1971). These studies have shown that the late mortality of those who survive a stroke is much higher than that observed in the general population. This is clearly

Table 2.2 Discharge rates by domestic structure.

	Household composition	No. of patients	Mean age (years)	Discharged home Number	%
Males	Living with spouse	102	62.4	89	87.3
	Living with relatives	14	70.7	12	85.7
	Living alone	24	67.9	19	79.2
Females	Living with spouse	85	63.6	74	87.0
	Living with relatives	62	69.9	35	56.5
	Living alone	93	70.8	64	68.8

When seen in the global perspective, the most decisive factor influencing social readaptation after stroke is the general structure of the community of which the patients are members. Of particular importance are the patterns of family life and the prevailing attitudes towards handicapped people. It should thus be emphasised that the discharge rates given above are probably representative of the conditions in the highly industrialised and urbanised countries in Western Europe and in the U.S.A., but not of those in many other parts of the world. In the Far East, where large families live together as

demonstrated by means of life-table analysis, as shown in Figure 2.2. The excess mortality of the stroke patients is immediately apparent: for male patients, for example, the observed three-year survival rate is only 54 per cent, as compared with an expected rate of 88 per cent; after five years the actual number of survivors is one-half of that expected, after 10 years a mere one-fourth. The median survival time—i.e., the length of time required for 50 per cent of the individuals to have died—is less than four years for patients of either sex, whereas in the general population it exceeds 10 years. It is further noted

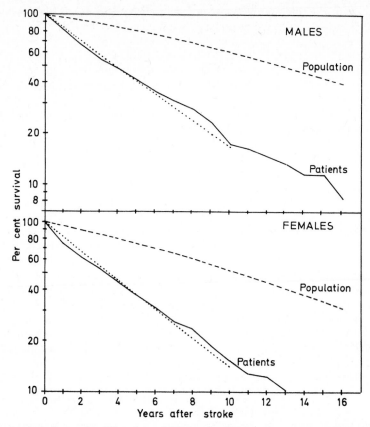

Fig. 2.2   Long-term survival after stroke, 150 males and 257 females (Marquardsen, 1969). (The dotted lines represent the average annual probabilities of dying.)

that the accelerated rate of death is found not only in the first year after the stroke, but throughout the period of observation. In fact, the annual death rate of the patients — represented by the slope of the survival curve — remains almost constant, irrespective of the time that has elapsed since the stroke. It is therefore convenient, for purposes of comparison, to describe the long-term mortality in any particular group of stroke patients by simply giving the average annual death rate observed over a specified period of time. Thus in the series on which Figure 2.2 is based the number of survivors decreased at an average annual rate of 16 per cent in males, 18 per cent in females.

The conclusion to be drawn from the course of the survival curves shown in Figure 2.2 is that

the excess mortality of patients who have recovered from stroke is not due to the effects of the cerebral lesion, but reflects the steady progression of underlying vascular disease. This is borne out by an analysis of the causes of death: in the follow-up studies referred to above the most frequent causes of death were recurrent stroke (accounting for 20 to 50 per cent of the deaths), myocardial infarction, congestive heart failure, and renal disease. At least three-quarters of all the deaths were caused by such vascular diseases.

Factors influencing the long-term mortality

As expected, the age of the patient is an important prognostic factor. Thus for each successive year after the stroke the annual death rate is twice as high for patients aged 70 to 79 years as for those 20 years younger. The *excess* mortality, on the other hand, is highest in the younger groups. Thus, stroke patients aged 50 to 60 years die at an annual rate equal to that which, according to official life-tables, is expected for persons 25 years older, whereas the survival of patients aged 70 to 79 years is similar to that of persons only 15 years older. The explanation of this trend must be that in the general population, with which the stroke patients are to be compared, the incidence of vascular disease rises steeply with advancing age. With respect to vascular mortality, therefore, old patients with cerebrovascular disease differ less from their 'normal' contemporaries than do young ones.

Cardiovascular disease. Evidence of pre-existing *heart disease*—whether obtained by history-taking, by observation of relevant clinical signs, or by electrocardiography—is an adverse factor in the long-term prognosis after stroke. A comparison of the survival curves for patients with and without abnormal ECGs thus shows that the presence of any type of ECG abnormality reduces the patient's chances of surviving for three years by nearly 50 per cent; after that time, however, the survival curves become nearly parallel. The reason for this may be that most of the patients with severe heart disease die within a few years of the stroke, leaving a group of survivors with a more benign type of cardiac disorder. The prognostic implications of all types of heart disease, but particularly of coronary artery disease, is more marked in males than in females.

Arterial hypertension. The role of hypertension in the prognosis after cerebrovascular accidents has been the subject of many discussions and the cause of some controversy. As is well known from the vast literature on hypertension, no definite answer can be given to such basic questions as where to draw the dividing line between normal and elevated blood pressure; whether to base the assessment on the systolic or the diastolic pressure; and whether to prefer resting or 'casual' pressures. For patients with cerebrovascular accidents the issue is further confused by the fact that a stroke may

produce considerable changes in the blood pressure level; in the period of convalescence after stroke it is therefore particularly difficult to classify patients as either hypertensives or normotensives. Nevertheless, most workers who have published follow-up studies of patients with stroke, although using different definitions of hypertension, seem to agree that patients with blood pressures exceeding a given level fare much worse than those with lower pressures (Marshall and Kaeser, 1961; Carter, 1964; Marquardsen, 1969). The only studies that have failed to demonstrate an adverse prognostic influence of raised blood pressure are those based on patients in geriatric units (Adams, 1965; Droller, 1965). The obvious conclusion is that the significance of hypertension varies with age. In fact, Figure 2.3 shows that not only the age but also the sex of the patient must be taken into consideration. It appears that at ages under 70 patients with blood pressures over 180/100 survive for a shorter time than those with lower pressures; at ages over 70 the difference between the two categories, although less marked, is still present in males, but almost absent in females. The remarkable immunity of old women to the effects of hypertension has been observed in numerous studies of the prognosis in essential hypertension.

The height of the blood pressure influences not only the actual length of survival but also the eventual cause of death. In particular, a close relationship exists between the presence of hypertension at the time of the original stroke and the risk of dying from recurrent cerebrovascular accident. In the author's series the proportion of late deaths due to recurrent stroke rose from 18 per cent in patients with diastolic blood pressures below 100 mm to 41 per cent in those whose pressures were 120 mm or over. Moreover, in the group with low pressures the recurrent accidents were more often infarcts than haemorrhages, whereas in the hypertensive group the reverse was the case. It should be noted that certain causes of death were found to be inversely related to the blood pressure level; for example, fatal pulmonary embolism occurred almost exclusively in patients whose diastolic pressures were under 100 mm.

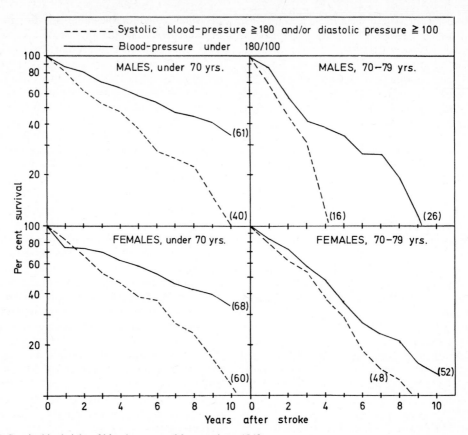

Fig. 2.3   Survival by height of blood pressure (Marquardsen, 1969).

Valuable prognostic information is gained by taking both blood pressure and ECG findings into consideration. Figure 2.4 shows that the ECG findings were particularly important in the estimation of the patients' chances of surviving for one or two years, whereas the long-term outlook seemed to depend more on the blood pressure level. Patients in whom both blood pressure and ECG were normal had a remarkably favourable prognosis, the three-year survival rate being almost equal to that of the general population. In contrast, patients with abnormal ECGs and high blood pressures fared badly: about 60 per cent of these patients died within three years of the stroke.

Characteristics of the cerebral lesion. Once the acute phase of the stroke is over, the anatomical type of the cerebral lesion is no longer a prognos-

tic factor of major importance. Available evidence indicates that the late prognosis of survivors from cerebral haemorrhage is similar to, or maybe even better than, that of patients with cerebral infarction (Eisenberg, 1964; Whisnant *et al.*, 1971). Reservation must be made for certain categories of patients who present specific problems: in survivors from subarachnoid haemorrhage, for example, the prognosis depends mainly on whether or not recurrent bleeding from an aneurysm will occur; when no aneurysm can be demonstrated by angiography, the prognosis is excellent (Pakarinen, 1967). In patients with cerebral infarction the angiographical findings seem to have some bearing on the prognosis; patients with normal angiograms survive longer than those who present arteriosclerotic stenosis or occlusion (Shenkin

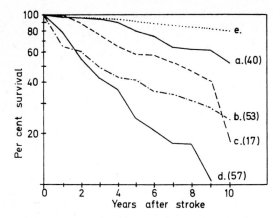

Fig. 2.4   Survival by height of blood pressure and electro-cardiographic findings (Marquardsen, 1969). (Patients under 70 years; both sexes.) a. BP < 180/100; ECG normal (mean age 59.2 years). b. BP < 180/100; ECG abnormal (mean age 59.3 years). c. BP = 180/100; ECG normal (mean age 57.7 years). d. BP ≧ 180/100; ECG abnormal (mean age 60.5 years). e. Sample of general Danish population, age 59 years.

et al., 1965; Acheson *et al.*, 1969). This seems to be in keeping with the view that the extent of arterial disease is the dominating prognostic factor.

The natural history of occlusion of the internal carotid artery or other extracranial arteries has attracted particular attention because of the possibility that vascular surgery might improve the long-term prognosis in cases of this type. A difficulty arises from the fact that most published series of patients with carotid occlusion comprise highly selected groups of relatively young patients admitted to neurological or neurosurgical departments; such series are of course not directly comparable with the ordinary types of patients with strokes. Nevertheless, it should be noted that in the 'Joint Study of Extracranial Arterial Occlusion' (Bauer *et al.*, 1969) the three-year survival rate observed in the 'non-surgical group' was exactly the same as that experienced by the patients of similar age in the author's series of unspecified stroke cases. It seems, therefore, that the late mortality of patients with extracranial arterial occlusion conforms to the general pattern seen in cerebral infarction.

The *extent* of the cerebral lesion is a reliable

indicator not only of the immediate prognosis for life, as already mentioned, but also of the late survival. A convenient, although indirect, measure of the extent of permanent cerebral damage is the resulting physical disability of the patient. Figure 2.5 illustrates the relevance of this factor. Patients who regained the ability to walk un-aided fared much better than those who could walk only with assistance. Patients who became permanently bedfast or chairfast experienced a strikingly high mortality, the median survival time being less than one year.

Combinations of prognostic factors. An analysis of the author's series gave the result that for patients who have recovered from the immed-iate effects of a stroke the probability of surviv-ing for five years can be estimated with fair reliability on the basis of only three factors: age at onset, a history of cardiac symptoms, and blood pressure level. Thus, irrespective of the severity of the stroke, the following proportions of patients under 70 years of age were alive after five years: three-fourths of those who had neither cardiac symptoms nor blood pressure over 180/100 mm; half of those in whom only one of these factors was present; one-fourth of those with both cardiac symptoms and hyper-tension. Such prognostic criteria are useful in

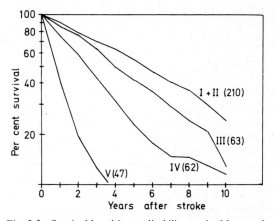

Fig. 2.5   Survival by ultimate disability grade (Marquard-sen, 1969). (Patients under 80; both sexes.) I & II. Indepen-dent in self-care (mean age 63.4 years). III. Requires some help, but walks without assistance (mean age 68.5 years). IV. Dependent on others; can walk only with assistance (mean age 67.8 years). V. Bedfast or chairfast (mean age 76.5 years).

the ordinary type of arteriosclerotic or hypertensive stroke but are not applicable to specific categories of stroke such as cerebral embolism from rheumatic endocarditis or subarachnoid haemorrhage from intracranial aneurysm or angioma.

RECURRENCE RATE

Many clinicians concerned with the management of cerebrovascular disease have been puzzled by the observation that some survivors from stroke suffer very early recurrences, whereas others remain free from further attacks for many years. It is of obvious clinical importance to obtain statistical information about the risk of recurrences in different types of stroke, and to study the factors that influence the recurrence rate. In series of patients with cerebral infarction, or with unspecified stroke, recurrent episodes have been reported in 15 to 38 per cent of the individuals, about half of the recurrences being fatal (Marshall and Kaeser, 1961; Baker et al., 1962; Carter, 1964; Droller, 1965; Marquardsen, 1969). The differences in these overall rates clearly reflect the widely varying lengths of observation. The influence of this factor can be eliminated by calculating, for each series, the number of recurrences observed in 100 patient-years; when this is done, the results of different studies are remarkably similar, with recurrence rates ranging from 8 to 11 per 100 patient-years.

It seems to be a widespread belief that recurrent attacks are particularly frequent in the first year after the original stroke and that the risk decreases in later years. However, in the author's series the annual rate of recurrence remained at the initial level for at least 10 years after the stroke, the average annual rate being 8.9 per cent for males, 10.6 for females. An annual recurrence rate of this magnitude means that, in the absence of deaths from causes other than cerebrovascular accident, 75 per cent of the patients can be expected to have a recurrent episode within 15 years of the original stroke. It is suggested, therefore, that any stroke patient who survives long enough is likely to have a further cerebral accident. It is evident, however, that

with a relatively low annual risk of recurrence and a high mortality from other causes, the majority of the patients will die from intercurrent disease before having had another attack. This explains why the overall recurrence rate observed in follow-up studies rarely exceeds 30 per cent, and why few patients actually suffer more than two recurrences.

There is some evidence that recurrent attacks are more often fatal than are initial strokes, but the difference may be a statistical artefact, since non-fatal recurrences are more likely to escape notice than fatal ones. An analysis of the author's series showed that recurrent lesions of the previously affected hemisphere carried a lower fatality rate than contralateral lesions. The difference results from the fact that cerebral haemorrhages, which constituted about half of the recurrent lesions, tended to occur in the hitherto unaffected side of the brain. A possible explanation of this trend is that occlusions or arteriosclerotic stenoses in the proximal part of the carotid arterial system may to some extent protect the ipsilateral hemisphere against the effects of systemic hypertension. Such an explanation is supported by the observation, made by several vascular surgeons, that cerebral haemorrhage sometimes occurs as a postoperative complication of carotid endarterectomy.

Factors influencing the recurrence rate

Type of initial cerebral lesion. Particularly high recurrence rates have been observed in patients with cerebral embolism from rheumatic heart disease. According to Carter (1964), such patients have at least a 50 per cent chance of recurrence, especially if atrial fibrillation is present; recurrent emboli are more often in the same hemisphere as the original episode than in the contralateral one. The same author felt that emboli tend to come in showers, the rate being highest in the first few months after the first attack; this was ascribed to some change of consistency in an atrial or auricular mural thrombus, or to some alteration in cardiac rhythm.

Arteriosclerotic occlusion or stenosis of the

internal carotid artery as demonstrated by angiography seems to be associated with a higher recurrence rate than occlusion of the middle cerebral artery. The cause of this difference may be that the former type of lesion remains a potential source of emboli that may enter the intracranial circulation, whereas an occlusion of the middle cerebral artery effectively blocks the path of any future emboli to that territory.

Survivors from cerebral haemorrhage are too few to justify any statements concerning the risk of recurrence in this type of stroke. It is interesting, however, that in most of the above-mentioned cases of secondary haemorrhagic strokes the original accident has been diagnosed as cerebral infarction. This gives some support to the view that recurrent cerebrovascular accidents, whether infarcts or haemorrhages, may have a common aetiology, the underlying diseases being arteriosclerosis and hypertension.

Clinical factors. The risk of sustaining further strokes is inversely related to the severity of the neurological deficit caused by the primary lesion. Recurrences are thus rarely seen in patients who are completely and permanently disabled after their first stroke; this is hardly surprising, since in this category of patients a new vascular episode, at least when affecting the ipsilateral hemisphere, can add little to the damage already done, and may therefore be clinically 'silent'.

In the author's series a history of heart failure or the presence of ECG abnormalities at the time of the first stroke were associated with an annual recurrence rate of about 15 per cent, which is twice the rate found in survivors without indication of heart disease. Patients with atrial fibrillation had only slightly higher recurrence rates than those with other types of ECG abnormality. An analysis of the fatal recurrences verified by necropsy showed that recurrent strokes suffered by patients with antecedent heart failure were most likely to be cerebral infarctions; cerebral haemorrhages occurred almost exclusively in patients without clinical signs of heart disease.

As expected, the risk of recurrences increases with the height of the blood pressure. In the personal series the patients whose diastolic pressures at the time of the initial stroke were over 120 mm presented recurrence rates exceeding 20 per cent per year; all the fatal recurrences in this group were haemorrhages.

Combination of factors. Particularly high recurrence rates are observed in patients who present a combination of two or more of the above prognostic factors. For example, in patients with both hypertension and atrial fibrillation the risk of having a further stroke within one year is about 50 per cent. It should be realised, however, that such associations, although statistically significant, are of limited value in the assessment of the prognosis in individual cases. No investigator has hitherto succeeded in making a sharp distinction between patients who are likely to have recurrences and those who are not.

CONCLUSIONS

Even with modern standards of medical care, cerebrovascular accidents often result in death or permanent disability, and even those patients who have apparently recovered from the stroke experience a high excess mortality and excess morbidity, which remain remarkably constant over the subsequent years. The obvious explanation is that a stroke, apart from being in itself a serious brain disorder, is a more or less incidental manifestation of a steadily progressing generalised vascular disease, most often of the arteriosclerotic or hypertensive type. This statement refers particularly to the natural history of cerebral infarction, but may be true also of cerebral haemorrhage, with the exception of bleeding aneurysms or other strictly local defects.

It has been demonstrated in the survey that in most cases of stroke a reliable assessment of the prognosis can be made on the basis of two categories of clinical signs, reflecting the extent and site of the cerebral lesion and the severity of generalised cardiovascular disease, respectively. Reservation must be made for the minority of patients whose strokes are complications of diseases other than arteriosclerosis or hypertension, e.g., rheumatic heart disease, blood dyscrasias, various types of arteritis, etc.

In view of the serious consequences of cerebrovascular accidents, both for the individual and for the community, it is important to decide whether it is possible, by eliminating some of the adverse prognostic factors, to improve the outlook. In the acute phase of cerebral infarction, for example, the immediate treatment of cerebral oedema, heart failure, and respiratory distress can probably limit the extent of hypoxic brain damage and thus improve the patient's chances of surviving and recovering. A corresponding effect may be achieved by administering certain vasoactive drugs, e.g., aminophylline, which in some cases may increase the blood supply of the ischaemic area of the brain. In the phase of convalescence, when the extent of cerebral damage is finally established, rehabilitation procedures help the patient to make the best use of the spontaneous recovery that has occurred, thus counteracting contractures, bed sores, thrombophlebitis, and other potentially dangerous complications. When the patient has reached the ultimate grade of recovery, the object of further treatment must be to prevent recurrent cerebrovascular accidents and to delay the progress of co-existing cardiovascular disease in general. With this in mind, the methods of choice must be treatment of hypertension and heart failure, together with the elimination of sources of emboli, either by vascular surgery or by anticoagulant therapy.

Although the above therapeutic activities seem commendable on theoretical grounds, it should be remembered that even a highly significant association between a certain factor and an unfavourable prognosis does not necessarily mean that elimination of that factor will improve the prognosis. It is a regrettable fact that very little is known about the actual prognostic consequences of admission to hospital, of many drugs, of surgical operations, of special rehabilitation techniques, etc. Hence, controlled trials of various types of management of stroke are urgently needed. It is to be hoped that the results of such trials will provide a basis for large-scale therapeutic endeavours that may contribute to a more effective control of cerebrovascular disease in the community.

REFERENCES

Acheson, J., Acheson, H. W. K. & Tellwright, J. M. (1968) The incidence and pattern of cerebrovascular disease in general practice. *Journal of the Royal College of General Practitioners*, **16**, 428.

Acheson, J., Boyd, W. N., Hugh, A. E. & Hutchinson, E. C. (1969) Cerebral angiography in ischaemic cerebrovascular disease. *Archives of Neurology*, **20**, 527.

Acheson, R. M. & Fairbairn, A. S. (1970) Burden of cerebrovascular disease in the Oxford Area in 1963 and 1964. *British Medical Journal*, i, 621.

Adams, G. F. (1965) Prospects for patients with strokes. *British Medical Journal*, ii, 253.

Adams, G. F. (1974) *Cerebrovascular Disability and the Ageing Brain*. London; Churchill Livingstone.

Adams, G. F. & Hurwitz, L. J. (1963) Mental barriers to recovery from strokes. *Lancet*, ii, 533.

Adams, G. F. & Merrett, J. D. (1961) Prognosis and survival after strokes. *British Medical Journal*, i, 309.

Baker, R. N., Broward, J. A., Fang, H. C., Fisher, C. M., Groch, S. N., Heyman, A., Karp, H. R., McDevitt, E., Scheinberg, P., Schwartz, W. & Toole, J. F. (1962) Anticoagulant therapy in cerebral infarction. *Neurology*, **12**, 823.

Bauer, R. B., Meyer, J. S., Fields, W. S., Remington, R., Macdonald, M. C. & Callen, P. (1969). Joint study of extracranial arterial occlusion. *Journal of the American Medical Association*, **208**, 509.

Blackwood, W., Hallpike, J. F., Kocen, R. S. & Mair, W. G. P. (1969) Atheromatous disease of the carotid arterial system and embolism from the heart in cerebral infarction: a morbid anatomical study. *Brain*, **92**, 897.

Boyle, R. W. & Reid, M. (1965) What happens to the stroke victim? *Geriatrics*, **20**, 949.

Brown, M. & Glassenberg, M. (1973) Mortality factors in patients with acute stroke. *Journal of the American Medical Association*, **224**, 1493.

Carter, A. B. (1964) *Cerebral Infarction*. London: Pergamon Press.

Carter, A. B. (1965) Prognosis of cerebral embolism. *Lancet*, ii, 514.

Droller, H. (1965) The outlook in hemiplegia. *Geriatrics*, **20**, 630.

Eisenberg, H., Morrison, J. T., Sullivan, P. & Foote, F. M. (1964) Cerebrovascular accidents. *Journal of the American Medical Association*, **189**, 883.

Feldman, D. J., Lee, P. R., Untereker, J., Lloyd, K., Rusk, H. A. & Toole, A. (1962) A comparison of functionally oriented medical care and formal rehabilitation in the management of patients with hemiplegia due to cerebrovascular disease. *Journal of Chronic Diseases*, **15**, 297.

Fisher, C. M. (1967) A lacunar stroke. *Neurology*, **17**, 614.

Gowers, W. R. (1888) *A Manual of Diseases of the Nervous System*. London: Churchill.

Haerer, A. F. (1973) Visual field defects and the prognosis of stroke patients. *Stroke*, **4**, 163.

Hatano, S. (1974) Multicentre stroke registration. Personal communication.

Isaacs, B. & Marks, R. (1973) Determinants of outcome of stroke rehabilitation. *Age and Ageing*, **2**, 139.

Katz, S., Ford, A. B., Chinn, A. B. & Newill, W. A. (1966) Prognosis after strokes. *Medicine* (Baltimore), **45**, 236.

Kelly, R. (1958) Discussion of spontaneous cerebral haemorrhage. *Proceedings of the Royal Society of Medicine*, **51**, 213.

Marquardsen, J. (1969) *The Natural History of Acute Cerebrovascular Disease: A Retrospective Study of 769 Patients*. Copenhagen: Munksgaard.

Marshall, J. & Kaeser, A. C. (1961) Survival after non-haemorrhagic cerebrovascular accidents. *British Medical Journal*, ii, 73.

Marshall, J. & Shaw, D. A. (1959) The natural history of cerebrovascular disease. *British Medical Journal*, i, 1614.

McKissock, W., Richardson, A. & Taylor, J. (1961) Primary intracerebral haemorrhage. *Lancet*, ii, 221.

McKissock, W., Richardson, A. & Walsh, L. (1960) Spontaneous cerebellar haemorrhage: a study of 34 consecutive cases treated surgically. *Brain*, **83**, 1.

Moskowitz, E., Lightbody, F. E. H. & Freitag, N. S. (1972) Long-term follow-up of the poststroke patient. *Archives of Physical Medicine and Rehabilitation*, **53**, 167.

Ng, L. K. Y. & Nimmannitya, J. (1970) Massive cerebral infarction with severe brain swelling. *Stroke*, **1**, 158.

Pakarinen, S. (1967) *Incidence, Aetiology, and Prognosis of Primary Subarachnoid Haemorrhage*. Copenhagen: Munksgaard.

Plum, F. & Posner, J. B. (1972) *The diagnosis of Stupor and Coma*. 2nd edn. F. A. Davis: Philadelphia.

Rankin, J. (1957) Cerebral vascular accidents in patients over the age of 60. Part II, Prognosis. *Scottish Medical Journal*, **2**, 200.

Robinson, R. W., Cohen, W. D., Higano, N., Meyer, R., Lukowsky, G. H., McLaughlin, R. B. & MacGilpin, H. H. (1959) Life-table analysis of survival after cerebral thrombosis, ten-year experience. *Journal of the American Medical Association*, **169**, 1149.

Rompel, K. & Wiedenmann (1970) Restitution und Letalitat bei Verschlussen zerebraler Gefasse. *Medizinische Klinik*, **65**, 1334.

Rout, M. W., Lane, D. J. & Wolner, L. (1971) Prognosis in acute cerebrovascular accidents in relation to respiratory pattern and blood gas tensions. *British Medical Journal*, iii, 7.

Shafer, S. Q., Bruun, B. & Richter, R. W. (1973) The outcome of stroke at hospital discharge in New York City blacks. *Stroke*, **4**, 782.

Shenkin, H. A., Haft, H. & Somach, F. M. (1965) Prognostic significance of arteriography in nonhaemorrhagic strokes. *Journal of the American Medical Association*, **194**, 612.

Thygesen, P., Christensen, E., Dyrbye, M., Eiken, M., Frantzen, E., Gormsen, J., Lademann, A., Lennox-Buchthal, M., Rønnov-Jessen, V. & Therkelsen, J. (1964) Cerebral apoplexy. *Danish Medical Bulletin*, **11**, 233.

Whisnant, J. P., Fitzgibbons, J. P., Kurland, L. T. & Sayre, G. P. (1971) Natural history of stroke in Rochester, Minnesota, 1945 through 1954. *Stroke*, **2**, 11.

3. Pathology of Degenerative Cerebral Arterial Disease

M. Rufus Crompton

Cerebral arterial disease is one of the most perplexing subjects a pathologist can study. This is not only because of the vagaries of vascular disease but because of the complexity of the brain and the selective vulnerability of its many parts to ischaemia. Diseases of the cerebral arterial system usually occur late in life against a background of widespread long-standing vascular changes in many body organs. Often the function of the heart, kidney, and limb vessels is impaired by disease, and hypertension is an added feature in many cases.

Atheromatous cerebral arterial disease, even more than coronary artery disease, is but one facet of a generalised disorder. The prognosis of myocardial ischaemia in a man in his mid-50s is usually that of his coronary arteries; the prognosis of a man suffering a stroke in his early 70s is not necessarily that of his cerebral arteries. It is equally that of his renal, coronary, or peripheral arteries. Similarly, the pathology in his cerebral arteries may depend on the functioning and pathology of his heart, and the treatment of his neurological deficit may be best directed towards his heart or kidneys.

This account is limited to arterial atheroma, hypertensive arterial disease, and cerebral berry aneurysms. These often co-exist and account for the bulk of cerebral arterial disease. It is not a comprehensive review of current knowledge but a personal interpretation of the mechanisms considered to underlie the pathology of stroke.

CEREBRAL ARTERIAL ATHEROMA

This chapter is not concerned with discussing the essential nature and pathogenesis of atheroma (Crawford, 1964) but only with the different types of atheroma, the changes they may undergo, and how they affect the cerebral arteries.

Atheroma of any type is almost always associated with loss of muscle and elastic tissue, thus resulting in an inelastic, rigid artery which can neither constrict nor dilate. The *fibrous* type of disease, concentric or eccentric, usually involves the vertebral arteries (Hutchinson and Yates, 1957) which may be narrowed, especially at the origins and termination. It is a relatively static form of the disease and seldom proceeds to occlusion or embolisation. Its significance is in the continuing narrowing with resultant reduction of blood flow. However, a solitary, short stenosis has to reduce the lumen very considerably before there is a reduction in flow (Brice, Dowsett, and Lowe, 1964). Stenoses of this type are often multiple and affect more than one artery. For example, both vertebral arteries may be stenosed not only at origin and termination, but also along their course through the cervical vertebrae by tortuosity due to cervical spondylosis. Significant fibrous stenosis may also be present in the internal carotid arteries or more commonly in the cortical branches of the cerebral arteries, but in these sites the purely fibrous type of atheroma is rare.

The mainly *lipid* type of disease occurs in the cervical carotid and cerebral arteries. It tends to produce stenosis at the origins of branches, notably the subclavian and innominate arteries, the internal carotid arteries, and the intracerebral arteries. It is most often stenotic in the branches of the cerebral arteries. Atheroma commences in the carotid arteries earlier than it does in the cerebral arteries. However, the latter are of much narrower lumen, so that stenosis of one or both carotid arteries even if mild may be accompanied by significant multiple stenoses of the cerebral arteries, and also by stenosis of collateral branches between the cerebral arteries, between internal and external carotid fields of supply, and between external carotid and vertebral branches. It is this fact that makes atheromatous carotid disease so prone to cause brain damage, whereas carotid occlusion from other causes, such as surgery, usually does not result in cerebral infarction.

Lipid atheroma tends to ulcerate. This may be due to the rupture of lipid-laden phagocytes into the lumen or result from haemorrhage into the plaque. This occurs especially at the origin of the internal carotid arteries, in the basilar artery, and occasionally at the origin of the subclavian or innominate arteries. The result of this ulceration is initially the discharge of atheromatous debris, including cholesterol crystals, into the cerebral or retinal circulation where they may be observed ophthalmoscopically.

Later fibrin-platelet mural thrombi appear. These too may embolise into the cerebral and retinal circulations, or the mural thrombus may enlarge and larger emboli be thrown off. Mural thrombosis may progress to total thrombotic occlusion. If the subject survives, the thrombus will retract and re-canalisation will occur. If a mural thrombus shrinks back to the vessel wall it will be organised and will eventually be transformed into an atheromatous stenosis. It may become endothelialised, thus ending any embolisation that may have been occurring. This is the result that it is hoped to achieve by administering anticoagulants to patients with transient cerebral ischaemia.

Lipid atheroma also tends to become calcified. This is especially so at the origin of the internal carotid arteries, in the carotid canal, and terminal internal carotid artery, and in the basilar artery. In the basilar artery dilatation and elongation occurs, as it does in the aorta. And, as in the aorta, a fusiform serpiginous atheromatous aneurysm may result. This seldom ruptures but may exert pressure on cranial nerves and the brain stem. In addition to the generalised dilatation of the vessel, localised atheromatous ectasias may occur. The rupture of one of these may be the basis of spontaneous carotico-cavernous fistula in the aged, although it is practically impossible to exclude trauma or the rupture of a small berry aneurysm at the origin of an internal carotid meningeal branch.

CEREBRAL HYPERTENSIVE ARTERIAL DISEASE

The vascular changes associated with arterial hypertension are quite definite. However, atheroma very commonly co-exists since it is exacerbated by both age and hypertension. Nevertheless, the severe hypertensive does have a distinct type of arterial disease which produces characteristic occlusive and haemorrhagic lesions in the brain.

Sustained arterial hypertension results in the loss of muscle and its replacement by inelastic collagen in the cerebral arteries. The internal elastica fragments, splits, and degenerates. The result is an artery, often of enlarged lumen, with rigid non-collapsable walls. This is usually seen in the Circle of Willis and the larger branches of the cerebral arteries. In the smaller cerebral branches and in the perforating arteries, the collagenous walls undergo hyaline degeneration. They tend to become stenosed or they dilate to form small microaneurysms. These occur typically at the sites where hypertensive haemorrhage is usually seen and also at the sites where small cystic, old infarcts are common. This can be explained by their propensity either to thrombose or to leak and rupture. Microaneurysms of this type, which are not limited to arterial branchings as are berry aneurysms, were first demonstrated by Charcot and Bouchard (1868) by the simple expedient of separating the arterial supply from a brain allowed to decompose in a bucket of water. Russell (1963a) later demonstrated these small arterial blow-outs by the more refined technique of post-mortem angiography. There is little doubt that these microaneurysms are of prime importance in the production of hypertensive intracerebral haemorrhage, and as they may also be found in the subarachnoid space on cortical branches, they may explain some cases of spontaneous subarachnoid haemorrhage in which no berry aneurysm can be demonstrated. (Crawford and Crompton, 1965).

CEREBRAL BERRY ANEURYSMS

The structural basis of the pathogenesis of berry aneurysms was first suspected by Turnbull

(1914–1915) and established by Forbus (1930).

All the arteries of the body have a defect or gap in the media at the apex of their bifurcations or branchings. In the majority of organs this defect is covered by the single layer of the internal elastica, the multiple layers of the external elastica, and the parenchyma of the organ. In the cerebral and ovarian arteries there is no external elastica, and in the cerebral subarachnoid arteries there is no organ parenchyma, only the waterbath of the cerebrospinal fluid. As a result the integrity of the cerebral subarachnoid arteries at the apical defects depends almost completely on the internal elastica. It is at these defects that berry aneurysms form. Factors associated with their formation are age and arterial hypertension. The two, often co-existent, probably exert their effect by disrupting the internal elastica. The effect may be one somewhat akin to metal fatigue, whereby the longitudinal stretching of the artery with each pulse exerts a maximum strain on the internal elastica at the apices of the bifurcations. On the other hand it may be haemodynamic, depending on turbulence at the bifurcations replacing the normal arterial axial flow. This is probably the basis of the endothelial pads that form on either side of the apex, and it is noteworthy that within these pads the internal elastica is re-duplicated, its lacunae enlarged, and granular disintegration appears. It may also be significant that it is within these pads that atheroma first appears with all its disruptive effects on elastic tissue (Crompton, 1966a).

Age, arterial hypertension, and atheroma, all of which are inter-related, are associated with disruption of the arterial internal elastica and are undoubtedly of importance in the formation of berry aneurysms. It might then be expected that berry aneurysms would form in the second half of life. This is indeed the case. The aneurysms themselves are not congenital; the congenital feature (which is not an abnormality) is the arterial medial defect, present in most of the cerebral arteries of all individuals. Arterial hypertension is common among persons who suffer from a ruptured cerebral aneurysm, being present in about 60 per cent of an autopsied population of such individuals. Asymmetry of the vessels of the Circle of Willis is more frequent in persons with berry aneurysms. This is probably associated with increased local forces, whether pulsatile or haemodynamic, which are deleterious to the internal elastica. The mechanism is almost certainly similar in persons with large arteriovenous anomalies or angiomas who develop one or more berry aneurysms on the enlarged cerebral arteries feeding the anomaly. These vessels, carrying considerably more blood than the other cerebral arteries and having increased turbulence and pulsation, invariably show more and larger endothelial pads, atheroma, and internal elastic degeneration than the other cerebral arteries. These aneurysms not infrequently rupture, and it cannot be assumed that, in a patient displaying an angioma on angiography, it is the angioma that has produced the subarachnoid haemorrhage. Aneurysms on the tortuous, enlarged feeding arteries may not be seen on the angiogram.

It is universal experience among clinicians and pathologists that berry aneurysms do occur and rupture in young adults in whom none of the above factors or circumstances are present. This raises the question of why these young persons develop berry aneurysms. There are undoubtedly other factors in the production of these aneurysms. That it is some abnormality of mesoderm is suggested by the fact that berry aneurysms are of increased incidence in persons with polycystic disease of the kidneys. This is as true of those cases in whom the renal disease exhibits itself as slow renal failure without hypertension as it is of the cases with arterial hypertension. Examination of the cerebral arteries in normotensive individuals with polycystic renal disease who have ruptured a cerebral berry aneurysm shows that there appears to be an increased amount of collagenous fibrous tissue among the medial muscle. This may result in a more rigid arterial wall in which elongation during pulsation is impaired with resultant increased longitudinal strain on the internal elastica over the apical medial defects. This could disrupt the elastica at these sites with resultant aneurysm formation. This also may be one of the mechanisms by which arterial hypertension, which also produces rigid arterial walls, damages the internal elastica.

There is little doubt that factors other than age, arterial hypertension, and atheroma play a part in the formation of berry aneurysms. It might be thought that these are operative in multiple cases of ruptured berry aneurysms occurring in a single family. However, great care should be taken before coming to this conclusion. Arterial hypertension is known to run in families, and it need not be severe or sustained for it to be effective in producing cerebral berry aneurysms.

A histological study of the cerebral arteries in a variety of mammals ranging from badgers to horses to deer was undertaken (Crompton, 1966b) in the hope that it might shed some light on the pathogenesis of cerebral aneurysms in man, for these lesions do not occur in animals. Even the relatively large brain of the dolphin, approaching in size to that of man, was examined. It was surmised that it was the enlargement of man's forebrain, resulting in an increasing obtuseness of the apical angle at the arterial branches, which opened up or enlarged the medial defects.

It was found that all the mammals examined had medial defects as frequently as man. They were smaller, which is perhaps not surprising, but the most significant finding was that in all there was an appreciable external elastica, and in many there was also elastic tissue among the medial muscle fibres. Endothelial pads occurred, but atheroma was not seen.

It is probable that in man, the absence of any elastic tissue other than the internal elastica, together with longevity and the accompanying factors of hypertension and atheroma, are responsible for cerebral berry aneurysms in over 1 per cent of routine autopsies.

In conclusion it is of interest, in view of the frequency with which multiple cerebral berry aneurysms are symmetrical on the Circle of Willis, that a study of the Circle of Willis in persons with no aneurysms shows that the larger medial defects are also symmetrical. Therefore the unfortunate possession of one or more large medial defects in the cerebral arteries may be one factor predisposing to aneurysm formation.

The cerebral berry aneurysm having been initiated, its structure and mechanisms of growth and rupture must be considered (Crompton, 1966c). The wall of the aneurysm consists of attenuated adventitia, which is very sparse in the cerebral arteries, and intimal endothelium. Quite often vestiges of degenerate internal elastica are present in the neck of the aneurysm. There is usually intimal fibrous tissue or frank atheroma beneath the endothelium. Thus the wall of the aneurysm is inelastic and cannot expand with pulsation. Angiography shows that there is a relative stasis of blood in aneurysm sacks. After the contrast medium has passed into the venous phase, residual amounts are still present in the aneurysm. This may result in mural fibrin deposition, which can become endothelialised and converted into atheromatous material thickening the wall of the aneurysm.

The cerebral arteries, unless atheromatous, possess no vasa vasorum and depend on oxygen diffusion from the lumen. This means that they will be rendered anoxic by any slowing or stasis of the blood flow. It is also a fact that vasa vasorum are not seen in the walls of berry aneurysms unless significant atheroma is present, and it is doubtful if these vessels could contribute to oxygenating the endothelium. The constant state of relative stasis in aneurysms, by lowering the oxygen tension and predisposing to fibrin and platelet deposition, may damage the endothelium with consequent loss of its continuity and structural integrity. Plasma can then pass into the aneurysm wall, further impairing the oxygenation and nutrition of the wall with resulting degenerative changes and decrease in the strength of the structure. The wall then bulges locally and may rupture, or it may hold and eventually be organised into a patch of atheroma. This is probably the mechanism of formation of the small bulges or blisters, often with atheroma in their wall, which are part of the structure of cerebral berry aneurysms (Fig. 3.1). They are usually at the fundus where the aneurysm is mechanically weakest, and represent episodes of bulging which have stopped short of rupture. This is supported by the observation that ruptures are usually fundal and usually at one of these blisters. Their formation is one mechanism of enlargement of the

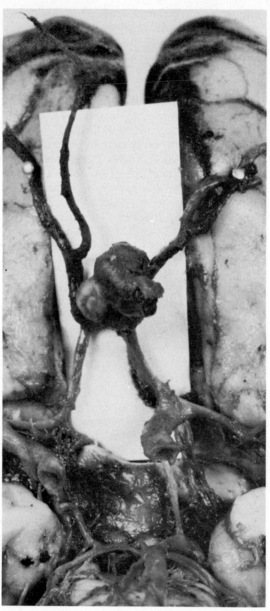

Fig. 3.1 Anterior communicating aneurysm with a pale bulge or blister. The pallor is due to atheroma in the wall of the blister.

are multiloculated (Fig. 3.2). The loculi represent continued enlargement of a blister. It would appear that at 4 mm diameter the stasis and mural fibrin deposition in an aneurysm becomes significant in producing endothelial damage and fibrin insudation into the wall.

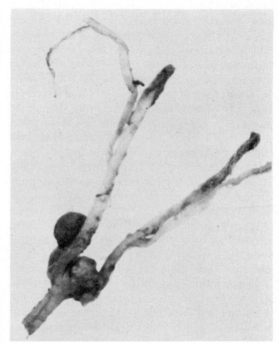

Fig. 3.2 Multiloculated middle cerebral aneurysm.

aneurysm, the other being a gradual stretching of the whole structure.

Many aneurysms, especially if over 4 mm in diameter, which is the optimum size for rupture,

This fibrin can be specifically stained in small bulges in the wall of an aneurysm. It is also invariably present around the margin of a rupture, being one of the criteria of identifying a true rupture histologically, and suggesting that fibrin insudation into the aneurysm wall is the precursor of bulging or of rupture of the wall. It is very doubtful if the fibrin is deposited deep in the wall after rupture.

A great deal of controversy has raged as to what predisposes to the rupture of a cerebral berry aneurysm. It has been suggested that physical activity might cause rupture, but there is little to support this. Hypotensive therapy has been given a considerable trial in persons surviving their first rupture, so as to prevent the common and often fatal second bleed. It was not effective, perhaps because thus increasing the intra-aneurysmal stasis had the exact opposite to the desired effect. It does, however, appear that the Valsalva effect and coughing, which raise both the arterial and the venous pressure, may play some part in initiating rupture. In a personal series, a large number of cases were found dead on the toilet seat and there appeared to be an association between aneurysmal rupture and chronic bronchitis. The sudden rise in arterial pressure might initiate the dissection of plasma into the wall of the aneurysm; in addition the arterial oxygen tension in the chronic bronchitic may be lower than normal.

Investigators have suggested that there is a connection between head injury and the rupture of cerebral berry aneurysms. The negative pressure pockets occurring in closed head injury have been indicated as predisposing to rupture (Overgaard, 1966), and Simonsen (1967) states that injuries at the level of the base of the skull are more likely to damage arterial structures. This is indeed the case as far as the internal carotid arteries are concerned, and provides the basis for some cases of carotico-cavernous fistula and delayed internal carotid occlusion due to thrombosis forming on intimal tears and post-traumatic dissecting aneurysms. It may well be the case also in the rupture of some internal carotid aneurysms, but no analysis of figures, including the author's, has proved this to be so.

Alcohol has been cited as a factor predisposing to aneurysmal rupture, either in its own right or through its association with head injury. However, here again no one has either proved or disproved the contention. It has been suggested that the bounding pulse of inebriation might tend towards rupture of the aneurysm. The pathologist is aware of the cases in which a ruptured berry aneurysm is unexpectedly found in persons who collapsed during or after a fracas. Alcohol is often present in the blood of the deceased. Head injury is also present in many of these cases. In spite of the lack of statistical evidence in favour of alcohol or head injury contributing to aneurysm rupture, the author and many other pathologists with a coroner's

practice remain impressed by the apparent associations. There are many interlinked factors in the complex problem of the pathogenesis of aneurysmal rupture, and care must be taken not to correlate positively factors which really only co-exist through their common linkage with a third factor and have no direct cause or effect relationship with each other. Furthermore a factor must not be assumed to be present unless proved. The deceased may be found in the lavatory because he went there to vomit after the aneurysm ruptured. It cannot be assumed that he had been straining at stool. The aneurysm may not rupture immediately after some effort or trauma. Dissection or insudation of fibrin into its wall may be initiated by such a factor and result in actual rupture sometime later. The reader may by now be aware of the confused body of evidence and opinion associated with the problem of aneurysmal rupture, and also aware of the lack of definite facts on cause and effect. Certainly in criminal rather than civil cases there must be a certainty beyond all reasonable doubt, and this we do not possess as far as the pathogenesis of aneurysmal rupture is concerned.

When an aneurysm ruptures the clinical evidence would suggest that often there is a leakage followed by massive haemorrhage. Almost certainly the bleeding ceases as a result of spasm of the artery bearing the aneurysm, although this may not occur until later, a fall in systemic blood pressure, a rise in intracranial pressure, and the formation of laminated thrombus as a crescentic, cap-like structure over the rupture (Fig. 3.3). This thrombus does not extend far out from the aneurysm, unless in a fissure like the Sylvian fissure, for the cerebrospinal fluid appears to inhibit thrombus accumulation. However, it does extend back into the aneurysm and may fill it, very seldom extending back into the parent vessel. Alternatively it may fill about two-thirds of the aneurysm or less. In all events it will result in the aneurysm appearing to be smaller on an angiogram than it really is.

With the passage of time in the next fateful six weeks or so, the clot will tend to retract. It may also lyse near the lumen and undergo cystic breakdown. Organisation takes place

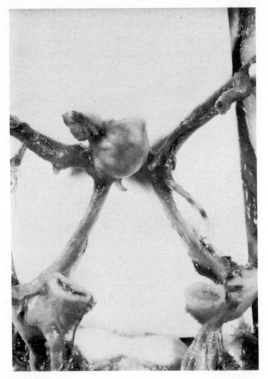

Fig. 3.3   Anterior communicating aneurysm with a fibrin cap or plug over a rupture on the fundus.

from all sides, and if all is well the rupture is healed and eventually appears as a patch of atheroma in a bulge or bubble. However, if not so fortunate, as the thrombus retracts, blood may dissect between it and the aneurysmal wall and eventually bursts out again through the original rupture.

The practical application of these facts is in the methods employed by surgeons to prevent re-bleeding from a ruptured aneurysm which has ceased bleeding. These methods, such as ligation of the carotid in the neck, firing pig bristles into the aneurysm, attracting iron filings into it, or electrocoagulating it, may aim to induce thrombosis within the aneurysm. Other methods, such as wrapping the aneurysm in hammered muscle or cotton gauze or acrylic resin, aim to induce thrombus and fibrosis around the aneurysm. Others such as clipping the neck attempt to isolate it from the circula-

tion (Fig. 3.4). Undoubtedly the latter is the best for obvious reasons. Of the other two methods, the induction of thrombus and organisation around the aneurysm appears to be more effective than the initiation of intra-aneurysmal thrombosis, possibly because, as stated above, the natural history of such thrombus in an aneurysm is for it to contract or retract; blood tends to dissect between it and the wall and rupture out again through the original rupture.

THE PATHOGENESIS OF STROKES

Ischaemic or occlusive strokes are characterised by three distinct pathological processes reflected in the clinical occurrence of transient ischaemic attacks or little strokes, developing major strokes, and established major strokes with some degree of eventual recovery to a relatively static end result.

Transient ischaemic attack, in which there is repetitive occurrence of almost identical neurological or visual deficit with complete recovery between episodes, has been the basis of considerable argument as to its pathogenesis. It was originally considered that the most likely explanation for these attacks was a lowering of blood pressure resulting in depression of cerebral perfusion, the site of particular atheromatous stenoses deciding the regions of the brain rendered most ischaemic and therefore accounting for the almost identical neurological deficit of each attack. Variations in blood pressure may indeed produce variations in cerebral perfusion, and in a hypertensive individual with high peripheral resistance, a high blood pressure is necessary to maintain adequate cerebral perfusion. However, when the pressure is lowered in such persons by hypotensive drugs, the effect is of generalised cerebral ischaemia rather than the focal neurological symptoms which occur in a true transient ischaemic attack. Likewise sudden tilting of elderly arteriosclerotic patients from the horizontal to the vertical position seldom produces symptoms of a transient ischaemic attack, nor does the somewhat dangerous procedure of pressing on the carotid sinus. Although

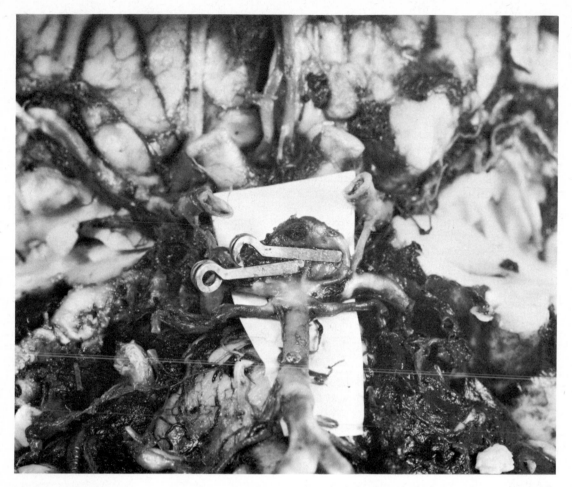

Fig. 3.4   Basilar bifurcation aneurysm with two clips applied to isolate the dark coloured apical rupture from the circulation.

cerebral perfusion may be impaired by episodes of heart block or paroxysmal tachycardia, it is the level of consciousness which is affected rather than a focal, visual, motor, sensory, or psychic function. In some conditions such as following a myocardial infarct or in aortic stenosis, there may be two factors, reduction of overall cerebral perfusion and embolisation to the brain and retina. It may be difficult to decide which factor predominates.

Small fibrin-platelet mural thrombi, containing very few red cells, form on damaged endothelium from the heart to the intracranial cerebral arteries. They may form on the endocardium over necrotic heart muscle, on rheuma-tic mitral and aortic valves, or on calcific or congenitally abnormal valves. They may form on apparently normal valves in persons with carcinoma, especially carcinoma of the pancreas. Arterial sites where ulcerative and calcific atheroma occur, such as at the origin of the internal carotid artery, the origins of the innominate and subclavian arteries, and the intra-cranial vertebral and basilar arteries, are frequently the source of minute fibrin-platelet emboli which may pass into the circulation in showers impacting in the cerebral and retinal arterioles (Ashby, Oakley, Lorentz, and Scott, 1963: Russell, 1961). They do not produce spasm in the arterioles, and as a result mainly of rapid fibrinolysis and moulding, they pass quickly through the capillary bed and into the venous system. These emboli may be seen in the retinal arteries ophthalmoscopically during a transient ischaemic attack or after manipulation of the carotid sinus. This mechanism adequately explains the transient nature of ischaemic attacks with almost complete recovery. However, there have been those who doubted whether it could explain the almost stereotyped repetitiveness of the attacks. They doubted that the emboli would impact at the same fork in the same vessel each time. In fact it is seen that in a unique and complex haemodynamic system such as occurs in branching arteries involved by stenotic atheroma, the flow takes particles of the same size along exactly the same course. A similar process can be seen in a river flowing fast over rapids. Leaves dropped in at the same spot, follow an almost identical path and often end up at the same spot on the bank downstream. It is therefore feasible that fibrin-platelet emboli, which are of fairly uniform size, will end up impacted in the same arteriolar bifurcations each time that they are released.

The current acceptance of the embolic theory of the production of transient ischaemic attacks has led to forms of medical and surgical treatment based on the prevention of mural thrombus formation and embolisation. These include the use of heparin and the practice of carotid endarterectomy. These treatments are aimed not so much at the prevention of the transient ischaemic attacks themselves as at the prevention of the frequent progression of these small attacks towards major strokes with permanent brain damage.

Mention should be made of arterial spasm, which has been cited as a factor in transient cerebral ischaemia. This has never been demonstrated, either in the retinal or cerebral arteries, and it would appear most unlikely in the rigid, muscle-depleted arteries and arterioles of the arteriopath. Apart from angiographic demonstration following cerebral aneurysm rupture, and resulting from local stimulation or trauma during surgery, spasm is not unequivocally established in human arteries. It has been shown beautifully in the cerebral and retinal arteries of rats (Byrom, 1954 and 1963) as a response to raising the arterial pressure, and it may account for the episodes of hypertensive encephalopathy in chronic nephritics, many of whom are young with adequately muscled cerebral arteries and arterioles. The symptoms of this encephalopathy and the pathological cerebral oedema often produced certainly bears little resemblance to the symptoms or pathological sequelae of transient ischaemic attacks.

Transient ischaemic attacks may terminate with the occurrence of established stroke, but common though this sequence is, it is not the sole outcome. The transient attacks may cease, in which case the friable mural fibrin-platelet thrombi will have been endothelialised and will eventually be incorporated into the intima of the artery. Further disruption of the endothelium by the underlying processes of atheroma may result in the resumption of mural thrombus formation and the recurrence of transient ischaemic attacks.

Developing major strokes may follow on transient ischaemic attacks or they may present *de novo*. In the former case the progression of the developing fibrin-platelet mural thrombus outstrips the rate of endothelialisation by peripheral endothelium and monocytes from the blood, and red cells begin to be incorporated in a laminated thrombus. This sends off considerably larger emboli than the original fibrin-platelet thrombus. In addition eruption and ulceration of underlying atheroma may result in atheromatous material, including crystals of cholesterol esters, being thrown into the circulation. (Sturgill and Netsky, 1963). Such crystals may occasionally be seen in the retinal circulation (Russell, 1963b).

The large emboli pass into the cerebral circulation and usually impact early in the branchings of the middle cerebral arteries, as these are the direct continuation of the axial flow of the internal carotid arteries. Occasionally, the emboli lodge at the termination of the internal carotid artery, but usually they are small enough to continue beyond this. In the vertebro-basilar system the emboli appear to be less stereotyped in their route and may end up in any arteries from the pons to occipital cortex.

The arteries narrow beyond a birfurcation, making it the obvious point for emboli to impact. As a result of the fall in intra-arterial pressure distal to the impacted embolus, the branches dilate. In addition fibrinolysis both within the embolus itself and also from the surrounding blood eventually fragments it. These fragments then pass on, probably up different branches until they impact again at a birfurcation whose narrowing will not allow them to proceed (Luessenhop *et al.*, 1962). It is evident that such a mechanism will give a developing stroke a definite sequence. The initial impaction of the embolus results in a large pale or ischaemic infarct. The endothelium of the arterioles and capillaries in this region will also be damaged as a result of the vascular stasis. When the embolus breaks up and moves on, blood will reflow into damaged arterioles and capillaries with resultant haemorrhage into the necrotic brain. This accounts for the haemorrhagic nature of embolic infarcts, the haemorrhages of which are usually confined to the grey matter. One frequently seen pattern is a large, pale infarct in the cortical distribution of a middle cerebral artery, combined with haemorrhagic infarction in the ganglionic distribution of the same artery. This is patently due to an embolus initially impacting proximal to the origin of the perforating ganglionic branches and then breaking up and passing on beyond them to impact permanently in cortical branches.

A large embolus can impact at one of the first main bifurcations of a middle cerebral artery permanently and thrombus may propagate distally and also proximally back to the origin of the middle cerebral artery. The appearance, then, is of middle cerebral thrombosis as described by the early neurologist-neuropathologists, who did not examine the neck vessels. A similar appearance may accompany internal carotid artery occlusion at its origin and be based on stasis in the middle cerebral artery rather than embolisation. It is seldom that thrombosis *in situ* occurs in the middle cerebral artery without proximal disease. However, there are exceptions, especially inexplicable instances in young adults of both sexes, and also in the pancerebral arterial thrombosis that occurs in the

swollen brains of persons, maintained on artificial ventilation, in whom angiographic contrast medium gets no further than the base of the skull.

The mural thrombus in the cervical carotid or basilar artery may, instead of or after throwing off emboli, enlarge to occlude the vessel (Fig. 3.5). This occlusive thrombosis *in situ*, especially if it is at the origin of the internal carotid artery,

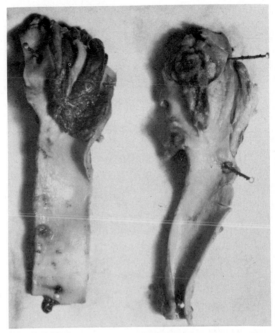

Fig. 3.5 The bifurcation of each common carotid artery. On one side thrombus occludes the origin of both internal and external carotid arteries. A tongue of thrombus extends up the internal carotid artery.

may propagate upwards until it meets the retrograde collateral flow from other arteries. It may propagate beyond these into the middle cerebral artery, and if the anterior communicating artery is vestigial, it may continue into the anterior cerebral artery. As already mentioned, the internal carotid thrombus may not propagate, but because of poor collateral flow around the Circle of Willis, thrombosis due to stasis may take place in the terminal internal carotid and middle cerebral artery (Fig. 3.6). Occasionally, there is an occlusive local thrombus at the origin

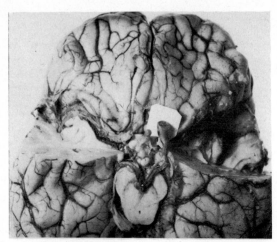

Fig. 3.6 Thrombus occluding the termination of the left internal carotid artery.

of the internal carotid artery and an embolic occlusion of the middle cerebral artery. It is in fact apparent that many combinations of embolisation and thrombosis *in situ* may occur.

Once the occlusive lesion has reached a state of equilibrium, the extent to which infarction is going to proceed depends on a number of factors.

The anatomical factors of importance are the adequacy of the Circle of Willis and the presence of other collateral connections, such as those between the external and internal carotid supplies at points like the ophthalmic arteries, numerous meningeal branches of both internal and external carotid arteries, carotico-tympanic and spheno-palatine arteries, connections between occipital branches of the external carotids, and similar branches of the vertebral arteries and vertebral branches with the thyrocervical trunks. For example, an arrangement in which the posterior cerebral arteries receive most of their blood from the internal carotid arteries, which is a not uncommon anomaly, will spare the occipital lobes in vertebro-basilar occlusion, but probably result in a larger parietal infarct in the event of internal carotid occlusion.

The presence, site, and multiplicity of atheromatous stenosis is another factor of great importance and, like the anatomical factor, influences the adequacy of collateral blood supply to the region of brain deprived of its blood supply. Unfortunately atheroma can be shown to affect the collaterals in most cases of occlusive carotid or basilar disease. In addition the small calibre collateral branches between the cerebral arteries on the surface of the brain are nearly always severely narrowed by the time significant disease of the carotid or vertebrobasilar system has taken place. In many instances the presence of intracranial arterial atheroma is more significant in the production of cerebral infarction than is stenosis of the extracranial arteries.

An adequate cerebral perfusion depends on a well-maintained blood pressure, and if this drops in the presence of cerebral emboli or atheroma such as may accompany a myocardial infarct, then cerebral infarction will be more extensive. Hypertension does not worsen the prognosis of a cerebral infarct; in fact, the opposite may be true.

All the factors mentioned above, together with the rate of formation and extent of propagation of the occlusive thrombus, may take hours or longer to decide the actual size of the resulting cerebral infarct. At the periphery of the infarct, the phenomenon of luxury perfusion takes place as collateral arteries enlarge. In places this flow exceeds the local metabolic demand so that red blood appears in the veins possibly through arterio-venous connections. The swelling of the infarct and adjacent oedema raise the intracranial pressure with resultant impairment of small collaterals.

The swelling infarct displaces the cingulate gyrus of the brain to the opposite side beneath the falx cerebri and also the temporal lobe down around the edge of the tentorium cerebelli with lateral compression and anteroposterior elongation of the midbrain, which is also displaced downwards. The paramedian mesencephalic arteries may, if this displacement is too extreme or rapid, rupture to produce the characteristic secondary midbrain haemorrhages in the midline and along the substancia nigra, which almost invariably accompany fatal cerebral infarction. Also seen in the fatal cases, although its presence in surviving cases is questionable, is haemorrhagic secondary occipital infarction involving the visual cortex. The mechanism is intermittent occlusion of posterior cerebral branches to this region against the edge of the tentorium resulting from impaction of the temporal lobe or lobes in the tentorial hiatus. It is intermittent because following impaction the cerebrospinal fluid pressure beneath the impacted hiatus builds up until the temporal lobes are lifted clear to allow the cerebrospinal fluid to flow up through the hiatus to equalise the pressure above and below. During this instant of disimpaction blood reflows through the posterior cerebral branches to brain and arteries devitalised by previous ischaemia. Haemorrhage into infarcted occipital brain occurs. The process then repeats itself.

These midbrain and pontine changes, together with the mechanisms around the tentorial hiatus which accompany them, are of course no different to identical processes accompanying cerebral tumours, intracranial haemorrhage, oedema due to head injury, or any other expanding supratentorial space occupying lesion. Whether they proceed to midbrain or pontine haemorrhage or merely get no further than a third nerve palsy decides of course whether our developing stroke is going to become an established and then a regressing stroke or whether death intervenes.

The established stroke clinically represents the maximum degree of neurological impairment present. This will partially regress. Pathologically it represents the maximum quantity of dead brain present when the processes of occlusion and collateral revascularisation have reached an equilibrium. This swollen, maximum infarct will shrink as the process of partial recovery of function takes place. The cerebral herniations across the midline to the opposite side and down through the tentorial hiatus will revert to the normal anatomical position, and eventually as the infarct becomes a contracted, cystic lesion, the mid-line will be drawn across to its own side and the ipsilateral ventricle will enlarge instead of being compressed and distorted towards the opposite side.

Initially the established infarct consists of a region of brain which has undergone coagulative necrosis (Fig. 3.7) The neuropil becomes rather homogeneous, losing its usual fibrillary

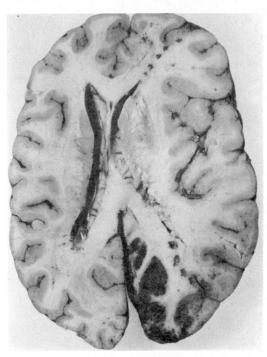

Fig. 3.7 Massive pale infarction of the territory of the left middle cerebral artery (*dotted*) with shift of the mid-line to the right and secondary left occipital haemorrhagic infarction.

character. The neurones lose their Nissl substance, the cytoplasm becoming uniformly eosinophilic and the nucleus becoming shrunken and darkly basophilic. The glial nuclei similarly shrink and the capillaries disintegrate. This necrosis represents, among other things, the breakdown of long protein chains into shorter polypeptides and eventually individual amino-acids, the whole process multiplying enormously the number of molecules present. In addition, at the periphery of the necrotic area, the glia and small blood vessels, being less vulnerable to anoxia than the neurones, may survive. However, the capillary endothelium, basement membrane, and astrocytic footplates, which make up the capillary wall and the blood-brain barrier, are damaged by ischaemia and as a result are permeable to fluid and large molecules. Thus the central portion of the infarct swells from osmosis and the peripheral portion from oedema. The result is that initially a cerebral infarct is a very rapidly enlarging space occupying lesion, enlarging much faster than any tumour and almost as fast as some haemorrhages. It is this rapid enlargement which proves fatal from the secondary brain stem haemorrhages described above. The peripheral oedema and compression also impair function in uninfarcted brain around it. When the infarct eventually shrinks, some of this function will return.

It is at the periphery of the infarct that vital changes take place representing reparative processes from which the age of the infarct can be deduced. Basically these changes are no different from the formation of granulation tissue elsewhere in the body, the only important addition being the astrocytic reaction which accompanies the usual mesodermal one. Within 12 hours the dilated capillaries are filled with polymorphonuclear leucocytes. These diapedese out into the surrounding tissues and may be present in very large numbers, making the biopsy diagnosis of infarction as against abscess very difficult. In fact the presence of micro-organisms is necessary for the confident diagnosis of the latter. This early polymorph reaction may also make itself apparent in the cerebrospinal fluid, as may red cells from a haemorrhagic infarct. Thus red cells do not necessarily imply a subarachnoid haemorrhage nor polymorphonuclear leucocytes a meningitis.

At about three days the polymorphonuclear leucocytes have been replaced by a mononuclear white cell reaction and there appears to be an increase in the number of capillaries, the endothelium of which is swollen and multiplying with mitoses as an indication of activity. Four days after the inception of the infarct, if it is a haemorrhagic one, the red cells break down into haemosiderin and haematoidin. A haemorrhagic infarct begins to look brown to the naked eye. After five days to a week, the mesodermal microglia have proliferated and lost their resting rod-like form, becoming phagocytic and taking up large amounts of cholesterol esters from the disintegrating myelin sheaths to convert themselves into compound granular corpuscles. This process continues with the breakdown of the central coagulated material as it is progressively removed by phagocytes into the blood and probably also the cerebrospinal fluid. Cystic spaces appear which are crossed by proliferating capillaries and young mesodermal fibrous tissue. Around three weeks after the infarct commenced, the astrocytes are seen to have acquired abundant eosinophilic cytoplasm and thick processes in which fibrils can be demonstrated by special stains. The astrocytes also proliferate by amitotic division, and binucleated forms may be seen. This fibrillary gliosis is complementary to the fibrovascular mesodermal reaction. There is nothing specific to infarction about it. It is identical to that seen in young plaques of multiple sclerosis, and axon impregnation may be necessary to distinguish the two on some occasions, when surviving axons can be seen in the multiple sclerotic plaque. After two or three months the infarct has shrunk and the resultant multicystic scar is smaller than the original mass of the brain that was destroyed, with a resultant depression on the surface of the brain and enlargement of the ipsilateral ventricle as described above.

Strokes due to primary intracerebral haemorrhage occur most frequently in persons afflicted with arterial hypertension. A proportion of those occurring in non-hypertensive individuals may be explained by small angiomatous malformations, tumours, leukaemia, and other blood dyscrasias and are not considered here.

The hypertensive arterial changes already described underlie the great majority of cases of intracerebral haemorrhage. They are present in hypertensives, and those involving the perforating arteries are present at the sites where haemorrhage most frequently occurs. These sites are the putamen, where the lenticulostriate arteries lie (Fig. 3.8), the basis pontis, the thalamus, the cerebellar hemispheres, the midbrain, the caudate nucleus, and subcortically, especially in the parieto-occipital regions (McKissock, Richardson, and Taylor, 1961).

The basis of such intracerebral haemorrhages is arterial bleeding from a small vessel. As such, it not infrequently is arrested before forming a haemorrhage adequate to give immediate clinical signs. The small haemorrhage produced is eventually re-absorbed leaving a slit-shaped, golden mesodermal and glial scar. The bleeding

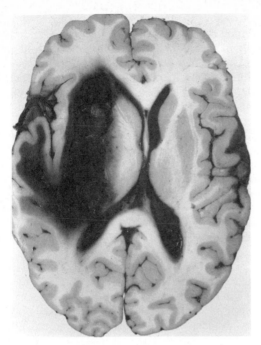

Fig. 3.8 Hypertensive external capsular haemorrhage. It is about to rupture into both the trigone and frontal horn of the lateral ventricle.

artery is almost certainly occluded as a result of the event, and thus every haemorrhage that is survived is accompanied by a small infarct, so that small cystic softenings in the basal ganglia, internal capsule, and brain stem frequently co-exist with the yellow scars of haemorrhage in the brains of hypertensives. Indeed, the process of occlusive thrombosis in the micro-aneurysms may predominate with the result that haemorrhage is not the dominant feature, but the brain is afflicted by multiple small, cystic infarcts in the basal ganglia or pons. This is the characteristic form of occlusive disease in the hypertensive, whereas the large cortical infarct is more typical of the cerebral atherosclerotic. Occasionally the small infarcts predominate in the parietal white matter of the centrum semiovale and in the internal capsules. Such an appearance used to be considered the pathological basis of pseudo-bulbar palsy. Alternatively large regions of poorly defined white matter degeneration may be present in the cerebral white matter, with sparing of the subcortical association fibres. This

was termed Binswanger's hypertensive subcortical encephalopathy. In the author's experience such a change is associated with the hypertensive type of disease that usually involves the perforating arteries, also involving the small cortical arteries and thus possibly explaining the white matter lesions as being due to endartery involvement. A similar appearance can occur in subacute bacterial endocarditis in which there is white matter atrophy and ventricular enlargement. The so-called cerebral Beurger's disease may be based on a similar pathogenesis, possibly showers of emboli to the cortical vessels. Certainly the appearance of the end result of organisation and retraction of small cortical emboli is very similar to the small arterial and arteriolar changes of hypertension. Small, crescentic, subcortical golden scars are very frequent in hypertensive brains. The rupture of one of these through the cortex might account for some cases of subarachnoid haemorrhage in which no berry aneurysm is found. Alternatively the typical hypertensive micro-aneurysm, which may occur on small cortical arteries, may underlie such haemorrhages. Although most of these subarachnoid haemorrhages are eventually, after meticulous dissection, explained by very small berry aneurysms, there is a residue which is probably accounted for by factors such as trauma or the possibilities discussed above.

When the hypertensive patient develops a major stroke, then if he is to survive, the haemorrhage will take place in the putamen or external capsular region, the cerebellum, or one of the lobes of the cerebrum. Haemorrhages at other sites such as the pons and thalamus, both of which are prone to spread into the midbrain, tend to end up in the public mortuary without reaching hospital first. Those in the external capsule split the fibres to form a lens-shaped haemorrhage that may rupture through the anterior or posterior limb of the internal capsule. into the lateral ventricle (Fig. 3.8). Haemorrhage into the ventricles can be survived as long as the bleeding into the ventricles is not faster than the rate at which it can escape from the fourth ventricle exit foramina. If a capsular, subcortical, or cerebellar haemorrhage is survived, then as a result of the fibre-separating rather than fibre-destroying mode of enlargement of the haemorrhage, the eventual removal of the blood will result in the walls of the cavity coming together to produce a linear pigmented scar with considerable recovery of function.

Strokes due to ruptured cerebral berry aneurysms take place in the same age group as those due to primary hypertensive haemorrhages. Also, about 60 per cent of ruptured aneurysm cases in an autopsy series are hypertensive, and a high proportion of hypertensive intracerebral haemorrhages reach the cerebrospinal fluid. Thus the clinical differentiation is basically angiographic.

Seldom in forensic practice does one see a bruised scalp in a person dying from a hypertensive cerebral haemorrhage, whereas this is very common in coronary artery disease and quite common with ruptured cerebral berry aneurysms, indicating that with a ruptured berry aneurysm the patient may fall as if pole-axed, but seldom does with primary hypertensive haemorrhage. The explanation probably lies with the site of the bleeding. The majority of berry aneurysms bleed into the basal subarachnoid space and blow it up like a bladder, suddenly stretching and distorting the perforating branches passing into the hypothalamus, subthalamus, and midbrain. The tension on these very fine vessels may even kink and obliterate them at their angled entrance through the pial surface. The effect is diencephalic ischaemia as suggested by Dott (1960). The upper end of the reticular substance is involved and rapid coma ensues. In a large number of subarachnoid haemorrhages, the suddenly raised pressure in the basal cisterns abates, blood reflows into the diencephalon, possibly with some residual arterial spasm, and consciousness returns. Permanent neurological deficit will be slight.

In addition to the intracranial occurrence, the patient not infrequently feels pain in the neck, back, abdomen, or limbs. Examination of the dorsal root ganglia shows that there is an actual interstitial haemorrhage in these structures (Crompton, 1965). The mechanism in these cases is difficult to determine, for they are some distance from any ruptured cerebral aneurysm.

Berry aneurysms at the base of the brain may not only cause diencephalic ischaemia due to a sudden rise in the pressure in the basal cisterns, they may result in blood being forced along the perivascular sheaths of the perforating vessels and then rupturing out to form small microhaemorrhages in sites such as the hypothalamus. The supraoptic and paraventricular nuclei of the hypothalamus are particularly prone to these haemorrhages (Crompton, 1963). Venous obstruction may also be a factor in producing the haemorrhages in these highly vascular neurosecretory centres. It is of course logical to deduce that interference with the blood flow in any cerebral perforating arteries will, if sustained, result in infarction. Such is the case (Crompton, 1964a), and in fatal subarachnoid haemorrhages patchy ischaemic necrosis may be seen in the midbrain and thalamus, especially with basilar aneurysms, in the corpus striatum and hypothalamus, especially with anterior and posterior communicating aneurysms, in the globus pallidus, especially with posterior communicating aneurysms, and in the putamen, especially with proximal middle cerebral aneurysms.

Aneurysms which lie deeply in cerebral fissures, such as anterior communicating and middle cerebral aneurysms, tend either to bleed directly into the brain (Crompton, 1962a) or to distend the fissure with a subarachnoid haematoma. The middle cerebral aneurysms may bleed into the external capsule to form a lens-shaped intracerebral haematoma indistinguishable from a primary hypertensive haemorrhage unless the aneurysm is found. This direct intracerebral rupture is more common in men, possibly because their aneurysms tend to be larger and therefore embedded in the brain (Crompton, 1962b). The internal carotid bifurcation aneurysm, if large and embedded in the brain, ruptures straight up into the corpus striatum. The posterior communicating aneurysms may rupture into the temporal horn, but usually bleeding is confined to the basal cisterns. The anterior communicating aneurysms, being in the fissure between the frontal lobes, may rupture directly into one or other frontal horn. However, the most characteristic behaviour for the fissure-embedded aneurysms is to first form a subarachnoid haematoma, Sylvian with middle cerebral and interfrontal with anterior communicating aneurysms, and then rupture into the brain. The Sylvian haematoma either extends directly into a lateral ventricle or forms an external capsular haematoma first. The interfrontal haematoma extends into one frontal horn or up into the cavum of the septum pellucidum, which then ruptures into one or both frontal horns. These subarachnoid haematomata are practically pathognomonic of ruptured aneurysms, seldom being seen in any other circumstance, and the haematoma in the cavum is almost diagnostic of a ruptured anterior communicating aneurysm. The author has seen it associated with no other condition.

Intracerebral rupture is a serious and usually fatal sequel of aneurysmal rupture. It is seen more often with second and subsequent bleeds, possibly due to restricting subarachnoid adhesions confining these bleeds and rendering them more likely to burst into the brain (Crompton, 1966d). However, the significance of subarachnoid haematomas is not limited to rupturing into the brain. The sudden distension of the Sylvian fissure lengthens and often angulates and distorts the middle cerebral branches as they enter the brain. The result is to slow down and possibly arrest the blood flow in these vessels. Evidence of this can be seen in the subintimal polymorphonuclear permeation of the arteries (Crompton, 1964b). This is practically identical to the changes in the renal arteries seen after postpartum haemorrhage (Sheehan and Moore, 1952) and in experiments on rabbits. Interstitial oedema of vein walls indicates the same stasis. If flow is re-established relatively soon these vessels are only partly damaged and survive as arteries with thickened endarteritic walls which may be seen years later. If flow does not return soon enough, then fibrinoid necrosis of the wall takes place. If flow then returns, haemorrhage can occur from these necrotic arteries, enlarging the subarachnoid haematoma without any further bleeding from the aneurysm. It is apparent what a dangerous place one of these subarachnoid haematomas is for a surgeon to explore or attempt to evacuate. He will almost certainly produce both haemorrhage and infarction. It is obvious that the arterial necrosis described will produce considerable infarction, and indeed Sylvian haematomas often are surrounded by infarcted insula cortex.

Infarcts may involve large regions of the brain following the rupture of a berry aneurysm. Apart from the damage to the perforating arteries and cortical branches in a subarachnoid haematoma, already described, the angiographically demonstrable arterial spasm, together with the rise in intracranial pressure which embarrasses collateral flow, and any drop in systemic arterial pressure may all contribute to the formation of large infarcts. It appears that there is usually a combination of at least two such factors before infarction takes place. Certainly infarction does not follow in every case with angiographic demonstration of spasm, and it may be absent around some subarachnoid haematomas. However, it is very frequent when a combination of the two can be shown to have taken place, and it is a common cause of death following aneurysmal rupture.

In conclusion it may be mentioned that apart from obvious neurological damage due to infarction and intracerebral haemorrhage, persons surviving aneurysmal rupture for a long period may rarely develop hydrocephalus (Kibler, Couch, and Crompton, 1961).

REFERENCES

Ashby, M., Oakley, M., Lorentz, I. & Scott, D. (1963) Recurrent transient monocular blindness. *British Medical Journal*, ii, 894.

Brice, J. G., Dowsett, D. J. & Lowe, R. D. (1964) The effect of constriction on carotid blood-flow and pressure gradient. *Lancet*, i, 84.

Byrom, F. B. (1954) The pathogenesis of hypertensive encephalopathy and its relation to the malignant phase of hypertension. Experimental evidence from the hypertensive rat. *Lancet*, ii, 201.

Byrom, F. B. (1963) The nature of malignancy in hypertensive disease. Evidence from the retina of the rat. *Lancet*, i, 516.

Charcot, J. M. & Bouchard, C. (1868) Nouvelles recherches sur la pathogenie de l'hemorrhagic cerebral. *Archive de Physiologie Normale et Pathologique*, **1**, 110, 643, and 725.

Crawford, T. (1963) Article (p. 279) in *Evolution of the Atherosclerotic Plaque*, ed. Jones, R. J., Chicago and London: University of Chicago Press.

Crawford, T. & Crompton, M. R. (1965) The pathology of strokes. In *The Management of Cerebrovascular Disease*, ed. Marshall, J. London: Churchill.

Crompton, M. R. (1962a) Intracerebral haematoma complicating ruptured cerebral berry aneurysm. *Journal of Neurology, Neurosurgery and Psychiatry*, **25**, 378.

Crompton, M. R. (1962b) The pathology of ruptured middle cerebral aneurysms. *Lancet*, ii, 421.

Crompton, M. R. (1963) Hypothalamic lesions following the rupture of cerebral berry aneurysms. *Brain*, **86**, 301.

Crompton, M. R. (1964a) Cerebral infarction following the rupture of cerebral berry aneurysms. *Brain*, **87**, 263.

Crompton, M. R. (1964b) The pathogenesis of cerebral infarction following the rupture of cerebral berry aneurysms. *Brain*, **87**, 491.

Crompton, M. R. (1965) Subtentorial changes following the rupture of cerebral aneurysms. *Brain*, **88**, 75.

Crompton, M. R. (1966a) The pathogenesis of cerebral aneurysms. *Brain*, **89**, 797.

Crompton, M. R. (1966b) The comparative pathology of cerebral aneurysms. *Brain*, **89**, 789.

Crompton, M. R. (1966c) Mechanism of growth and rupture in cerebral berry aneurysms. *British Medical Journal*, i, 1138.

Crompton, M. R. (1966d) Recurrent haemorrhage from cerebral aneurysms and its prevention by surgery. *Journal of Neurology, Neurosurgery and Psychiatry*, **29**, 164.

Dott, N. M. (1960) Brain, movement and time. *British Medical Journal*, ii, 12.

Forbus, W. D. (1930) On the origin of miliary aneurysms of superficial cerebral arteries. *Bulletin of the Johns Hopkins Hospital*, **47**, 239.

Hutchinson, E. C. & Yates, P. O. (1957) Carotico-vertebral stenosis. *Lancet*, i, 2.

Kibler, R. F., Couch, R. S. C. & Crompton, M. R. (1961) Hydrocephalus in the adult following spontaneous subarachnoid haemorrhage. *Brain*, **84**, 45.

Luessenhop, A. J., Gibbs, M. & Velasquez, A. C. (1962) Cerebrovascular response to emboli. *Archives of Neurology*, **7**, 264.

McKissock, W., Richardson, A. & Taylor, J. (1961) Primary intracerebral haemorrhage. A controlled trial of surgical and conservative treatment in 180 unselected cases. *Lancet*, ii, 221.

Overgaard, J. (1966) Congress of the German Society of Neurosurgery, *Medical Tribune*, p. 2.

Russell, R. W. R. (1961) Observations on the retinal blood vessels in monocular blindness. *Lancet*, ii, 1422.

Russell, R. W. R. (1963a) Observations on intracerebral aneurysms. *Brain*, **86**, 425.

Russell, R. W. R. (1963b) Atheromatous retinal embolism. *Lancet*, ii, 1354.

Sheehan, H. L. & Moore, H. C. (1952) *Renal Cortical Necrosis and the Kidney of Concealed Accidental Haemorrhage*. Oxford: Blackwell.

Simonsen, J. (1967) Fatal subarachnoid haemorrhage in relation to minor head injuries. *Journal of Forensic Medicine*, **14**, 146.

Sturgill, B. C. & Netsky, M. G. (1963) Cerebral infarction by atheromatous emboli. *American Association Archives of Pathology*, **76**, 189.

Turnbull, H. M. (1914–1915) Alterations in arterial structure, and their relation to syphilis. *Quarterly Journal of Medicine*, **8**, 201.

4. Experimental Studies concerned with the Pathogenesis of Cerebral Ischaemia and Infarction

John Stirling Meyer, Vinod D. Deshmukh, and K. M. A. Welch

In recent years, a vast amount of knowledge on various aspects of cerebral ischaemia and infarction has been obtained using many different animal models and methods for measurement of cerebral blood flow, brain function, and metabolism. Some of the animal models provided improved understanding of the pathogenesis of cerebral ischaemia, while others were helpful in evaluating therapy. In order to obtain certain kinds of information, animal models are indispensible since such information cannot be obtained from human beings for ethical reasons.

This chapter is intended to correlate scattered facts available in the literature concerned with cerebrovascular research and thereby provide a more integrated view of the pathogenesis of cerebral ischaemia and infarction. Throughout the chapter, an attempt will be made to emphasise the possible relevance of these experimental findings to clinical situations.

Cerebral ischaemia may be defined as an impairment of blood supply to the brain which temporarily jeopardises neuronal function but produces no permanent change. By contrast, cerebral infarction may be defined as the result of a more severe and prolonged cerebral ischaemia with at least some irreversible functional and structural change. The potential for maximal recovery, however, may be ensured to some extent by controlling brain oedema, improving collateral circulation, and possibly correcting disorders of neurotransmission. The study of the latter factors, which have therapeutic implications, is of considerable importance in designing experimental animal models.

EXPERIMENTAL ANIMAL MODELS

Experimental cerebral ischaemia or infarction can be produced by various techniques in different animal preparations. The commonest technique is temporary clamping or permanent occlusion of the main artery supplying the area of the brain under study. Various cerebral arteries alone or in combination, such as one or both common carotid arteries, both carotid and vertebral arteries, the middle cerebral artery (MCA) or its branches, and the anterior cerebral plus the MCA, have all been ligated and their effects studied. In order to render the regional ischaemia more severe, vascular ligation has also been combined with hypotension, hypoxia, and exsanguination. Total or segmental vascular occlusion has also been produced by embolisation with moulded silicone cylinders, plastic microspheres, and blood clot. The brain can also be rendered ischaemic by excessive increases in intracranial cerebrospinal fluid pressure. A few investigators have studied haemorrhagic infarction produced by regional freezing of the brain, while others have studied brain metabolism following decapitation or isolating the brain as a perfused organ (isolated brain preparation).

Primates, including the baboon, rhesus monkey, and squirrel monkey, have provided the best experimental models for cerebral vascular research. The general pattern of cerebral vasculature in primates is essentially similar to but not identical with that of man. The major difference in the cerebral vasculature is the presence of a common anterior cerebral artery in primates.

This work was supported by Grant NS 09287 from the National Institute of Neurological Diseases and Stroke, and in part by Grant RR 00350 from the General Clinical Research Cènter Branch, Division of Research Resources, National Institutes of Health, Bethesda, Maryland, U.S.A.

The authors would also like to acknowledge the editorial assistance of Mrs Kathy Tucker in the preparation of the manuscript.

This, fortunately, does not offer much of a problem in designing the experimental model, because the two middle cerebral artery territories are quite separate and can be independently tested in each hemisphere. The primates also have relatively large brains. The average brain weight of a baboon or a rhesus monkey is about 100 g, which is approximately one-fifteenth of the human brain weight. The general configuration of the primate brain is also similar to that of man.

The most commonly used animal model for studies of cerebral infarction has been occlusion of the MCA. The first work using this model was reported from the Montreal Neurological Institute (Petersen and Evans, 1937). Meyer and Denny-Brown (1957) were the first to occlude temporarily or permanently the MCA to study its circulatory and metabolic effects in both closed and open skull preparations and in both acute and chronic monkey preparations. In the closed skull preparations after occlusion of the MCA the craniotomy defect was closed and observations were made of the leptomeningeal circulation through a skull window. In the open skull preparation, regional oxygen tension was measured with polarographic electrodes, regional blood flow studied with thermistors, and pH and P_{CO_2} were studied with microelectrodes.

This model of occluding the MCA in baboons and monkeys has been further developed by approaching the MCA through the orbit (Hudgins and Garcia, 1970; Symon, 1970). MCA occlusion in primates has now become the standard animal model for the study of infarction. It is recommended that the MCA be occluded by transorbital approach using an operating microscope, since there is minimal trauma to the brain and the skull remains closed (Hudgins and Garcia, 1970). This approach was originally used in squirrel monkeys in which an extensive infarction could be produced due to relatively poor collateral circulation. In baboons, likewise, occlusion of the main trunk of the MCA just proximal to the striate branches produces a highly predictable infarction in the opercular region of the Sylvian fissure including the adjacent parts of the temporal, frontal, and parietal lobes.

The baboon, as an experimental animal model, has also been extensively used for cerebrovascular research (Harper et al., 1972; Sengupta, Harper, and Jennett, 1974; Strandgaard, et al., 1974). The squirrel monkey model was used extensively by Sundt and his colleagues (Sundt and Michenfelder, 1971–1972; Michenfelder and Sundt, 1971; Little, Kerr, and Sundt, 1974a, b, c). They studied haemodynamic, biochemical, and ultrastructural effects of cerebral ischaemia following middle cerebral artery occlusion.

Recently, Molinari and his colleagues (1974) described a technique for producing segmental middle cerebral artery occlusion in primates by injecting specially moulded silicone cylinders through the internal carotid artery. This embolic technique has the advantage of producing cerebral infarction while preserving the integrity of the skull and the intracranial collateral circulation.

Brierley and his colleagues (1969) studied the effects of profound hypotension by ganglion blockade, tilting head up, and bleeding, on cerebral haemodynamics, intracranial pressure, and cortical evoked responses, along with histological structure of the brain in rhesus monkeys.

Historically, the dog was the first animal model for the study of infarction. Sir Ashley Cooper (1836) ligated all four major arteries supplying the brain in the dog and was unable to find any neurological manifestations. He demonstrated the development of a rich anastomotic circulation at necropsy. The dog model was also used by Rapela and Green (1964) for the measurement of cerebral venous outflow via a cannula placed in the torcula Herophili after ligation of the cerebral veins. They measured the outflow by the electromagnetic flowmeter, but the values of cerebral outflow were low possibly because of extracranial contamination.

The dog has also been used in the experiments designed by Zwetnow and his colleagues in studying the effects on CBF of changing the intracranial pressure and intracranial volume (Zwetnow, 1970; Lofgren and Zwetnow, 1973; Lofgren, von Essen, and Zwetnow, 1973).

Fluorescein angiography and photographic recordings were used by Shibata and his colleagues (1974) to study microcirculatory effects of MCA occlusion in dogs. Ross Russell (1971) used the fluorescein microangiographic technique for the study of experimental cerebral ischaemia and autoregulation in rabbits.

A cat is a less satisfactory model for cerebral vascular studies because of the presence of a *rete mirabile*, poor differentiation of the MCA, and variations of venous outflow with a large vertebral venus plexus. Thus, torcular flow in the cat does not predictably represent the entire cerebral venous outflow. Waltz and his group have used the cat more consistently than others as an experimental model for the study of cerebral ischaemia following middle cerebral artery occlusion (O'Brien and Waltz, 1973; O'Brien, Jordan, and Waltz, 1974; O'Brien, Waltz, and Jordan, 1974; Hoppe *et al.*, 1974). The reversibility of ischaemic brain damage in cats was shown by Hossmann and Kleihues (1973). The cat brain has also been used for ultrastructural studies after MCA occlusion (Nelson, 1974; Williams and Grossman, 1969) as well as histochemical changes measured in the ischaemic zone (MacDonald, Sundt, and Winkelmann, 1972).

The gerbil has recently become a popular animal model for the study of cerebral infarction since larger numbers can be used to advantage for statistical analysis at reasonable cost and minimal surgical preparation. Levine and Payan (1966) showed that mongolian gerbils are highly susceptible to ligation of the common carotid arteries, which predictably results in cerebral infarction. Bilateral ligation is uniformly lethal, while unilateral carotid ligation produces ischaemia of one hemisphere and/or the ipsilateral eye in approximately 50 per cent of animals. Some variability in mortality from one laboratory to another can be accounted for by the anaesthetic used. Later it was shown that the mortality in gerbils following unilateral carotid ligation is significantly reduced by the daily administration of dexamethasone in the first 48 hours after surgery (Harrison *et al.*, 1973; Harrison and Russell, 1972). This reduction in mortality is attributed to reduction in cerebral

oedema in the infarcted hemispheres. This protective effect of dexamethasone has not been universally confirmed in other laboratories using other animal models possibly due to reasons already discussed. In the same ischaemic model, metabolic studies have been carried out (Wexler, 1972).

The rat has long been used as an experimental model for studies of hypertensive encephalopathy since Byrom first produced experimental hypertensive encephalopathy in his classical work (1954). Recently, rats have been used for studies of the innervation of the cerebral blood vessels (Peerless, Yasargil, and Kendall, 1972), ultrastructural changes in cerebral ischaemia (Kogure *et al.*, 1974; Clendenon *et al.*, 1971), and neurophysiological and metabolic studies by Scremin *et al.* (1973) and by Siesjö and Plum (1972).

The so-called 'Levine' preparation has been widely used as an ischaemic anoxic model. In this preparation, the rat is subjected to ligation of one carotid artery and this is combined with anoxic anoxia. Utilising this model Plum (1966) showed electrolyte changes in the 'ischaemic hemisphere' in which sodium and water moved intracellularly causing regional oedema. There was an accompanying extracellular displacement of potassium. The disadvantage of the Levine model is that it is not one of pure ischaemia but of anoxic ischaemia, and the so-called 'control hemisphere' is not a true control as it is exposed to anoxia.

The mouse has been rarely used as an experimental animal model. Rosenblum (1970) studied the effects of blood viscosity on the cerebral transit time using fluorescein angiography and rapid serial photography. Edvinsson and his colleagues (1972) used mice for the study of adrenergic influences on brain blood volume. Nelson (1974) produced cold haemorrhagic infarction by freezing part of the cortex ('cold lesion') and studied any modifying effects of various drugs on the brain.

The rabbit has been utilised as an experimental animal model for the study of neurogenic factors influencing cerebral blood flow in at least three different studies: those concerned with stimulation of the bulbar vasomotor center and its effect on cerebral blood flow (Molnar and Szanto, 1964), the study of cholinergic influences on autoregulatory vasodilation (Mchedlishvili and Nikolaishvili, 1970), and studies of the effects of superior cervical sympathectomy on intracranial pressure (Edvinsson et al., 1972). Recently, Fieschi and his colleagues (1974) developed a useful experimental model for the study of platelet aggregation as a cause of ischaemia. He injected adenosine diphosphate (ADP) into the carotid artery of rabbits and measured the subsequent formation of platelet aggregates, thrombi and microemboli to the pial circulation, regional reduction in cerebral blood flow in the microembolic zones of ischaemia, and subsequent increase in lactate and oedema formation. Despite the above haemodynamic and biochemical changes, there were no morphological changes on light microscopy. Similar observations regarding platelet aggregation, red cell clumping, stasis, and haemoconcentration were made (Meyer, 1958a) in monkeys after middle cerebral artery occlusion, utilising the skull window and microphotography originally proposed by Forbes (1928).

EXPERIMENTAL METHODS

The effects of cerebral infarction can be classified into the following approaches to study: (1) changes in cerebral electrical activity, (2) cerebral haemodynamic effects, (3) metabolic changes and, (4) morphological changes. All of these effects have been studied by different investigators, depending upon the stage of development and the availability of suitable measurement techniques. The experimental methods will be described under these four broad headings.

CEREBRAL ELECTRICAL ACTIVITY

Electroencephalography was one of the first techniques to be used for the assessment of experimental ischaemia. Corday, Rothenberg, and Putnam (1953) induced EEG slowing after ligation of the carotid artery and lowering the systemic blood pressure (MABP) in the monkey, and showed that the failure was due to poor collateral circulation producing regional ischaemia.

Brierley et al. (1969) used somatosensory cortical evoked potentials in addition to electroencephalography in the study of brain damage due to profound arterial hypotension produced by ganglionic blockade, head-up postural tilting, and exsanguination. They showed good correlation between survival time, amplitude of cortical evoked responses, and the degree of brain damage.

Recently, regional cerebral blood flow was measured by the hydrogen clearance technique and local somatosensory evoked potentials before and after MCA occlusion in the baboon (Branston et al., 1974). They found that following MCA occlusion, the amplitude of the cortical evoked potential diminished steadily at a rate correlating with the reduction of local blood flow. The degree and rate of depression of the amplitude of the cortical evoked potentials was highly and significantly correlated with residual blood flow. There was a threshold type of relationship between the evoked potential amplitude and the local blood flow. They also demonstrated that cortical evoked potentials are reduced when regional blood flow is reduced below 16 ml/100 g brain/min and are abolished below 12 ml/100 g brain/min. The zone of flow was later shown histologically to be infarcted.

MEASUREMENT OF CEREBRAL BLOOD FLOW AND HAEMODYNAMICS

Various methods for measuring cerebral blood flow and cerebral haemodynamics have been reviewed (Purves, 1972; Meyer and Welch, 1972; Olesen, 1974). Here only the methods that have been used for the study of experimental cerebral ischaemia will be briefly discussed. For technical details, the original reviews should be consulted.

One of the first methods for observation of the cerebral circulation was direct visual observation and/or photographic recording of pial vessels by means of a skull window. The technique was originally used by Donders as early as 1849. Using an elaborated design of this technique, Meyer (1958a, 1961) made observations on the cerebral haemodynamic changes following middle cerebral artery occlusion in cats and monkeys. Cyanosis of pial vessels with slowing of blood circulation was observed in animals with transient hemiplegia following middle cerebral artery occlusion. In animals with severe hemiplegia, clumping, segmentation, and stasis of red cells within the pial vessels were seen. Effects of experimental cerebral emboli of different types were studied, and different zones of ischaemia and collateral circulatory hyperaemia were recognised.

The skull window technique has also been successfully utilized in evaluating neurogenic influences on cerebral blood flow (Mchedlishvili and Nikolaishvili, 1970; Langfitt and Kassell, 1968) as well as the effects of profound hypotension (Brierley et al., 1969). The disadvantages of the skull window technique are that only gross changes in the diameter of the leptomeningeal vessels can be appreciated and that the normal physiology of intracranial pressure may be disturbed if CSF leaks or the window compresses the brain.

Visual observations and photographic recording of the pial circulation in an 'open skull' preparation was further refined by the use of fluorescein angiography (Feindel, Yamamoto, and Hodge, 1967; Shibata et al., 1974). The zone of ischaemia following MCA occlusion was clearly demarcated. Recently they have added carbon black particles perfused through the heart for further delineation of the ischaemic areas. Fluorescein angiography has also been used by Ross Russell (1971) to demonstrate loss of autoregulation in the leptomeningeal arteries of rabbits following regional vascular occlusion. Fluorescein was also used for measurement of mean transit time in the cerebral microcirculation of the mouse (Rosenblum, 1970).

Electromagnetic flowmeters have been used to advantage for continuous measurement of blood flow through the large arteries and veins of the brain (Meyer, Yoshida, and Sakamoto, 1967b; Deshmukh et al., 1971–1973; D'Alecy, 1973; Rapela and Green, 1964; McDowall et al., 1971). The electromagnetic flow probes of a suitable size are applied over the exposed internal carotid and vertebral arteries or both jugular veins or the torcula Herophili. The column of blood moving through that vessel acts as a moving conductor between two small electromagnets located in the probe. The change in electromagnetic field is proportional to the change in the velocity of blood flow.

The advantages of this technique are that (1) it is a continuous measure of blood flow through the vessel, (2) the brain tissue supplied by the vessel is left undisturbed, and (3) it is relatively simple and inexpensive. The disadvantages are that it does not represent brain tissue perfusion under certain circumstances, e.g. local spasm of the vessel or effects of unusual development of collateral circulation (Deshmukh and Harper, 1973). It also necessitates surgical exposure of the vessels. Collapse of the thin walled internal jugular veins and drifting of the zero base line can be additional technical problems.

Diffusible indicator clearance techniques are probably the most reliable and well-accepted methods for measurement of CBF at present. There is a large accumulation of scientific literature on the subject especially those concerned with Xenon[133] clearance technique. The principle of this technique is simple and is a modification of the Fick principle. The freely diffusible indicator is delivered by intracarotid injection and saturation of the brain as a simple step function. The clearance or washout of the indicator from brain tissue is directly proportional to the blood flow through the brain tissue over the ensuing 10 minutes, the faster or greater the blood flow, the faster will be the washout of the tracer, while the slower or smaller the blood flow, the slower will be the clearance of indicator from the brain tissue.

The advantages of the method are that one can obtain a reliable and reproducible measure of actual brain tissue perfusion from multiple regions of interest depending on the number of sensors used. The disadvantages are that it is a discontinuous method of measurement of cerebral blood flow and the equipment is large and relatively expensive. It also involves puncture of the carotid artery for the administration of Xenon[133] in the most commonly used technique.

The most commonly used diffusible indicator at present is the inert radioactive gas Xenon[133]. It was first used by Glass and Harper (1963) in man for the measurement of regional cerebral blood flow (rCBF). The method was further elaborated and standardised by Harper and his colleagues in Glasgow and by Lassen and Ingvar in Scandinavia. The method has been described in detail by Hoedt-Rasmussen (1967).

Krypton[85], which emits beta radiations, has been used as an indicator since 1955, but it is not generally used at present, the main disadvantage being that it necessitates exposure of the cerebral cortex for measurement of cerebral blood flow.

Hydrogen clearance method was originally described by Aukland, Bower, and Berliner (1964) and is still being used by several authors (Branston et al., 1974; Gotoh, Meyer, and Tomita, 1966; Rovere et al., 1973; Scremin et al., 1973). The advantage is that CBF can be measured in very small localised areas. The disadvantage is that it needs insertion of fine platinum electrodes into the brain parenchyma.

Less commonly used methods are: Carbon[14] labelled antipyrine autoradiographic method (Dinsdale, Robertson, and Haas, 1974; Reivich, Jehle, Sokoloff, and Kety, 1969); thermistor heat clearance techniques (Molnar and Szanto, 1964); radioactive oxygen (O^{15}) clearance technique (Grubb et al., 1974); the 'pulse index' method-ratio of arterial and venous pulse heights as a measure of regional circulation (Symon, 1970); and the nitrous oxide method of Kety and Schmidt (1945) (Hoyer et al., 1974).

INTRACRANIAL PRESSURE AND BRAIN OEDEMA

Cerebral infarction and cerebral haemorrhage are regularly accompanied by increased intracranial pressure (ICP) and brain oedema, depending on the severity of the lesion. The changes in ICP have been assessed by monitoring epidural, subdural, intraventricular, and cisternal magna pressures, as well as by monitoring superior sagittal sinus wedge pressure and brain tissue pressure (Johnson et al., 1971; McDowall et al., 1971; O'Brien and Waltz, 1973; Reulen and Kreysch, 1973; Tulleken et al., 1975; Zwetnow, 1970). Measurement of local brain tissue pressure by using fine cotton wick catheters has been used for measuring tissue pressure. Trauma due to the catheter tip has been

minimised by the use of fine drawn glass catheters.

Ischaemic cerebral oedema can also be assessed by measurement of cerebral water content (Harrison et al., 1973; O'Brien et al., 1974; Shibata et al., 1974; West and Matsen, 1972). Net weight of brain less the dry weight (tissue density) gives an estimate of brain oedema (Nelson, 1974). The greater the water content of the brain tissue, the greater is the brain oedema.

Experimental brain oedema can be induced in localised areas by local freezing of the brain (Frei et al., 1973; Reulen and Kreysch, 1973). In this model, using the cotton wick technique, a pressure difference of as much as 13 mmHg has been shown between the oedematous and undamaged cerebral hemisphere in cats. Global brain oedema can be induced by graded water intoxication (Meinig, Reulen, and Magawly, 1973), with generalised increases in the intracranial pressure and brain water content.

MORPHOLOGICAL STUDIES

Structural changes following cerebral ischaemia and infarction have been studied and documented in detail (Meyer, 1958b), using photography, special staining techniques, and microscopy. Regional experimental infarction was produced in the rhesus monkey by MCA occlusion associated with lowering and raising the blood pressure with various pharmacological agents. The infarcted tissue was stained by haematoxylin and eosin, giemsa stain, phloxin, and methylene blue, cresyl violet, and phosphotungstic acid haematoxylin. With this technique, neuronal and glial swelling in the infarcted zone with pallor of Nissl bodies was confirmed, and clumping of platelets in the venules and arterioles was established.

Brierley and his colleagues (1969) studied brain damage following profound arterial hypotension. In order to prepare the brain for neuropathological studies, it was perfused in vivo with FAM (40 per cent formaldehyde glacial acetic acid –absolute methanol, 1:1:8, 1500–2000 ml) prior to fixation and sectioning. Paraffin sections were stained by the method of Nissl using cresyl fast violet, luxol fast blue, and haematoxylin and eosin. Celloidin sections were stained with Mallory's phosphotungstic acid hematoxylin (for fibrous glia) and Woelde's modification of Heidenhain's method (for myelin sheaths). They observed ischaemic brain damage when the cerebral perfusion pressure was reduced to less than 25 mmHg.

Recently, several detailed ultrastructural studies of the ischaemic cerebral cortex have been published. Williams and Grossman (1969) studied the fine structure of cerebral cortical synapses during failure of synaptic transmission produced by ischaemia. Likewise, Little and Sundt (1974c) showed early changes in the synaptosomes within a few minutes of middle cerebral artery occlusion in the monkey. Following 3.5 to 4 minutes of ischaemia, presynaptic afferent fiber terminal activity was abolished and the distribution of synaptic vesicles was altered (Williams and Grossman, 1969). Clump-

ing of vesicles was seen adjacent to but removed from the synaptic cleft in at least 10 per cent of synaptic endings and there was more than a two-fold increase in the number of presynaptic profiles devoid of vesicles in ischaemic cortex.

Ultrastructural studies also revealed reduction in the size of the capillary lumen, by swollen endothelial and perivascular astrocytes, and severe tissue destruction with rupture and dissolution of cell membranes, swelling of cell organelles, and apical dendrites (Hossman and Kleihues, 1973).

Dodson and his colleagues (1974) studied the ultrastructural changes following MCA occlusion in normotensive and hypotensive baboons. The morphological changes were greater in the latter group. In both groups, the changes were maximum in the ischaemic basal ganglia. The ultrastructural changes consisted of vacuolar formation within the mitochondria, endoplasmic

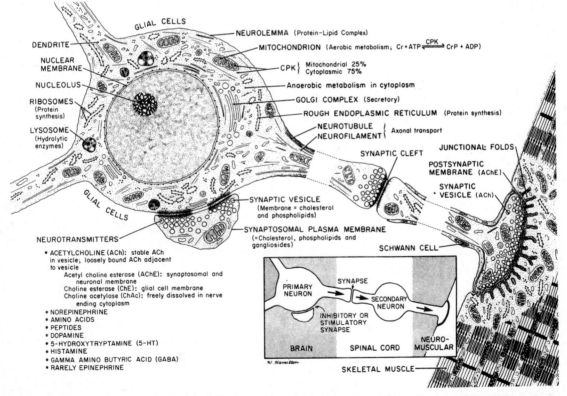

Fig. 4.1   Diagram of the morphophysiological relationships of a typical neuronal chain. (*Courtesy of* Ronald F. Dodson, Ph.D., Assistant Professor, Department of Neurology, Baylor College of Medicine.)

reticulum, and Golgi elements (Fig. 4.1). They also point out the importance of these elements to intracellular metabolism and neurotransmission.

The lysosomes have been shown to be less susceptible to ischaemia and do not appear to play a major role in early ischaemic changes (Little *et al.*, 1974b). The same group of investigators (Little *et al.*, 1974a) also showed two patterns of neuronal degeneration—shrinkage and swelling. Neuronal shrinkage, however, was by far the predominant response. Axosomatic synapses appeared to be more vulnerable to ischaemia than axodendritive synapses. They also observed a later decrease in the number of synaptic vesicles and suggested that some release of neurotransmitter substances occurred as an early consequence of ischaemia.

EXPERIMENTAL EMBOLISM

A critical and extensive study of cerebral circulatory and metabolic changes following different kinds of emboli was carried out by Meyer, Gotoh, and Tazaki (1962). Amongst other things, these authors wished to verify whether cerebral vasospasm followed cerebral embolisation, the evidence for which was derived from the work of Villaret and Cachera (1939) in dogs. Meyer's group compared the effects of plastic, oil, air, and pumice emboli in cats and monkeys. Emboli of less than 15 microns in size passed through cerebral capillary networks without any spasm or morphological changes. However, they produced transient slowing of the pial circulation. Oil emboli injected into the carotid artery resulted in multiple oil droplets causing arteriolar obstruction for 3 to 10 minutes. No spasm was seen. Air emboli (1.2 ml of air injected into the carotid artery) produced more lasting (2 to 4 hours) circulatory slowing, but no spasm or thrombosis. Powdered pumice particles were found to be most effective in producing fibrinoplatelet thrombi, a moderate (less than 20 per cent) reduction in the arteriolar diameter was seen. Brain oedema was also commonly observed following embolisation.

Pumice embolisation also produced severe reduction in cortical blood flow (measured by the thermistor technique, Po_2 and pH with an increase of cortical Pco_2 in the ischaemic area (Fig. 4.2). Ischaemic anoxia, hypercarbia, and acidosis of the cortex were rapid in onset and more severe than those seen after occlusion of the carotid or middle cerebral arteries. This was considered most likely to be due to the failure of the collateral circulation as a result of multiple emboli lodging in the collateral network of arterioles. Cortical ischaemic anoxia resulted in a cellular influx of sodium and an efflux of potassium with slowing and eventual suppression of EEG.

The effects of air embolism were also studied in dogs by Danis and Willman (1963). They found no change in the water content of the ischaemic hemisphere, but tissue serotonin levels were significantly elevated, especially in the thalamus.

Recently, Kogure and his colleagues (1975) investigated the effects of cerebral embolisation due to intracarotid injection of carbon microspheres (35.5 microns in diameter) in rats. They found that the embolisation resulted in sudden cerebral ischaemia. This was accompanied by a transient but significant depression of cerebral energy metabolism, not only in the infarcted focus but also throughout the non-infarcted cerebral mass. Excess of lactate in the brain was probably used as the immediate substrate for cellular oxidation during the recovery from ischaemia. Two types of cerebral oedema were observed: an early, reversible, and localised oedema, and a late, generalised, cerebral oedema. The cerebrospinal fluid did not reflect the tissue metabolic events reliably at the time intervals studied up to 24 hours.

Molinari *et al.* (1974) recently described a model in primates for segmental occlusion of the middle cerebral artery. They claim to produce cerebral infarction in all experimental animals preserving consciousness, integrity of skull, and collateral circulation. The procedure involves exposure and cannulation of the carotid artery under local anaesthesia with sedation and the injection of specially moulded silicone cylinders (Microfil) into the internal carotid artery. Thus,

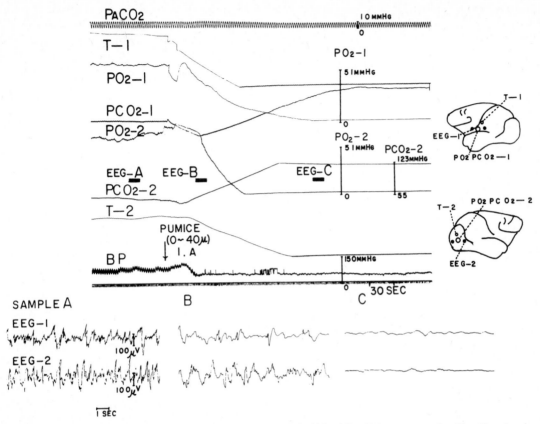

Fig. 4.2   Monkey. Slow speed records of alveolar CO_2 ($P\,CO_2$), cortical blood flow T-1, oxygen tension (PO_2-1), and carbon dioxide tension (PCO_2-1) from the left Sylvian region and corresponding measurements made from the right occipital region (T-2, PCO_2-2, PCO_2-2). EEG records were made at conventional speed from the same areas of brain, and points at which EEG samples were made are noted on the slow speed records. Large boluses of pumice particles (measuring 0–40 μ) were injected into the left carotid artery at arrow. Note that severe ischaemic anoxia and hypercarbia occurred in both hemispheres and that EEG s owing and suppression resulted. No recovery occurred. (*From* Meyer, J. S., Gotoh, F. & Tazaki, Y. (1962) *Journal of Neuropathology and Experimental Neurology*, **21**, 12.)

the effects of acute cerebral infarction can be studied in sedated, conscious animals.

EXPERIMENTAL INFARCTION

As the pathophysiology of cerebral infarction is complex and dynamic, various aspects of experimental infarction have been studied in detail by different investigators. For the convenience of description, the subject is subdivided into the following subtitles: (1) changes in cerebral blood flow and vascular reactivity,

(2) ischaemic brain oedema, and (3) neurochemical changes.

CHANGES IN CEREBRAL BLOOD FLOW AND VASCULAR REACTIVITY

One of the early studies on this aspect of infarction was by Meyer (1958a). He studied the effects of transcranial occlusion of the middle cerebral artery with or without clipping of the collateral vessels, in 23 monkeys, as chronic preparations. Brain blood flow was assessed by stereo microscopic observations and photography through a skull window. Cortical PO_2 and EEG were also monitored.

Occlusion of the middle cerebral artery resulted in a functional deficit ranging from transient hemiparesis with recovery to severe persistent hemiplegia. Lowering the blood pressure below 70 mmHg or occlusion of principal collateral vessels, in addition to occluding the MCA, consistently produced severe hemiplegia. Transient hemiplegia was accompanied by cyanosis of the pial vessels with slowing of circulation but restoration of flow by collateral vessels. When collateral circulation failed, severe hemiplegia developed and was accompanied by intravascular clumping, segmentation, and stasis of red blood cells. Ischaemic anoxia produced vascular endothelial damage and oedema. Restoration of blood flow to damaged vessels resulted in perivascular haemorrhages. Heparin and dicoumerol tended to prevent aggregation of platelets and blood cells in collateral vessels.

In the animal recovered from occlusion of the MCA, transient hemiplegia could be provoked by reduction of the systolic blood pressure, resulting in temporary collapse of the collateral circulation. It could also be precipitated by anoxic anoxia or by spontaneous seizures.

Brierley and his colleagues (1969), in an elaborate study, demonstrated the cerebral circulatory effects of profound arterial hypotension in 15 rhesus monkeys. Pial circulation was studied by means of a cranial window. Electrocorticogram and somatosensory evoked potentials were recorded. Neuropathological observations were made. They concluded that brain damage occurred only when cerebral perfusion pressure fell rapidly to below 25 mm-Hg and was sustained at this level for at least 15 minutes. The amplitude of the somatosensory evoked cortical response correlated well with the severity of neuronal dysfunction and brain damage.

Symon, Pasztor, and Branston (1974) more recently made some important observations using the hydrogen clearance technique for measurement of local cortical blood flow and measuring the cortical evoked potentials. On · occlusion of the middle cerebral artery by subtemporal or transorbital approach in baboons, they found diffuse reduction of hemispheric blood flow with 25 per cent reduction in the opercular areas and a 20 per cent decrease in the deeper nuclei, particularly the putamen. Reactivity to carbon dioxide was reduced, and paradoxical responses or intracerebral steal or 'squeeze' was found in the most densely ischaemic opercular region.

In the most recent publication (Branston et al., 1974) excellent correlation was demonstrated between the rate of depression of the evoked potential amplitude (expressed in units of per cent of control potential per minute) with the regional local blood flow during different degrees of cerebral ischaemia. They also observed a threshold type of relationship between regional blood flow and cortical evoked potential amplitude. If regional blood flow was greater than 16 ml/100 g/min, the evoked potential was unaltered, but at flows less than about 12 ml/100 g/min, the evoked potential was abolished.

ISCHAEMIC BRAIN OEDEMA

Epidural, subdural, and intraventricular pressures were studied bilaterally in cats following unilateral middle cerebral artery occlusion (O'Brien and Waltz, 1973). Despite some technical difficulties, increases in intracranial pressures, directly related to neurological deficits, were shown on the side of vascular occlusion with slight or no change over the opposite hemisphere. The intracranial pressure gradients gradually disappeared as the cerebral ischaemia and brain oedema resolved over a period of several days.

Ischaemic cerebral oedema can also be assessed by serial estimations of brain water content in the infarcted and the normal cerebral hemispheres. Harrison et al. (1973) demonstrated in mongolian gerbils that after carotid artery ligation, fatal cerebral infarction develops in 60 per cent of their cases. This mortality rate could be reduced by intraperitoneal injections of dexamethasone. The authors attribute this reduced mortality to a significant reduction in brain oedema following dexamethasone.

The mechanism of action of dexamethasone in experimental ischaemic cerebral oedema has been further elaborated by Hoppe et al. (1974). Large parenteral doses of dexamethasone lessen the extravascular distribution of water and pertechnetate in cerebral tissue which was made necrotic by arterial occlusion for two days. However, the drug has little or no effect on the water content of brain/blood ratio of pertechnetate in ischaemic cerebral tissue that does not become necrotic. Dexamethasone prevents the development of oedema in the non-ischaemic, relatively normal brain, opposite the cerebral infarction.

NEUROCHEMICAL CHANGES

The neurochemical changes in the anoxic-ischaemic encephalopathy in the rat (Levine and Payan, 1966) have been well studied and the data summarised (Clendenon et al., 1971). Nicotinamide adenine dinucleotide (NAD) shifts to the reduced form which favours reduction of pyruvate to lactate. In the decapitated mouse brain, lactate immediately begins to accumulate and reaches a five-fold increase in concentration within 10 minutes. Within 30 seconds of ischaemia, a shift of sodium into the intracellular compartment is seen, and glucose drops to about 15 per cent of control value. The latter approaches zero levels and glycogen becomes undetectable after about 10 minutes. Adenosine triphosphate (ATP) and triphosphoinositide are reduced, and phosphofructokinase is disinhibited. These processes are potentially reversible if substrate and oxygen can be restored within the first hour or so.

Sundt and his colleagues clearly demonstrated serial changes in brain ATP, lactate levels, and lactate/pyruvate ratios in squirrel monkeys following unilateral occlusion of the MCA (Sundt and Michenfelder, 1971–1972; MacDonald et al., 1972). The ATP concentrations were progressively reduced to 55, 35, and 20 per cent of normal, while the lactate levels progressively increased to 7, 8, and 10 times normal after two, three, and four hours of occlusion. The lactate/pyruvate ratio also gradually increased. These neurochemical changes could be reversed by restoring local blood flow by the collateral circulation. The authors attribute this loss of autoregulation and 'luxury perfusion' to localised areas of lactacidosis.

The same group of investigators also studied the various brain enzymes including ATP-ase, acid and alkaline phosphatase, succinic and lactic dehydrogenase, cytochrome oxidase, DPNH-diaphorase, indoxyl esterase, and phosphorylase by histochemical techniques at intervals between six hours and eight weeks after middle cerebral artery occlusion in cats. Unequivocal enzyme changes did not develop until 12 hours after occlusion, and no specific enzyme system was demonstrated to fail prior to others. After 12 hours of occlusion, relative activities of all enzymes tend to fall progressively in the infarction zone and to increase in marginal zones.

Cerebral energy metabolism during prolonged ischaemia was studied in a series of experiments in rats by Siesjö and his colleagues and their observations were recently summarised (Siesjö and Ljunggren, 1973; Siesjö and Plum, 1972). The overall ATP synthesis of the mitochondria of the brain is relatively resistant to hypoxia. For example, the arterial Po_2 can be lowered to below 20 mmHg and the cerebral venous Po_2 to below 10 mmHg without any significant changes in the brain ATP, ADP, or AMP contents, although lactate production is increased and the EEG is abnormal. Adenyl energy charge calculated as

$$\frac{ATP + 1/2ADP}{ATP + ADP + AMP}$$

remained relatively unchanged.

On the other hand, the cerebral extracellular and intracellular lactate rises at arterial Po_2 values below 50 mmHg and phosphocreatine (an important energy source) decreases when Po_2 is below 35 mmHg. In complete ischaemia produced by increasing the cerebrospinal fluid pressure greater than systemic arterial pressure, the energy production is severely reduced after three minutes of total ischaemia. After 5 to 7.5 minutes of total ischaemia, minimal values for energy charge are observed.

Recently, Yatsu (1974) briefly reviewed the changes in membrane lipids in brain ischaemia. Global cerebral ischaemia was produced by combined arterial hypotension and hypoxia (4 per cent oxygen). Yatsu concluded that ATP synthesis in isolated mitochondria is unimpaired at a time when functional ischaemic brain damage occurs. Thus, the energy synthesising machinery is less vulnerable to ischaemia than energy dependent functions. He concluded from studies of brain phospholipids that the mitochondria elsewhere in the brain were relatively resistant to ischaemia. No significant changes were found in phospholipids in brain mitochondria, microsomes, and synaptosomes. However, the ability of isolated synaptosomes to synthesise inositide glycerophosphatide (IGP) was impaired. The last observation together with studies of synaptosomal mitochondria suggest that neurotransmission may be primarily vulnerable to ischaemia.

Cerebral ischaemia has also been shown to induce lipolysis and markedly to increase the free fatty acid pool (Bazan, 1970). The enlargement of the total pool was mainly due to the production of arachidonic, stearic, oleic, and palmitic acids. Free fatty acids of the 16 to 18C lengths are known to be uncouplers of oxidative phosphorylation.

Dysautoregulation

Different aspects of cerebral vascular autoregulation have been recently reviewed (Olesen, 1974; Purves, 1972). Only the features of autoregulation pertinent to cerebral ischaemia are discussed here.

The intrinsic ability of cerebral vessels to maintain cerebral blood flow (CBF) constant despite changes in cerebral perfusion pressure (CPP) has been defined as 'autoregulation'. Autoregulation is frequently impaired in ischaemia of the brain so that CBF passively follows changes in CPP, which is termed 'dysautoregulation' (Symon, 1970; Symon, Held, and Dorsch, 1972). Dysautoregulation is caused by vasoparalysis due to local brain tissue lactacidosis and/or neurogenic influences (Hoedt-Rasmussen, 1967; Ott et al., 1975).

Meyer et al. (1972) tested cerebral autoregulation in an infarction model in baboons. Cerebral ischaemia was produced by temporary (10 minutes) occlusion of both carotid and both vertebral arteries. CBF was measured by the venous outflow technique. Systemic arterial blood pressure was increased by clamping of the abdominal aorta or by rapid infusion of levarterenol bitartrate. Dysautoregulation or impaired autoregulation was demonstrated in all animals following cerebral ischaemia. Both rapid and slow phases of autoregulation were impaired.

Dysautoregulation in ischaemic cerebral cortex was also demonstrated by Sundt and Waltz (1971) in squirrel monkeys. Cerebral blood flow was measured by the Krypton[85] clearance technique and cerebral ischaemia was produced by a temporary occlusion of the middle cerebral artery. During MCA occlusion, cortical blood flow in core areas of ischaemia decreased 20 to 50 per cent of preocclusion values and became pressure dependent with failure of autoregulation. On releasing the occluding clip, cortical blood flow was restored.

Recently, Ott and his colleagues from this laboratory (1975) showed good correlation between dysautoregulation and increased acetylcholinesterase levels in infarcted cortical gray matter and basal ganglia. They also found that the time course of onset of dysautoregulation correlated with increased cholinesterase uptake by the brain. Intravenous infusion of scopolamine, a cholinergic neurotransmitter blocker, restored autoregulation to the ischaemic zones. In this study in baboons, infarction was produced by occlusion of the middle cerebral artery and cerebral blood flow was measured by the intracarotid injection of Xenon[133] technique using the gamma camera. Hypertensive phase of autoregulation was tested by increasing the systemic arterial pressure by intravenous infusion of metaraminol or angiotensin. It was concluded that displacement of acetylcholine into brain from cholinergic synapses after cerebral ischaemia causes dysautoregulation.

Etiology of hypertensive encephalopathy—the question of 'breakthrough' versus spasm

Byrom (1954) was the first to study experimental hypertensive encephalopathy. He produced renal hypertension in rats by the use of a modified Goldblatt clamp placed around the renal artery. Pial circulation was observed through a skull window. As the blood pressure rose to extremely high levels, segmental arterial and arteriolar spasm was observed. At first, localised waist-like arteriolar constrictions were seen, which became more diffuse in later stages as well as zones of sausage-like vasodilation. These spasmodic changes were originally thought by Byrom to cause multifocal haemorrhages and infarcts, and zones of damage to the blood brain barrier. In later years he considered the zones of vasodilation might be responsible for the lesions. Meyer (1961) confirmed these observations in cats and presented a unified concept about the pathogenesis of hypertensive encephalopathy in which the vasospasm was thought to be the initial triggering event (Fig. 4.3).

chain of events in hypertensive encephalopathy are: systemic arterial pressure rises to a critical point or upper limit at which the cerebral vessels can no longer compensate by autoregulatory vasoconstriction; this results in forced vasodilation or 'breakthrough' of autoregulation with resultant damage to blood brain barrier and increase in cerebral blood flow. The latter is probably transient and multifocal. It leads to extravasation of fluids, periarterial haemorrhages, and multifocal brain damage, which later leads to reduced metabolism and blood flow (Ekstrom-Jodal, Häggendal, Linder, and Nilsson, 1972; Häggendal and Johansson, 1972; Olesen, 1974). This upper limit of autoregulation was found to be at blood pressures 30 to 40

HYPERTENSIVE ENCEPHALOPATHY

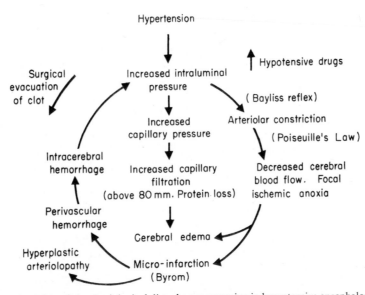

Fig. 4.3 Schematic representation of the physiological disturbance occurring in hypertensive encephalopathy and hypertensive intracerebral haemorrhage. (*From* Meyer, J. S. (1961) In *Pathogenesis and Treatment of Cerebrovascular Disease*, ed. Fields, W. S. Springfield, Illinois: Charles C. Thomas.)

Recently, the concept of vasoconstriction as the initial event has been questioned and an alternative hypothesis of 'breakthrough' or forced vasodilatation has been put forward (Lassen and Agnoli, 1972; Strandgaard *et al.*, 1974). Probably both mechanisms play a part. According to the 'breakthrough' concept, the

per cent above the resting values in baboons and it is apparently not influenced by unilateral sympathetic denervation (Strandgaard *et al.*, 1974).

In an important recent publication by Dinsdale *et al.* (1974), it was demonstrated that angiotensin-induced hypertension in rabbits led to cerebral hyperperfusion at the time of maximum systolic blood pressure followed by multifocal areas of hypoperfusion five minutes later and subsequently for the following 60 minutes. These areas of low flow were mainly clustered in the arterial boundary zones where damage to the blood brain barrier was also demonstrated. Thus, they suggest that intense vasoconstriction and passive vasodilatation ('breakthrough') may co-exist with decreased blood flow in the hyperpermeable areas.

It is possible that both excessive cerebral vasoconstriction and patchy zones of 'breakthrough' play a role in the pathogenesis of hypertensive encephalopathy. In a recent study this was the conclusion when hypertension was induced in hypertensive and normotensive patients by infusion of metaraminol. In these patients, Meyer and his colleagues (1975c) observed excessive autoregulatory cerebral vasoconstriction and patchy areas of high flow gray or fast component on Xenon[133] clearance.

NEUROGENIC AND CHEMICAL CONTROL

This controversial but important subject has aroused much interest among investigators all over the world. Four full sections, including 32 papers were devoted to this subject in the last International CBF Conference at Philadelphia (Langfitt et al., 1973). Two reviews on the subject have also recently been presented (Lassen, 1974; Meyer, 1975a).

Effects of electrical stimulation of the brain stem vasomotor centers on CBF were first reported by Molnar and Szanto (1964). Detailed studies were later carried out by Langfitt and Kassell (1968) and Meyer et al. (1969a and 1971). Langfitt and Kassell observed a 40 per cent average maximum increase in cerebral blood flow within 1 to 4 seconds of brain stem stimulation, without changes in blood pressure in five of seven rhesus monkeys in whom the high cervical cord had been sectioned.

Consistent increases of 41 per cent in CBF and $CMRO_2$ were found in a group of monkeys who showed simultaneous EEG activation on brain stem stimulation (Meyer et al., 1971) (Fig. 4.4). In animals without EEG activation, the increases were smaller (24 per cent). The stimulated areas which caused increases in CBF were located in the pontine and midbrain reticular formations, the thalamus, and the hypothalamus. Stimulation of the cerebral cortex, the fifth and seventh cranial nerves did not produce any consistent changes.

There seems to be convincing evidence to suggest that the electrical stimulation of cervical sympathetic nerves reduces cerebral arterial inflow, tissue perfusion, and venous outflow. The effect is more pronounced during hypercapnia. Meyer et al. (1967b) demonstrated different degrees of vasoconstriction in the internal and external carotid arteries and the vertebral arteries on stimulation of the superior cervical ganglion, stellate ganglion, and the cervical sympathetic chain in monkeys (Fig. 4.5). Mean values for the percent decrease of internal and external carotid and vertebral artery flows, as measured by the electromagnetic flowmeters during stimulation of the superior cervical ganglion, were 29.9, 67.7, and 17.6, respectively.

Reduction in gray matter flow (James et al., 1969) and mean cerebral blood flow as measured by Xenon[133] clearance technique during sympathetic stimulation in baboons were also demonstrated (Deshmukh et al., 1971–1972). The vasoconstrictor effect was more marked during hypercapnia.

However, the effects of surgical sympathectomy are not clear. James et al. (1969) reported that acute surgical sympathectomy caused an increase in CBF which was more marked at high P_aCO_2 values and also changed the cerebral autoregulatory response. These findings, however, have not been confirmed (Harper et al., 1972; Eklöf et al., 1971). Unilateral sympathectomy also does not seem to change the upper limit of the hypertensive phase of autoregulation (Strandgaard et al., 1974). There is some recent evidence that the pharmacological blockade with phenoxybenzamine reduces the vasoconstrictor tonus of cerebral vessels during hypocapnia and raised cerebral perfusion pressure, and also enhances the vasodilator response to

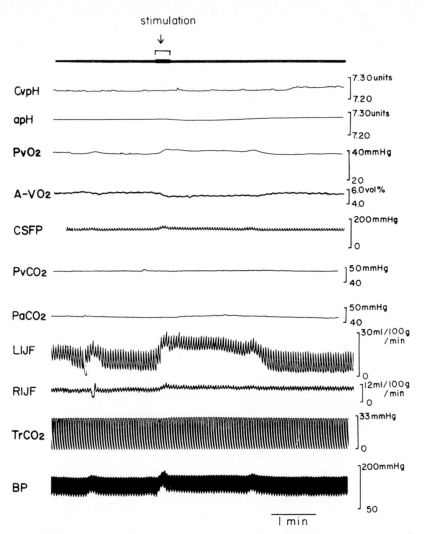

Fig. 4.4   Increase in CBF during stimulation of the left segmental reticular formation. The increase in flow within both internal jugular veins is well sustained during and following the period of stimulation. It was greater on the side stimulated. The change in blood pressure is small and brief. The CSFP showed a small increase. Apart from a sustained increase of P_{O_2} and decrease in A-V_{O_2} corresponding with the increase in blood flow, the other parameters showed little or no change. (*From* Meyer, J. S., *et al.*, (1971) *Neurology*, **21**, 255.)

carbon dioxide inhalation (Kawamura *et al.*, 1974).

The evidence for cholinergic influence on cerebral blood flow is currently being debated. James *et al.* (1969) reported that sectioning the carotid, vagus, and aortic nerves in the neck reduced the cerebrovascular dilatory response to hypercapnia and hypoxia, while central stimula-

tion of the aortic and vagus nerves increased brain blood flow independently of $P_a co_2$. These findings, however, could not be confirmed (Harper *et al.*, 1971). Mchedlishvili and Nikolaishvili (1970) suggested that cerebral autoregulatory vasodilatation in response to hypotension could be blocked by administration of atropine in rabbits. Atropine was shown to

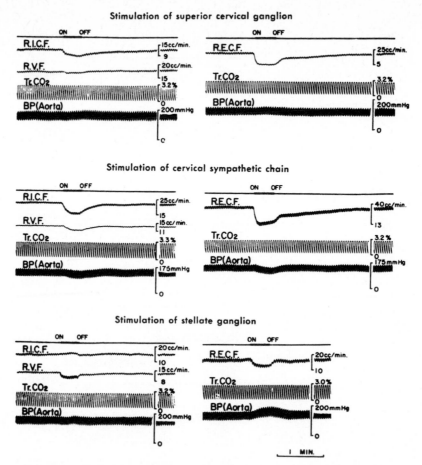

Fig. 4.5 Time relationships and difference in magnitude of the decrease in external and internal carotid and vertebral flow during stimulation of the superior cervical ganglion, sympathetic chain, and stellate ganglion. R.I.C.F. = right internal carotid flow; R.V.F. = right vertebral flow; Tr. CO_2 = tracheal carbon dioxide; BP (aorta) = blood pressure, aorta; R.E.C.F. = right external carotid flow. (*From* Meyer, J. S., *et al.* (1967b) *Neurology*, **17**, 640.)

block the increase in CBF (measured by hydrogen clearance method) in rats during a state of spontaneous EEG desynchronization (Scremin *et al.*, 1973) and also the CBF response to hypercapnia (Rovere *et al.*, 1973).

Substantial pharmacological evidence in favour of cholinergic influence is being accumulated. Stoica *et al.* (1973) showed that atropine blocks the increase in CBF and metabolism accompanying activation of brain stem reticular formation by pyrithioxin. Intravertebral administration did not change CBF under normal conditions but it did limit hypercapnic vasodilatation

and enhanced the hypocapnic vasoconstriction (Kawamura *et al.*, 1975). Intravertebral neostigmine, although ineffective under normal conditions, could increase the vasodilator response to CO_2 inhalation and reduce vasoconstriction in response to hypertension (Aoyagi *et al.*, 1975). Again, recently, acetylcholine by intravertebral route has been shown to produce 25 per cent rise in CBF and a 22 per cent increase in $CMRO_2$ in baboons (Matsuda *et al.*, 1974).

Brain extracellular pH is considered by some investigators as the main factor controlling cerebral blood flow (Lassen, 1968; 1974). There is no doubt that the cerebral vessels are extremely sensitive to changes in arterial $P\text{CO}_2$. Even a mmHg change in $P_a\text{CO}_2$ can change CBF by about 4 per cent. This CO_2 reactivity is mediated by variations in pH and bicarbonate concentration of cerebrospinal fluid around the arterioles (Wahl *et al.*, 1970).

The concensus of opinion, at present, seems to be in favour of a dual regulation by both the chemical and neurogenic mechanisms (Mchedlishvili and Nikolaishvili, 1970; Deshmukh *et al.*, 1971–1972; Harper *et al.*, 1972; Stoica *et al.*, 1973; Gotoh *et al.*, 1973; Moskalenko *et al.*, 1974). According to this view, the intraparenchymal vessels with relatively poor innervation are regulated by local brain metabolism and its

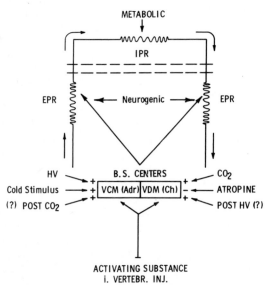

Fig. 4.6 Schematic diagram originally proposed by Deshmukh and associates (1971–1972) and presently supplemented by Stoica and colleagues (1973). The extraparenchymal resistance (EPR) is mediated principally by neurogenic control, whereas intraparenchymal resistance (IPR) is principally under chemical control. Brain stem vasodilator mechanisms (VDM) and vasoconstrictor mechanisms (VCM) are added, which influence the EPR vessels. Alterations in $P_a\text{CO}_2$ modulate the tonus of the dual mechanisms. For example, changes in $P\text{CO}_2$ influence cerebral blood flow not only by a direct effect on IPR but also by modifying the balance between VCM and VDM which controls EPR. VDM is considered to be primarily cholinergic, whereas VCM is primarily adrenergic. (*From* Stoica *et al.* (1973) *Neurology*, **23**, 696).

products, while the densely innervated large extraparenchymal vessels can be influenced by the autonomic activity. Recently, more evidence is accumulating about the neurogenic influences from the reticular activating system. A schematic diagram (Fig. 4.6) briefly summarises the main influences.

METABOLIC CHANGES FOLLOWING CEREBRAL ISCHAEMIA

The brain requires one-fifth of the cardiac output to maintain its high energy requirements. Energy derived from consumption of glucose and oxygen is converted by oxidative phosphorylation into high energy phosphate bonds, particularly creatine phosphate and adenosine triphosphate. Glucose is rapidly transported across the blood brain barrier and is probably stored to some extent in the cytoplasm of the astrocytes, as well as diffusing via the extracellular fluid to the nerve cells and other glia. The large amount of energy provided by oxidative phosphorylation is used almost exclusively for two important functions: (1) maintaining the low sodium and high potassium gradients within the parenchymal cells which are essential for neuronal conduction and brain function, and (2) synthesis, storage, release, and re-uptake of the neurotransmitters in the synaptosomes, which are likewise essential for normal brain function.

GLOBAL VERSUS REGIONAL ISCHAEMIA

Cerebral metabolic changes following global or regional ischaemia are similar except that in the global type of model the effects are generalised, tend to be more severe, and are technically easier to measure (e.g., by temporary cardiac arrest of occlusion of the carotid and vertebral arteries in the neck) (Ames *et al.*, 1968; Meyer *et al.*, 1968; Yatsu, 1974). Regional ischaemia tends to be better tolerated since a collateral circulation develops and blood flow is more or less restored. It is seldom reduced to zero (Meyer and Welch, 1972; Waltz and Sundt, 1967). Hence, the collateral flow may provide the deficient substrates and remove certain acid metabolites, the accumulation of which may impair brain function. Thus, viability of the ischaemic tissue may be maintained despite regional functional impairment. Regional functional recovery may ultimately result if sufficient collateral circulation is established. (Denny-Brown, Meyer, and Fang, 1953; Hudgins and Garcia, 1970; Michenfelder and Sundt, 1971; Meyer and Welch, 1972).

Animal models used for measuring effects of regional cerebral ischaemia include clamping or ligating the middle cerebral artery in the cat, dog, and primate, or occluding the carotid artery in the gerbil, rat, or rabbit. The latter two models require hypotension or anoxemia, in addition, in order to produce regional infarction (Levine and Payan, 1966; Plum, 1966; Zervas et al., 1974; Welch, Spira, Knowles, and Lance, 1974).

GROSS, MICROSCOPIC, AND ULTRASTRUCTURAL ANATOMY IN RELATION TO GRADIENTS OF RESISTANCE TO CEREBRAL ISCHAEMIA

There are gradients of resistance to ischaemia of the brain. These gradients appear to depend on regional metabolic rate, capillary density, and, at the ultrastructural level, regional differences in diffusion characteristics across membranes of neurons, glia, endothelium, pericytes, smooth muscle cells, and their organelles for gases and metabolites. Regions of higher metabolic rate are more vulnerable to ischaemia than regions of lower metabolic rate, e.g., grey matter of the cortex and basal ganglia are more susceptible to ischaemia than white matter. For example, following cardiac arrest, cerebral grey cortex tends to be more affected than the white matter. The brain stem is relatively resistant to ischaemia (Himwich, 1951).

Likewise, the different cells themselves that make up the brain parenchyma and its nutrient blood vessels show gradients of resistance to ischaemia. The astrocytes show the earliest change, consisting of swelling of the footplates around small blood vessels (Dodson et al., 1973). Furthermore, within the neurons, certain ultrastructural units are more susceptible to ischaemia than others (Fig. 4.1). The synaptosomal vesicles of the neurons are particularly susceptible to early damage (Williams and Grossman, 1969; Sundt and Waltz, 1971) while the mitochondria are more resistant. In the astrocyte, the cell membrane is affected early with swelling of the footplates, and in the cells of the vasculature, the pericyte likewise shows early swelling and dissolution.

SODIUM AND POTASSIUM TRANSPORT, CELL MEMBRANE INTEGRITY, OEDEMA AND NEUROTRANSMITTER FUNCTION

In metabolic terms, there are also gradients of resistance to ischaemia of the various metabolic pathways in the brain. The sodium and potassium transport system, which is Na^+ and K^+ ATPase dependent, of the cell membranes of the astrocytes and neurons are particularly susceptible to ischaemia. Movement of potassium into the extracellular space and cerebrospinal fluid with an accompanying movement of sodium and chloride into cells is an early sign of cerebral ischaemia and anoxia. This flux of sodium and potassium correlates with impaired neuronal activity as judged by slowing and loss of electroencephalographic (EEG) activity (Meyer and Welch, 1972) plus swelling of both neurons and astrocytes (Dodson et al., 1973). These morphological and functional correlates reflect failure of the sodium and potassium transport systems, which are highly dependent on rich supplies of energy from oxidative phosphorylation. As regional creatine phosphate and possibly adenosine triphosphate become depleted, sodium, chloride, and water move into the neurons and K^+ moves out of the cell into the cerebrospinal fluid with resultant brain oedema and impaired nerve conduction (Meyer and Welch, 1972; Siesjö and Plum, 1972)

As will be described later, synthesis, storage, release, and uptake of neurotransmitters, particularly norepinephrine, dopamine, serotonin, and GABA, are extremely sensitive to ischaemia. When these mechanisms are impaired, the neurotransmitters are released from the synaptosomes into the synaptic cleft where they are no longer taken up, they accumulate in excess, and diffuse into the extracellular space and cerebrospinal fluid (Meyer et al., 1973; Meyer, Welch, Okamoto, and Shimazu, 1974; Zervas et al., 1974; Kogure and Scheinberg, 1975). Thus, neurotransmission as well as neuroconduction become impaired, and the neuronal function fails as shown by slowing and flattening of the EEG and loss of evoked potentials.

THE PASTEUR EFFECT: EARLY EFFECTS ON GLUCOSE METABOLISM

Since one volume per cent of oxygen is required to oxidise 1.34 mg per cent of glucose, the glucose to oxygen ratio in the living brain should theoretically be 1:34 and the respiratory quotient unity. However, the actual values observed in patients have been consistently higher (Scheinberg and Stead, 1949; Gottstein, 1964; Meyer et al., 1967a). These studies, taken together, indicate that some degree of anaerobic glycolysis is normally present in the brain, an argument strengthened by the fact that more lactate and pyruvate are found in cerebral venous blood than in arterial blood in normal subjects (Meyer and Welch, 1972). In cerebral ischaemia and infarction, lactate accumulates rapidly in the ischaemic tissue and rapidly passes the blood-brain and cerebrospinal fluid barriers to appear in the cerebral venous blood and the cerebrospinal fluid. This has been shown to be due to a Pasteur effect, whereby brain oxygen availability (increases and decreases of brain tissue Po_2, intracellular Po_2, cerebral venous Po_2) regulates the balance between the normal efficient oxidative consumption of glucose (via the Krebs cycle) and the relatively inefficient emergency system of anaerobic glycolysis (via the Embden-Meyerhoff pathway). As ischaemia of the brain progresses, glucose consumption increases and oxygen consumption decreases; Po_2 values progressively reduce. Eventually, anaerobic glycolysis fails to supply sufficient energy which results in irreversible brain dysfunction.

ABNORMALITIES OF METABOLISM IN SEVERELY ISCHAEMIC BRAIN

As stated above, ischaemic brain is acidic. This stimulates increased collateral flow to the ischaemic area with potential for recovery. When permanent irreversible brain damage occurs, $CMRO_2$ is reduced and lactate production is no longer stimulated. In severe infarction, the brain destroys itself by metabolising its own lipids, ketoacids, and proteins as fuel (Yatsu, 1974;

Meyer et al., 1975b). In the brain recovering from ischaemia, elongation of free fatty acids (FFA) has been shown to occur (Yatsu, 1974). In recently infarcted human brain, release of inorganic phosphate, FFA, neurotransmitters and cyclic AMP has been shown. This probably effects a breakdown of phospholipids from cell membranes (Meyer et al., 1975b).

NEUROTRANSMITTER CHANGES FOLLOWING CEREBRAL ISCHAEMIA

In recent years, considerable interest has been directed towards investigation of the effects of cerebral ischaemia on central neurotransmission and on the metabolism of individual putative neurotransmitters. This has necessitated adaptation and application of recently developed techniques, such as histofluorescence (Hillarp, Fuxe, and Dahlstrom, 1966), to studies in experimental models of cerebral ischaemia. Histofluorescence, as well as immunofluorescence and electronmicroscopy (Bloom, 1972), indicate only qualitative changes in brain tissue distribution and content of neurotransmitter or related enzymes. Quantitative changes must be assessed by biochemical analysis of neurotransmitter levels, both in tissue and cerebrospinal fluid (Weil-Malherbe, 1971). Such changes can be indirectly supported by measurement of uptake from or release of neurotransmitters into the cerebral circulation (Welch et al., 1972).

In addition, altered neurotransmitter turnover and synthesis may be indicated by measurement of precursor uptake from the cerebral circulation (Wurtman and Fernstrom, 1972), by studying tissue enzyme kinetics (Lowry and Passoneau, 1972), and by measurement of the rate of neurotransmitter or metabolite accumulation in tissue or cerebrospinal fluid after administration of pharmacological agents that either inhibit neurotransmitter breakdown, such as monoamine oxidase inhibitors, or else prevent their removal from CSF, e.g., probenecid (Cramer, Ng, and Chase, 1972).

Information on possible pathophysiological changes brought about by disordered neurotransmitter function can be gained by introduction of exogenous neurotransmitters into the CNS either by intracisternal, intraventricular, or intracerebral injection, and then by assessing the effect of each on CBF, metabolism, EEG, and clinical state (Gessa *et al.*, 1970). Neurotransmitter release from brain tissue can also be observed by various ventricular perfusion techniques (Ashcroft *et al.*, 1968) or the use of cortical cups as refined by Mitchell (1963). Modification of the pathophysiological accompaniments of cerebral ischaemia by procedures which filter neurotransmitter synthesis, e.g., pretreatment with p-chlorphenylalanine or alpha-methyltyrosine or procedures which cause degeneration of neurotransmitter systems such as stereotaxic ablation or intraventricular 6-hydroxydopamine, may also serve to emphasise the importance of disordered neurotransmitter function in the progression of cerebral infarction.

Recent studies have shown consistent alteration in tissue biogenic amine content after cerebral ischaemia and hypoxia. Biogenic amines such as norepinephrine (NE), dopamine (DA), and serotonin (5-HT) may be regarded as putative neurotransmitters. They are synthesised intraneuronally and are found in high concentrations in the axon terminal synaptosomes of neuronal systems, which appear specific for the individual amine; they may be released as result of a physiological, electrical, or pharmacological stimulation. Measurement of cerebral arteriovenous differences for 5-HT during four-vessel occlusion in the baboon showed initial release of 5-HT from ischemic brain into cerebral venous blood (Welch *et al.*, 1972).

Subsequent accumulation of 5-HT in brain tissue was attributed to movement from blood into brain across a damaged blood-brain barrier. Subsequently, Zervas *et al.* (1974) have shown depletion of dopamine in the ischaemic hemisphere of both gerbils and squirrel monkeys. This work has been confirmed in our laboratory in the gerbil and in the same ischaemic model, depletion of serotonin, together with a less significant depletion of NE has also been observed. Kogure *et al.* (1975) have shown similar changes in the rat. Reviewed overall, results suggest that cerebral ischaemia promotes synaptosomal release with initial abnormal accumulation of neurotransmitters in the extraneuronal environment together with subsequent intraneuronal monoamine depletion. Normal presynaptic neurotransmitter re-uptake is also impaired under ischaemic conditions, either due to cell damage or reduced availability of oxygen and consequent depletion of energy reserves. Monoamine oxidases, which normally break down released monoamines, may also be rendered inactive under ischaemic hypoxic conditions (Pausescu, Lugojan, and Pausescu, 1970), thereby promoting the potency of the released neurotransmitters.

Physiologic presynaptic release of neurotransmitters such as NE and 5-HT stimulate adenyl cyclase in brain to promote enhanced post-synaptic intracellular synthesis of cyclic AMP (Klainer *et al.*, 1962). It therefore seems complementary to the above experimental studies that cyclic AMP becomes markedly elevated in brain tissue within seconds after induction of ischaemia (Steiner, Firendelli, and Goldberg, 1972), although the precise relationship of this event to monoamine change is undetermined. Anoxia and ischaemia also increase brain tissue concentrations of the putative inhibitory neurotransmitter, gamma-aminobutyric acid (GABA) (Tews *et al.*, 1963; Lovell, Elliott, and Elliott, 1963) in experimental animals. Studies of cholinesterase and acetylcholinesterase, referred to in an earlier section of this chapter, indirectly imply that ischaemia also influences acetylcholine levels, probably through similar mechanisms which lead to impairment of monoamine metabolism. Comprehensive studies concerning the effect of ischaemia on less well-established putative neurotransmitters such as the prostaglandins are still awaited.

Assuming that disorder of neurotransmitter function exists in ischaemic brain, what relationship does this have to the pathophysiological accompaniments of ischaemia and the progression of infarction? Monoamine leakage in abnormal amounts into the synaptic cleft may produce depolarisation or hyperpolarisation of postsynaptic cells, thereby impairing synaptic transmission. In addition, diffusion of such agents on to cells not normally receiving input from these specific neurotransmitters may evoke a false neurotransmitter effect on that particular cell. Such factors serve to make disruption of normal synaptic neurotransmission a likely event under ischaemic conditions.

Release of abnormal amounts of central neurotransmitters such as NE and serotonin, which are known to have a profound cerebral vasoconstrictor effect when administered exogenously, may also in part explain the areas of focal or spreading cortical pallor with associated vasoconstriction seen when the middle cerebral artery is occluded in the primate model. Studies by Welch, Hashi, and Meyer (1973) have suggested that release and accumulation of such agents impairs the collateral circulation surrounding ischaemic brain foci, thus contributing to the progression of infarction. Cerebral oedema of extracellular type may transpire from diffusion of monoamines such as 5-HT and NE on to the microvasculature, thereby increasing vasopermeability (Majno and Palade, 1961). On the other hand, intracellular oedema may result from the influence of excessive neurotransmitter overflow on neuronal metabolism and neuronal membrane ionic exchange (Osterholm and Pyenson, 1969).

When considering the relationship of disordered monoamine metabolism to alteration in cerebral metabolism during ischaemia, it is interesting to speculate that increase of cyclic AMP under ischaemic conditions may be responsible for increased glycolysis and tissue lactic acid accumulation (Eshler and Ammon, 1966; Lowry and Passoneau, 1966) since it is apparent that cyclic AMP has a regulative effect on phosphofructokinase activity. Perhaps this may indicate an explanation for the mechanism of the Pasteur effect, whereby reduced delivery of oxygen to cerebral tissue results in increased glycolysis and lactic acid formation (Meyer et al., 1969b).

The remote effect of depressed cerebral blood flow and metabolism that follows focal ischaemia, i.e. diaschisis (Hoedt-Rasmussen and Skinhoj, 1964) could also be explained on disordered neurotransmission and transneuronally mediated inhibition of function caused by neurotransmitter overflow and diffusion into contiguous non-ischaemic brain areas or into CSF for eventual re-uptake into brain areas remote from the original ischaemic lesion. Studies in man performed in this laboratory have also shown that increased CSF levels of serotonin measured during the early stages after acute cerebral hemispheric infarction correlate with bilateral reduction in hemispheric blood flow, reintroducing a possible vascular component in the etiology of diaschisis (Meyer et al., 1974).

Finally, having shown a relationship of disordered neurotransmitter function to the pathophysiological accompaniments of cerebral ischaemia, what effect does pharmacological manipulation of neurotransmitter function have on the pathogenesis of this disorder? Zervas and Hori (1973) have administered alpha methyltyrosine to squirrel monkeys and claim improvement in morbidity and mortality after unilateral cerebral hemispheric infarction has been produced by clipping the middle cerebral artery. Studies from this laboratory using the gerbil stroke model have shown that prior treatment of animals with p-chlorophenylalanine reduces the stroke incidence rate from 44 per cent to 26 per cent (p < 0.001), supporting the possibility that reduced availability of serotonin for release from ischaemic tissue on to collateral vessels limits the impairment of collateral vasocapacitance after focal cerebral ischaemia. Preliminary studies of this nature seem encouraging to the pursuit of further pharmacological agents, which may modify the pathophysiological accompaniments of experimental cerebral ischaemia.

EXPERIMENTAL SURGICAL
REVASCULARISATION PROCEDURES
FOR ISCHAEMIC BRAIN

In order to improve the inflow of arterial blood to zones of cerebral ischaemia, various surgical procedures have been tried. Some of these experimental approaches will be discussed since they are applicable to man.

Early experimental reconstructive work on the cerebral arteries of animals was reviewed by Donaghy and Yasargil (1967). Lingular to basilar artery segmental replacement, arteriotomy and patch grafting of cortical arteries, and extracranial to intracranial shunts between the superficial temporal and the middle cerebral arteries were successfully achieved. Preliminary reports on clinical experience with the superficial temporal to middle cerebral artery anastomosis in 20 patients have been published (Yasargil, Krayenbuhl, and Jacobson, 1970). In nine patients, an end-to-side anastomosis between the end of the superficial temporal artery and the side of the temporal division of the middle cerebral artery was performed. In 11 patients a direct arteriotomy with embolectomy or thrombectomy was performed on the middle cerebral artery. Some of the patients seem to have benefitted, though no definite conclusions can be drawn.

Reichman (1971) reported the results of a lingular-basilar artery microanastomosis in 33 dogs. Twenty-nine anastomoses were open after three months studied by arteriography or autopsy. In 24 dogs, the cerebral arterial inflow was isolated (by staged procedures) to the new lingual-basilar system in order to evaluate its functional capacity. The longest survival period was two years. Arteriography in the initial stages revealed arterial spasm which was found to be detrimental.

A more optimistic report was published by Crowell and Olsson (1973). They anastomosed the superficial temporal artery to a branch of the middle cerebral artery in 20 dogs two hours after occlusion of the middle cerebral artery. In another group of 11 animals, middle cerebral artery occlusion without any bypass grafting was performed. All animals were evaluated clinically and pathologically two weeks after the surgery. Animals with patent or occluded bypass grafts fared better than the control group.

A recent and more elaborate study of experimental microvascular anastomosis was published by Fein and Molinari (1974). An electromagnetic flow probe was chronically implanted over the superficial temporal artery for assessment of its flow. Regional CBF was measured by the intracarotid injection of Xenon[133] and regional clearance. Preoperative and postoperative assessment of cerebral autoregulation and CO_2 reactivity were carried out. Following clipping of the middle cerebral artery, a microvascular anastomosis between the superficial temporal and a cortical artery was performed. A significant reduction in CBF after clipping of the middle cerebral artery and an increase in regional CBF following cortical artery anastomosis were observed.

A different surgical approach to improve tissue perfusion in the ischaemic zone was utilized by Abraham et al. (1975). They performed bilateral ligation of the external carotid arteries, four hours after middle cerebral artery occlusion in baboons, and assessed regional cerebral blood flow by the Xenon[133] clearance technique. Flows in the ischaemic and nonischaemic areas were greatly enhanced, while the hyperemic areas showed reduction, thus indicating a favourable redistribution of blood supply.

REFERENCES

Abraham, J., Ott, E. O., Aoyagi, M., Tagashira, Y., Achari, A. N. & Meyer, J. S. (1975) Regional cerebral blood flow changes following bilateral external carotid artery ligation in acute experimental infarction. *Journal of Neurosurgery*, in press.

Ames, A. III, Wright, R. L., Kowada, M., Thurston, J. M. & Majno, G. (1968) Cerebral ischaemia. II. The no-reflow phenomenon. *American Journal of Pathology*, **52**, 437.

Aoyagi, M., Meyer, J. S., Deshmukh, V. D., Ott, E. O., Tagashira, Y., Kawamura, Y., Matsuda, M., Achari, A. N. & Chee, A. N. C. (1975) Central cholinergic control of cerebral blood flow in the baboon: Effect of cholinesterase inhibition with neostigmine on autoregulation and CO_2 responsiveness. *Journal of Neurosurgery*, submitted for publication.

Ashcroft, G. W., Crawford, T. B. B., Dow, R. C. & Guildberg, H. C. (1968) Homovanillic acid, 3,4-dihydroxyphenyl acetic acid and 5-hydroxyindol-3-acetic acid in serial samples of cerebrospinal fluid from the lateral ventricle of the dog. *Journal of Pharmacology and Chemotherapy*, **33**, 441.

Aukland, K., Bower, B. F. & Berliner, R. W. (1964) Measurement of local blood flow with hydrogen gas. *Circulation Research*, **14**, 164.

Bazan, N. G., Jr. (1970) Effects of ischaemia and electroconvulsive shock on free fatty acid pool in the brain. *Biochimica et Biophysica Acta*, **218**, 1.

Bloom, F. E. (1972) Localisation of neurotransmitters by electron microscopy. *Proceedings of the Society for Research on Nervous and Mental Disease*, **2**, 25.

Brierley, J. B., Brown, A. W., Excell, B. J. & Meldrum, B. S. (1969) Brain damage in the rhesus monkey resulting from profound arterial hypotension. I. Its nature, distribution and general physiological correlates. *Brain Research*, **13**, 68.

Branston, N. M., Symon, L., Crockard, A. & Pasztor, E. (1974) Relationship between the cortical evoked potential and local cortical blood flow following acute middle cerebral artery occlusion in the baboon. *Experimental Neurology*, **45**, 195.

Byrom, F. B. (1954) Pathogenesis of hypertensive encephalopathy and its relation to the malignant phase of hypertension: Experimental evidence in the hyptertensive rat. *Lancet*, ii, 201.

Clasen, R. A., Pandolfi, S. & Casey, D., Jr. (1974) Reserpine in experimental cerebral edema: Further observations. *Neurology*, **24**, 594.

Clendenon, N. R., Allen, N., Komatsu, T., Liss, L., Gordon, W. A. & Heimberger, K. (1971) Biochemical alterations in the anoxic–ischaemic lesion of rat brain. *Archives of Neurology*, **25**, 432.

Cooper, A. (1836) Some experiments and observations on tying the carotid and vertebral arteries and the pneumogastric, phrenic and sympathetic nerves. *Guy's Hospital Report*, **1**, 457.

Corday, E., Rothenberg, S. F. & Putnam, T. J. (1953) Cerebrovascular insufficiency. An explanation of some types of localized cerebral encephalopathy. *A.M.A. Archives of Neurology and Psychiatry*, **66**, 551.

Cramer, H., Ng, L. K. Y. & Chase, T. N. (1972) Effect of probenecid on levels of cyclic AMP in human cerebrospinal fluid. *Journal of Neurochemistry*, **19**, 1601.

Crowell, R. M. & Olsson, Y. (1973) Effect of extracranial-intracranial vascular bypass graft on experimental acute stroke in dogs. *Journal of Neurosurgery*, **38**, 26.

D'Alecy, L. G. (1973) Sympathetic cerebral vasoconstriction blocked by adrenergic alpha receptor antagonists. *Stroke*, **4**, 30.

Danis, R. K. & Willman, V. L. (1963) Cerebral air embolism effects on brain water and serotonin content. *Surgical Forum*, **14**, 63.

Denny-Brown, D., Meyer, J. S. & Fang, H. C. H. (1953) Effects of vascular occlusion on cortical oxygen tension. In *Proceedings of the 5th International Neurological Congress*, Lisbon.

Deshmukh, V. D. & Harper, A. M. (1973) The effect of serotonin on cerebral and extracerebral blood flow with possible implications in migraine. *Acta Neurologica Scandinavia*, **49**, 649.

Deshmukh, V. D., Harper, A. M., Rowan, J. O. & Jennett, W. B. (1971–1972) Studies on neurogenic control of the cerebral circulation. *European Neurology*, **6**, 166.

Dinsdale, H. B., Robertson, D. M. & Hass, R. A. (1974) Cerebral blood flow in acute hypertension. *Archives of Neurology*, **31**, 80.

Dodson, R. P., Aoyagi, M., Hartmann, A. & Tagashira, Y. (1974) Acute cerebral infarction and hypotension: An ultrastructural study. *Journal of Neuropathology and Experimental Neurology*, **33**, 400.

Donaghy, R. M. P. & Yasargil, M. G. (1967) *Micro-vascular Surgery*. Stuttgart: Georg Thieme Verlag.

Donders, F. C. (1849) De bewegingen der hersenen en de veranderingen der vaatvulling van de pia mater, ook bij gesloten onuitzet-beren schedel regtstreeks onderzocht. *Onderzoek. ged. inh. physiol. Lab. d. Utrecht, Hoogeoch*, ii, 97.

Edvinsson, L., Nielsen, K. C., Owman, C. & West, K. A. (1971) Sympathetic adrenergic influence on brain vessels or studied by changes in cerebral blood volume of mice. *European Neurology*, **6**, 193.

Ekström-Jodal, B., Häggendal, E., Linder, L. E. & Nilsson, N. J. (1972) Cerebral blood flow autoregulation at high arterial pressures and different levels of carbon dioxide tension in dogs. *European Neurology*, **6**, 6.

Eklöf, B., Ingvar, D. H., Kagström, E. & Olin, T. (1971) Persistence of cerebral blood flow autoregulation following chronic bilateral cervical sympathectomy in the monkey. *Acta Physiologica Scandinavia*, **82**, 172.

Eshler, C. J. & Ammon, H. P. T. (1966) The influence of the sympatheticolytic agent, propranolol, on glycogenolysis and glycolysis in muscle, brain and liver of white mice. *Biochemical Pharmacology*, **15**, 2031.

Fein, J. M. & Molinari, G. (1974) Experimental augmentation of regional cerebral blood flow by microvascular anastomosis. *Journal of Neurosurgery*, **41**, 421.

Feindel, W., Yamamoto, Y. L. & Hodge, C. P. (1967) Intracarotid fluorescein angiography: A new method for examination of the epicerebral circulation in man. *Canadian Medical Association Journal*, **96**, 1.

Fieschi, C., Battistini, N., Lenzi, G. L. Volante, F., Weber, R. G., Laghi Pasini, F. & Vittoria, A. (1974) Experimental and clinical observations on platelet aggregability in focal brain ischaemia. In *Platelet Aggregation in the Pathogenesis of Cerebrovascular Disorders*, Round Table Conference, Rome, October 30–31, 1974, pp. 31–33 (abstract).

Forbes, H. S. (1929) Cerebral circulation. I. Observation and measurement of pial vessels. *Archives of Neurology and Psychiatry* (Chicago), **19**, 751.

Frei, H. J., Wallenfang, T., Poll, W., Reulen, H. J., Schubert, R. & Brock, M. (1973) Regional cerebral blood flow and regional metabolism in cold induced oedema. *Acute Neurochirurgica*, **29**, 15.

Ganser, V. & Boksay, I. (1974) Effect of pentoxifylline on cerebral oedema in cats. *Neurology*, **24**, 487.

Gessa, G. L., Krischna, G., Forn, J., Tagliamonti, A. & Brody, B. L. (1970) Behavioral and vegetative effects produced by dibutyryl cyclic AMP injected into different areas of the brain. In *Advances in Biochemical Psychopharmacology*, ed. Greengard, P. & Costa, E. Vol. 3, pp. 371–381. New York: Raven Press.

Glass, H. I. & Harper, A. M. (1963) Measurement of regional blood flow in cerebral cortex of man through intact skull. *British Medical Journal*, i, 593.

Gotoh, F., Meyer, J. S. & Tomita, M. (1966) Hydrogen method for determining cerebral blood flow in man. *Archives of Neurology*, **15**, 549.

Gotoh, F., Muramatsu, F., Fukuuchi, Y. & Amano, T. (1973) Dual control of cerebral circulation. Separate sites of action in vascular tree in autoregulation and chemical control. *Stroke*, **4**, 327 (abstract).

Gottstein, U. (1964) Der Hirnkreislauf bie Hyperthyreose und Myxödem. *Verhandlungen der Deutschen Gesellschaft fur Innere Medizin*, **70**, 921.

Grubb, R. L., Raichle, M. E., Eichling, J. O. & Ter-Pogossian, M. M. (1974) The effects of changes in P_aCO_2 on cerebral blood volume, blood flow, and vascular mean transit time. *Stroke*, **5**, 630.

Haggendal, E. & Johansson, B. (1972) Pathophysiological aspects of the blood brain barrier change in acute arterial hypertension. In *Cerebral Blood Flow and Intracranial Pressure*. Proceedings of the 5th International Symposium on Cerebral Blood Flow Regulation, Acid-Base and Energy Metabolism in Acute Brain Injuries, Roma–Siena 1971. Pp. 24–28. Basel: S. Karger.

Harper, A. M., Deshmukh, V. D., Rowan, J. O. & Jennett, W. B. (1972) The influence of sympathetic nervous activity on cerebral blood flow. *Archives of Neurology*, **27**, 1.

Harper, A. M., Deshmukh, V. D., Rowan, J. O. and Jennett, W. B. (1971) Studies on possible neurogenic influences on the cerebral circulation. In *Brain and Blood Flow*. Proceedings of the Fourth International Symposium on the Regulation of Cerebral Blood Flow, London, September 1970, ed. Ross Russell, R. W. Pp. 182–186. London: Pitman.

Harper, A. M. & Glass, H. I. (1965) Effect of alterations in the arterial carbon dioxide tension on the blood flow through the cerebral cortex at normal and low arterial blood pressure. *Journal of Neurology, Neurosurgery and Psychiatry*, **28**, 449.

Harrison, M. J. G., Brownbill, D., Lewis, P. D. & Russell, R. W. R. (1973) Cerebral edema following carotid artery ligation in the gerbil. *Archives of Neurology*, **28**, 389.

Harrison, M. J. G. & Russell, R. W. R. (1972) Effect of dexamethasone on experimental cerebral infarction in the gerbil. *Journal of Neurology, Neurosurgery and Psychiatry*, **35**, 520.

Hillarp, N. A., Fuxe, K. & Dahlstrom, A. (1966) Demonstration and mapping of central neurons containing dopamine, noradrenalin, and 5-hydroxytryptamine and their reactions to psychopharmaca. *Pharmacological Review*, **18**, 727.

Himwich, H. E. (1951) *Brain Metabolism and Cerebral Disorders*. Baltimore: William & Wilkins.

Høedt-Rasmussen, K. (1967) Regional cerebral blood flow. The intra-arterial injection method. *Acta Neurologica Scandinavica*, **43** (suppl. 27), 1.

Høedt-Rasmussen, K. & Skinhoj, E. (1964) A transneuronal depression of the cerebral hemispheric metabolism in man. *Acta Neurologica Scandinavica*, **40**, 41.

Hoppe, W. E., Waltz, A. G., Jordan, M. M. & Jacobson, R. L. (1974) Effects of dexamethasone on distributions of water and pertechnetate in brains of cats after middle cerebral artery occlusion. *Stroke*, **5**, 617.

Hossmann, K. A. & Kleihues, P. (1973) Reversibility of ischaemic brain damage. *Archives of Neurology*, **29**, 375.

Hoyer, S., Hamer, J., Alberti, E., Stoeckel, H. & Weinhardt, F. (1974) The effect of stepwise arterial hypotension on blood flow and oxidative metabolism of the brain. *Pflügers Archives*, **361**, 161.

Huber, P., Meyer, J. S., Handa, J. & Ishikawa, S. (1965) Electromagnetic flowmeter study of carotid and vertebral blood flow during intracranial hypertension. *Acta Neurochirurgica*, **13**, 37.

Hudgins, W. R. & Garcia, J. H. (1970) Transorbital approach to the middle cerebral artery of the squirrel monkey: A technique for experimental cerebral infarction applicable to ultrastructural studies. *Stroke*, **1**, 107.

James, I. M., Millar, R. A. & Purves, M. J. (1969) Observations on the extrinsic neural control of cerebral blood flow in the baboon. *Circulation Research*, **25**, 77.

Johnson, I. H., Rowan, J. O., Harper, A. M. & Jennett, W. B. (1971) Cerebral blood flow in experimental intracranial hypertension. In *Cerebral Blood Flow and Intracranial Pressure*, Proceedings of the 5th International Symposium on Cerebral Blood Flow Regulation, Acid-Base and Energy Metabolism in Acute Brain Injuries, Roma–Siena, 1970, ed., Fieschi, C. Basel: S. Karger.

Kawamura, Y., Meyer, J. S., Hiromoto, H., Aoyagi, M. & Hashi, K. (1974) Neurogenic control of cerebral blood flow in the baboon. Effects of alpha adrenergic blocking agent phenoxybenzamine on cerebral autoregulation and vasomotor reactivity to changes in P_aCO_2. *Stroke*, **5**, 747.

Kawamura, Y., Meyer, J. S., Hiromoto, H., Aoyagi, M. & Ott, E. O. (1975) Neurogenic control of cerebral blood flow in the baboon. Effects of the cholinergic inhibitory agent, atropine, on cerebral autoregulation and vasomotor reactivity to changes in P_aCO_2. *Journal of Neurosurgery*, in press.

Kety, S. S. & Schmidt, C. F. (1945) Determination of cerebral blood flow in man by the use of nitrous oxide in low concentrations. *American Journal of Physiology*, **143**, 53.

Klainer, L. M., Chi, Y., Friedberg, S. L., Rall, T. W. K. & Sutherland, E. W. (1962) Adenyl cyclase. IV. The effect of neurohormones on the formation of 3′,5′ monophosphate by preparation from brain and other tissues. *Journal of Biochemistry*, **237**, 1239.

Kogure, K., Busto, R., Scheinberg, P. & Reinmuth, O. M. (1974) Energy metabolites and water content in rat brain during the early stage of development of cerebral infarction. *Brain*, **97**, 103.

Kogure, K., Scheinberg, P., Matsumoto, A., Busto, R. & Reinmuth, O. M. (1975) Caticholamines in experimental brain ischaemia. *Archives of Neurology*, **32**, 21.

Langfitt, T. W. & Kassell, N. F. (1968) Cerebral vasodilatation produced by brain-stem stimulation: Neurogenic control vs. autoregulation. *American Journal of Physiology*, **215**, 90.

Langfitt, T. W., McHenry, L. C., Reivich, M. and Wollman, H. (1973) Symposium Abstracts, Cerebral Circulation and Metabolism. Sixth International CBF Symposium, Philadelphia, June 6–9, 1973. *Stroke*, **4**, 321.

Lassen, N. A. (1968) Editorials. Brain extracellular pH: The main factor controlling cerebral blood flow. *Scandinavian Journal of Clinical and Laboratory Investigation*, **22**, 247.

Lassen, N. A. (1974) Control of cerebral circulation in health and disease. *Circulation Research*, **34**, 749.

Lassen, N. A. & Agnoli, A. (1972) The upper limit of autoregulation of cerebral blood flow—On the pathogenesis of hypertensive encephalopathy. (Editorial) *The Scandinavian Journal of Clinical and Laboratory Investigation*, **30**, 113.

Levine, S. & Payan, H. (1966) Effects of ischaemia and other procedures on the brain and retina of the gerbil (Meriones unguiculatus). *Experimental Neurology*, **16**, 255.

Little, J. R., Kerr, F. W. L. & Sundt, T. M. (1974a) Significance of neuronal alterations in developing cortical infarction. *Mayo Clinic Proceedings*, **49**, 827.

Little, J. R., Kerr, F. W. L. & Sundt, T. M. (1974b) The role of lysosomes in production of ischaemic nerve cell changes. *Archives of Neurology*, **30**, 448.

Little, J. R., Kerr, F. W. L. & Sundt, T. M. (1974c) Synaptic alterations in developing cortical infarction: An experimental investigation in monkeys. *Stroke*, **5**, 470.

Lofgren, J. & Zwetnow, N. N. (1973) Cranial and spinal components of the cerebrospinal fluid pressure-volume curve. *Acta Neurologica Scandinavica*, **49**, 575.

Lofgren, J., von Essen, C. & Zwetnow, N. N. (1973) The pressure-volume curve of the cerebrospinal fluid space in dogs. *Acta Neurologica Scandinavica*, **49**, 557.

Lovell, R. A., Elliott, S. J. & Elliott, K. A. C. (1963) The gamma aminobutyric acid and factor 1 content of brain. *Journal of Neorochemistry*, **10**, 479.

Lowry, O. H. & Passoneau, J. V. (1966) Kinetic evidence for multiple binding sites of phosphofructokinase, *Journal of Biochemistry*, **241**, 2268.

Lowry, O. H. & Passoneau, J. V. (1972) *A Flexible System of Enzymatic Analysis.* New York & London: Academic Press.

MacDonald, V. D., Sundt, T. M. & Winkelmann, R. K. (1972) Histochemical studies in the zone of ischemia following middle cerebral artery occlusion in cats. *Journal of Neurosurgery*, **37**, 45.

Majno, G. & Palade, G. E. (1961) Studies on inflammation. I. The effect of histamine and serotonin on vascular permeability: An electron microscopic study. *Journal of Biophysical and Biochemical Cytology*, **11**, 571.

Mathew, N. T., Meyer, O. S. & Hrastnik, F. (1975) *Vasospasm versus 'Breakthrough' in the Pathogenesis of Hypertensive Encephalopathy in Blood Flow and Metabolism in the Brain*, ed. Harper, M. *et al.* Edinburgh: Churchill Livingstone.

Matsuda, M., Meyer, J. S., Ott, E. O., Aoyagi, M. & Tagashira, Y. (1974) Cholinergic influence on autoregulation and CO_2 responsiveness of the brain. *Circulation*, **50**, III-90 (abstract).

McDowall, D. G., Fitch, W., Pickerodt, V. W. A., Coroneos, N. J. & Keaney, N. P. (1971) Haemodynamic effects of experimental intracranial space-occupying lesions in passively ventilated dogs and baboons. In *Cerebral Blood Flow and Intracranial Pressure*, Proceedings of the 5th International Symposium on Cerebral Blood Flow Regulation, Acid-Base and Energy Metabolism in Acute Brain Injuries, Roma–Siena, ed. Fieschi, C. Basel: S. Karger.

Mchedlishvili, G. I. & Nikolaishvili, L. S. (1970) Evidence of a cholinergic nervous mechanism mediating the autoregulatory dilatation of the cerebral blood vessels. *Pflügers Archives*, **315**, 27.

Meinig, G., Reulen, H. J. & Magawly, C. (1973) Regional cerebral blood flow and cerebral perfusion pressure in global brain oedema induced by water intoxication. *Acta Neurochirurgica*, **29**, 1.

Meyer, J. S. (1958a) Circulatory changes following occlusion of the middle cerebral artery and their relation to function. *Journal of Neurosurgery*, **15**, 653.

Meyer, J. S. (1958b) Importance of ischaemic damage to small vessels in experimental cerebral infarction. *Journal of Neuropathology and Experimental Neurology*, **17**, 571.

Meyer, J. S. (1961) Changes in cerebral blood flow resulting from vascular occlusion. In *Pathogenesis and Treatment of Cerebrovascular Disease*, ed. Fields, W. S. Pp. 1–25. Springfield, Illinois: Charles C. Thomas.

Meyer, J. S. (1975a) Evidence for neurogenic control of cerebral circulation. In *Proceedings of the Sixth International CBF Symposium on Cerebral Circulation and Metabolism*, Philadelphia, June 6–9, 1973, ed. Langfitt, T. *et al.* Berlin: Springer Verlag.

Meyer, J. S. & Denny-Brown, D. (1957) The cerebral collateral circulation. 1. Factors influencing collateral blood flow. *Neurology*, **7**, 447.

Meyer, J. S., Gotoh, F., Akiyama, M. & Yoshitake, S. (1967a) Monitoring cerebral blood flow, oxygen, glucose, lactate and ammonia metabolism. Experimental trials in animals. *Circulation Research*, **21**, 649.

Meyer, J. S., Gotoh, F. & Tazaki, Y. (1962) Circulation and metabolism following experimental cerebral embolism. *Journal of Neuropathology and Experimental Neurology*, **21**, 4.

Meyer, J. S., Itoh, Y., Okamoto, S., Welch, K. M. A., Mathew, N. T., Ott, E. O., Sakaki, S., Miyakawa, Y., Chabi, E. & Ericsson, A. D. (1975b) Circulatory and metabolic effects of glycerol infusion in patients with recent cerebral infarction. *Circulation*, in press.

Meyer, J. S., Nomura, F., Sakamoto, K. & Kondo, A. (1969a) Effect of stimulation of the brain-stem reticular formation on cerebral blood flow and oxygen consumption. *Electroencephalography and Clinical Neurophysiology*, **26**, 125.

Meyer, J. S., Ryu, T., Toyoda, M., Shinohara, Y., Wiederholt, I. & Guiraud, B. (1969b) Evidence for a Pasteur effect regulating cerebral oxygen and carbohydrate metabolism in man. *Neurology*, **19**, 954.

Meyer, J. S., Sawada, T., Kitamura, A. & Toyoda, M. (1968) Cerebral oxygen glucose, lactate, and pyruvate metabolism in stroke. Therapeutic considerations. *Circulation*, **37**, 1036.

Meyer, J. S., Stoica, E., Pascu, I., Shimazu, K. & Hartmann, A. (1973) Catecholamine concentrations in CSF and plasma of patients with cerebral infarction and haemorrhage. *Brain*, **96**, 277.

Meyer, J. S., Teraura, T., Marx, P., Hashi, K. & Sakamoto, K. (1972) Brain swelling due to experimental cerebral infarction: Changes in vasomotor capacitance and effects of intravenous glycerol. *Brain*, **95**, 833.

Meyer, J. S., Teraura, T., Sakamoto, K. & Kondo, A. (1971) Central neurogenic control of cerebral blood flow. *Neurology*, **21**, 247.

Meyer, J. S. & Welch, K. M. A. (1972) Relationship of cerebral blood flow and metabolism to neurological symptoms. In *Progress in Brain Research*. Vol. 35, pp. 285–347. Amsterdam: Elsevier.

Meyer, J. S., Welch, K. M. A., Okamoto, S. & Shimazu, K. (1974) Disordered neurotransmitter function. Demonstration by measurement of norepinephrine and 5-hydroxytryptamine in CSF of patients with recent cerebral infarction. *Brain*, **97**, 655.

Meyer, J. S., Yoshida, K. & Sakamoto, K. (1967b) Autonomic control of cerebral blood flow measured by electromagnetic flowmeters. *Neurology*, **17**, 638.

Michenfelder, J. S. & Sundt, T. (1971) Cerebral ATP and lactate levels in the squirrel monkey following occlusion of the middle cerebral artery. *Stroke*, **2**, 319.

Mitchell, J. F. (1963) The spontaneous and evoked release of acetylcholine from the cerebral cortex. *Journal of Physiology* (London), **165**, 98.

Molinari, G. F., Moseley, J. I. & Laurent, J. P. (1974) Segmental middle cerebral artery occlusion in primates: An experimental method requiring minimal surgery and anaesthesia. *Stroke*, **5**, 334.

Molnar, L. & Szanto, J. (1964) The effect of electrical stimulation of the bulbar vasomotor centre on the cerebral blood flow *Quarterly Journal of Experimental Physiology*, **49**, 184.

Moskalenko, Y. E., Demchenko, I. T., Krivchenko, A. I. & Fedulova, I. P. (1974) Dynamics and control mechanisms in maintenance of regional cerebral blood flow. *Stroke*, **5**, 461.

Nelson, S. R. (1974) Effect of drugs on experimental brain edema in mice. *Journal of Neurosurgery*, **41**, 193.

O'Brien, M. D., Jordan, M. M. & Waltz, A. G. (1974) Ischaemic cerebral edema and the blood-brain barrier. *Archives of Neurology*, **30**, 461.

O'Brien, M. D. & Waltz, A. G. (1973) Intracranial pressure gradients caused by experimental cerebral ischaemia and edema. *Stroke*, **4**, 694.

O'Brien, M. D., Waltz, A. G. & Jordan, M. M. (1974) Ischaemic cerebral edema. Distribution of water in brain of cats after occlusion of the middle cerebral artery. *Archives of Neurology*, **30**, 456.

Olesen, J. (1972) The effect of intracarotid epinephrine, norepinephrine and angiotensin on the regional cerebral blood flow in man. *Neurology*, **22**, 978.

Olesen, J. (1974) *Cerebral Blood Flow Methods for Measurement Regulation. Effects of Drugs and Changes in Disease*. Copenhagen: FADL Forlag.

Osterholm, J. L. & Pyenson, J. (1969) Experimental effects of free serotonin in the brain and its relation to brain injury. Part III. Serotonin induced cerebral edema. *Journal of Neurosurgery*, **31**, 417.

Ott, E. O., Abraham, J., Meyer, J. S., Achari, A. N., Chee, A. N. C. & Mathew, N. T. (1975) Disordered cholinergic neurotransmission and dysautoregulation after acute cerebral infarction. *Stroke*, **6**, 172.

Pausescu, E., Lugojan, R. & Pausescu, M. (1970) Cerebral catecholamine and serotonin metabolism in post-hypothermic brain edema. *Brain*, **93**, 31.

Peerless, S. J., Yasargil, M. G. & Kendall, M. J. (1972) The adrenergic and cholinergic innervation of the cerebral blood vessels. In *Proceedings of the Fourth European Congress of Neurosurgery. Present Limits of Neurosurgery*, ed. Fusek, I. & Kung, Z. Prague: Avicenum, Czechoslovak Medical Press.

Petersen, J. N. & Evans, J. P. (1937) Anatomical end results of cerebral arterial occlusion: Experimental and clinical correlation. *Transactions of the American Neurological Association*, **63**, 88.

Plum, F. (1966) Brain swelling and edema in cerebral vascular disease. In *Cerebrovascular Disease*, ed. Millikan, C. H. Ch. XXII, pp. 318–348. Baltimore: Williams & Wilkins.

Purves, M. J. (1972) *The Physiology of the Cerebral Circulation*. Cambridge: University Press.

Rapela, C. E. & Green, H. D. (1964) Autoregulation of canine cerebral blood flow. *Circulation Research* (suppl.), **15**, 205.

Reichman, O. H. (1971) Experimental lingular-basilar arterial microanastomosis. *Journal of Neurosurgery*, **34**, 500.

Reivich, M., Jehle, J. Sokoloff, L. & Kety, S. S. (1969) Measurement of regional cerebral blood flow with antipyrine-14C in awake cats. *Journal of Applied Physiology*, **27**, 296.

Reulen, H. J. & Kreysch, H. G. (1973) Measurement of brain tissue pressure in cold induced cerebral oedema. *Acta Neurochirurgica*, **29**, 29.

Rosenblum, W. I. (1970) Effects of blood pressure and blood viscosity on fluorescein transit time in the cerebral microcirculation in the mouse. *Circulation Research*, **27**, 825.

Rovere, A. A., Scremin, O. U., Bersei, M. R., Raynald, A. C. & Giardini, A. (1973) Cholinergic mechanism in the cerebrovascular action of carbon dioxide. *Stroke*, **4**, 969.

Russell, R. W. R. (1971) A microangiographic study of experimental cerebral ischaemia and of the effects of blood pressure changes. In *Brain and Blood Flow*, Proceedings of the Fourth International Symposium on the Regulation of Cerebral Blood Flow, London, September 1970, ed. Russell, R. W. R. London: Pitman.

Scheinberg, P. & Stead, E., Jr. (1949) Cerebral blood flow in male subjects as measured by the nitrous oxide technique. Normal values for blood flow, oxygen utilization, glucose utilization and peripheral resistence, with observation on effect of tilting and anxiety. *Journal of Clinical Investigation*, **28**, 1163.

Scremin, O. U., Rovere, A. A., Raynald, A. C. & Giardini, A. (1973) Cholinergic control of blood flow in the cerebral cortex of the rat. *Stroke*, **4**, 232.

Sengupta, D., Harper, M. & Jennett, B. (1974) Effect of carotid ligation on cerebral blood flow in baboons. II. Response to hypoxia and haemorrhagic hypotension. *Journal of Neurology, Neurosurgery and Psychiatry*, **37**, 578.

Shibata, S., Hodge, C. P. & Pappius, H. M. (1974) Effect of experimental ischaemia on cerebral water and electrolytes. *Journal of Neurosurgery*, **41**, 146.

Siesjö, B. K., Johannson, H., Ljunggren, B. & Norberg, K. (1974) Brain dysfunction in cerebral hypoxia and ischaemia. In *Brain Dysfunction in Metabolic Disorders*, ed. Plum, F. Vol. 53. New York: Raven Press.

Siesjö, B. K. & Ljunggren, B. (1973) Cerebral energy reserves after prolonged hypoxia and ischaemia. *Archives of Neurology*, **29**, 400.

Siesjö, B. K. & Plum, F. (1972) Pathophysiology of anoxic brain damage. In *Biology of Brain Dysfunction*, ed. Gaul, E. G. New York: Plenum Press.

Steiner, A. L., Firendelli, J. A. & Goldberg, D. M. (1972) Radioimmunoassay for cyclic nucleotides. III. Effects of ischaemic changes during development of regional distribution of adenosine 3′,5′ monophosphate and guanosine 3′,5′ monophosphate in mouse brain. *Journal of Biochemistry*, **247**, 1121.

Strandgaard, S., MacKenzie, E. T., Sengupta, D., Rowan, J. O., Lassen, N. A. & Harper, A. M. (1974) Upper limit of autoregulation of cerebral blood flow in the baboon. *Circulation Research*, **34**, 435.

Stoica, E., Meyer, J. S., Kawamura, Y., Hiromoto, H., Hashi, K., Aoyagi, M. & Pascu, I. (1973) Central neurogenic control of cerebral circulation: Effects of intravertebral injection of pyrithioxin on cerebral blood flow and metabolism. *Neurology*, **23**, 687.

Sundt, T. M. & Michenfelder, J. D. (1971–1972) Cerebral ATP and lactate levels with electrocorticogram correlation before, during and after middle cerebral artery occlusion in the squirrel monkey. *European Neurology*, **6**, 73.

Sundt, T. M. & Waltz, A. G. (1971) Cerebral ischaemia and reactive hyperemia: Studies of cortical blood flow and microcirculation before, during and after temporary occlusion of middle cerebral artery of squirrel monkeys. *Circulation Research*, **28**, 426.

Symon, L. (1970) Regional vascular reactivity in the middle cerebral arterial distribution. An experimental study in baboons. *Journal of Neurosurgery*, **33**, 532.

Symon, L., Held, K. & Dorsch, N. W. C. (1972) On the myogenic nature of the autoregulation mechanism in the cerebral circulation. *European Neurology*, **6**, 11.

Symon, L., Ishikawa, S., Lavy, S. & Meyer, J. S. (1963) Quantitative measurement of cephalic blood flow in the monkey. *Journal of Neurosurgery*, **20**, 199.

Symon, L., Pasztor, E. & Branston, N. M. (1974) The distribution and density of reduced cerebral blood flow following acute middle cerebral artery occlusion: An experimental study by the technique of hydrogen clearance in baboons. *Stroke*, **5**, 355.

Teraura, T., Meyer, J. S., Sakamoto, K., Hashi, K., Marx, P., Sterman-Marinchesu, C. & Shinmaru, S. (1972) Hemodynamic and metabolic concomitants of brain swelling and cerebral edema due to experimental cerebral infarction. *Journal of Neurosurgery*, **36**, 728.

Tews, J. K., Potter, S. H., Roa, P. D. & Stone, W. E. (1963) Free amino acids and related compounds in dog brain. Post mortem and anoxic changes. The effects of ammonium chloride infusion on levels during seizures induced by picrotoxin and pentylenetetrazol. *Journal of Neurochemistry*, **10**, 641.

Tulleken, C. A. F., Meyer, J. S., Ott, E. O., Abraham, J. & Dodson, R. F. (1975) Brain tissue pressure gradients in experimental infarction recorded by multiple wick-type transducers. In *Proceedings of the Second International Symposium on Intracranial Pressure*, Lund, Sweden, June 17–19, 1974, ed. Lundberg, N. *et al.* Berlin: Springer Verlag.

Villaret, M. & Cachera, R. (1939) In *Les embolies cerebrales*. Paris: Masson.

Wahl, M., Deetjen, P., Thurau, K., Ingvar, D. H. & Lassen, N. A. (1970) Micropuncture evaluation of the importance of perivascular pH for the arteriolar diameter on the brain surface. *Pflügers Archives*, **316**, 152.

Waltz, A. G. & Sundt, T. M. (1967) The microvasculature and microcirculation of the cerebral cortex after arterial occlusion. *Brain*, **90**, 681.

Weil-Malherbe, H. (1971) The chemical estimation of catecholamines and their metabolites in body fluids and tissue extracts. In *Methods of Biochemical Analysis*, ed. Glick, D. Supplemental Vol., p. 119. New York: Interscience Publishers.

Welch, K. M. A., Hashi, K. & Meyer, J. S. (1973) Cerebrovascular response to intracarotid injection of serotonin before and after middle cerebral artery occlusion. *Journal of Neurology, Neurosurgery and Psychiatry*, **36**, 724.

Welch, K. M. A., Meyer, J. S., Teraura, T., Hashi, K. & Shinmaru, S. (1972) Ischaemic anoxia and cerebral serotonin levels. *Journal of the Neurological Sciences*, **16**, 85.

Welch, K. M. A., Spira, P. J., Knowles, L. & Lance, J. W. (1974) Simultaneous measurement of internal and external carotid blood flow in the monkey. *Neurology*, **24**, 450.

West, C. R. & Matsen, F. A. (1972) Effects of experimental ischaemia on electrolytes of cortical cerebrospinal fluid and on brain water. *Journal of Neurosurgery*, **36**, 687.

Wexler, B. C. (1972) Pathophysiological responses of acute cerebral ischaemia in the gerbil. *Stroke*, **3**, 71.

Williams, V. & Grossman, R. G. (1969) Ultrastructure of cortical synapses after failure of presynaptic activity in ischaemia. *Anatomical Records*, **166**, 131.

Wurtman, J. & Fernstrom, J. D. (1972) L-tryptophane, L-tyrosine and the control of brain monoamine biosynthesis. In *Perspectives in Neuropharmacology*, ed. Synder, S. H., pp. 143–193. Oxford: University Press.

Yasargil, M. G., Krayenbuhl, H. A. & Jacobson, J. I. (1970) Microneurosurgical arterial reconstruction. *Surgery*, **87**, 221.

Yatsu, F. M. (1974) Membrane lipids and brain ischemia. *Current Concepts of Cerebrovascular Disease (Stroke)*, **9**, 19.

Zervas, N. T. & Hori, H. (1973) Effect of alpha methyltyrosine on cerebral infarction. *Stroke*, **4**, 331 (abstract).

Zervas, N. T., Hori, H., Negora, M., Wurtman, R. J., Laren, F., & Lavyne, N. H. (1974) Reduction in brain dopamine following experimental cerebral ischaemia. *Nature*, **247**, 283.

Zwetnow, N. N. (1970) Effects of increased cerebrospinal fluid pressure on the blood flow and on the energy metabolism of the brain. *Acta Physiologica Scandinavica* (suppl.), **339**, 5.

5. Cerebral Blood Flow Measurements in Stroke

Cesare Fieschi and Michel Des Rosiers

In the last 30 years there has been a growing interest in the physiology of cerebral blood flow (CBF) brought about by the development of new quantitative methods. The application of these methods to clinical as well as experimental investigations in man has gone through two phases and a third one is foreseen:

Phase 1, 1945–1960; invasive quantitative techniques for measurement of global CBF: the nitrous oxide method of Kety and Schmidt (1948) and its variants (Lassen and Munck, 1955).

Phase 2, 1961–1975; invasive quantitative techniques for measurement of regional blood flow (rCBF) by intracarotid injection of radioactive inert gases (Lassen *et al.*, 1963).

Phase 3, now in progress; non-invasive quantitative techniques for measurement of rCBF by inhalation (Obrist *et al.*, 1967) or intravenous injection (Agnoli *et al.*, 1969) of radioactive inert gases.

Other non-quantitative methods of clinical interest such as sequential scintiphotography (Heiss, Prosenz and Roszucky, 1972), intravenous technitium angiography (Planiol *et al.*, 1971), or intracarotid radioactive microsphere angiography (Blaudino, 1973) are also being used to study disturbances in brain perfusion, especially in patients with anomalies of the large extracranial arteries.

The disturbances in cerebral circulation following cerebrovascular diseases (CVD) to be summarised in this chapter will be limited to those observed with the invasive techniques for measurement of rCBF. For a more detailed and comprehensive analysis on the physiopathology of CBF the reader is referred to reviews such as those of Sokoloff (1959), Lassen (1959), Betz (1972), Olesen (1974), and Mosmans (1974).

METHODOLOGY

Principles of the rCBF method

The method for measurement of rCBF with radioactive inert gases was proposed by Lassen and Ingvar in 1961. Its principle is the assumption that the removal of a freely diffusible and inert indicator from a tissue is a function of the perfusion rate of that tissue. If one uses radioactive γ-emitting isotopes as indicators, it is then possible to record the clearance from various areas of the brain through the intact cranium by multiple detectors placed over the patient's scalp. The recording lasts from 10 to 15 minutes after the injection of the tracer, dissolved in physiological saline and administered as a single bolus in the internal carotid artery, during which time the patient is assumed to remain in a steady state.

The radioactive gas originally used was Krypton-85 (^{85}Kr). Its radioactive characteristics permit a good counting efficiency because of the high energy of its γ radiations (0.5 MeV). But the physical half-life of this isotope is rather long, 10.5 years, and only 0.4 per cent of its emissions are in the form of γ rays. Hence, if one is to record through the skull with this isotope, the quantity injected must be high (3 mCi) with a radiation dose to the brain reaching 29 mr/mCi (Høedt-Rasmussen 1967).

Because of these disadvantages investigators have turned to another radioactive inert gas, Xenon 133 (^{133}Xe). The latter is also a γ emitter (99 per cent of its incident radiations) with an energy of 0.081 MeV, permitting the administration of a lower dose with each intracarotid injection (0.5 to 1 mCi), with a radiation dose to the brain of 17 mr/mCi injected. Its physical half-life of 5.3 days precludes too long a storage after its preparation but reduces the hazards of its disposal in the atmosphere. However, because of the low energy of its gamma radiations, its usefulness is hampered by self-absorption in the tissues leading to a significant degree of Compton Scattering which accounts for 13 to 20 per cent of the total counts picked up by the probes over the scalp (Posner, 1973). Thus, opposite any given probe, the overlapping of radiations coming from adjacent regions of the brain constitutes a serious limitation for a method designed to evaluate the blood flow of circumscribed cerebral regions, and for that reason the use of a more efficient as well as safe radioactive tracer would be preferable.

Flow is not the only variable governing the rate of removal of a tracer from the brain tissue; the relative solubility of this tracer in brain and blood (brain:blood partition coefficient λ) is another important factor to be considered. In the case of Kr and Xe which are lipid soluble, the λ is above one, higher for white than for grey matter, and will vary with haematocrit of alteration in brain constituents as encountered in various types of pathology.

For a normal haematocrit and in normal brain tissue, the λ for Kr have been found to be equal to 1.32 for white matter and 0.97 for grey matter and for Xe, 1.57, and 0.84, respectively, with a weighted mean for whole brain of 1.11 for Kr and 1.13 for Xe (assuming a constant proportion of 60 per cent grey and 40 per cent white matter in each region to be measured). These are the standard values employed by most investigators although 'with some hesitation' (Høedt-Rasmussen, 1967). Indicators with a partition coefficient uniformly closer to 1, such as N_2O, H_2, or water, would be more reliable and allow more precise calculations.

Mathematical processing

From the data recorded by the probes rCBF can be calculated in several ways:

1. *Compartmental analysis* assumes that the clearance curve is the sum of two monoexponential components (Lassen *et al.*, 1963). This assumption is based on the existence of two compartments in brain, white, and grey matter, whose relative flows are known from autoradiographic studies to differ by a factor of 4 (Freygang and Sokoloff, 1959). By this approach the regional flow value for any given area of the brain is obtained from the biexponential analysis of the corresponding clearance curve as follows:

$$F_{BC} \text{ ml/100g/min} = (F_g \times W_g + F_w \times W_w)/ W_g + W_w$$

where F_{BC} represents the rCBF, F_g and W_g represent the flow and the relative weight of the rapidly perfused compartment, i.e.: the grey matter (frequently referred to as the 'fast phase' or the 'cortical flow') while F_w and W_w represent the flow and the relative weight of the slowly perfused compartment, i.e.: the white matter ('slow phase').

Although this bicompartmental analysis can provide the investigator with useful information, its results must be interpreted with caution; the weights of the two components vary in the same individual according to functional activity, the administration of sedative drugs, or the presence of pathology (Wilkinson and Browne, 1970). The 'fast phase' and 'slow phase' should thus be interpreted more on a physiological than purely anatomical basis.

In our own control series consisting of 10 cases without central nervous system diseases (mean age of 52 years), we obtained with this analysis the following values comparable to those reported in the literature for similar age groups: mean rCBF = 44.7 ± 6.2; F = 78.2 ± 18.3; $F_w = 20.8 \pm 2.7$; $W_g = 43\% \pm 6.3$; at a mean arterial CO_2 of 41.6 vol% (Table 5.1).

2. *Stochastic analysis*, or 'height-over-area equation' (Zierler, 1965), gives values for rCBF without compartmental estimates. It is based on the assumption that in any region with a perfusion of f, the mean transit time $\bar{t}$ of a tracer with a distribution volume of V is equal to:

$$\bar{t} = V/f \qquad (1)$$

If perfusion is expressed as flow per 100 g of tissue, as such:

$$F = f/w \times 100 \qquad (2)$$

where W represents the weight of the tissue in

Table 5.1 Mean rCBF values found in awake conscious control subjects without demonstrable organic brain disease.

Author	No. patients	No. probes	Mean age	Tracer	Compartmental analysis				Stochastic analysis F_{10}	Initial slope F(init.)	$P_a co_2$ mmHg
					F_g	F_w	$W_g\%$	F_{BC}			
Lassen et al. (1963)	6-Hosp.	2	45	85-Kr				60 ± 13			
Ingvar & Lassen (1965)	7-Normal	4	21–47	85-Kr	80 ± 11	21 ± 3	49 ± 4	50	50 ± 5	55 ± 6	38.6
Fieschi et al. (1966)	10-Hosp.	4	52	85-Kr	78 ± 18	21 ± 3	43 ± 6	45 ± 6	42 ± 5		41.6 (vol %)
Høedt-Rasmussen (1967)	9-Hosp.	1		85-Kr 133-Xe	81 ± 6	23 ± 4	48 ± 5	50	50 ± 8		40
Zingesser et al. (1968)	10-Normal	4	33	133-Xe				54 ± 6			
McHenry, Jaffe & Goldberg, (1969)	5-Hosp.	8		133-Xe	77 ± 6	22 ± 1	54 ± 6	52 ± 3	54 ± 3		39
Wilkinson et al. (1969)	10-Hosp.	16	46	133-Xe	87 ± 17	22 ± 4	46 ± 5	51 ± 9	53 ± 6	60 ± 14	45
Olesen, Paulson & Lassen (1971)	8-Hosp.	35	52	133-Xe					50 ± 5	64 ± 9	41
Sveindottir et al. (1971)	11-Hosp.	32	38	133-Xe	84 ± 12	22 ± 3	50 ± 7	53	51 ± 5	60 ± 10	39
				Mean	81	22	48	52	50	60	

grams, then equation (1) can be rewritten as follows:

$$\bar{t} = \frac{V}{W} \times \frac{100}{F} \qquad (3)$$

or

$$F = \frac{V}{W} \times \frac{100}{\bar{t}} \qquad (4)$$

Since $\bar{t}$ corresponds to the total area (A) under the clearance curve over the maximum height (H) reached by this curve, equation (4) will finally become

$$F_{10} = \frac{V}{W} \times \frac{H}{A} \times 100 \qquad (5)$$

where F_{10} (flow for a 10 min recording) represents the rCBF expressed in ml per 100 g of brain tissue per minute and (V/W) represents the distribution volume of the tracer per unit weight of tissue, that is its weighted λ which is assumed as for the bicompartmental analysis to be a known constant. Since as stated above the latter can vary and should be determined for any given condition, the stochastic analysis has essentially the same limitations as the bicompartmental approach without giving as detailed information. For practical purposes rCBF values obtained with either method are fairly similar, as computed from 6 data groups: $\Delta F_{BC} - F_{10} = 0.2\%$, N.S. (Table 5.1).

3. With the *initial slope analysis* or two minute-flow index, introduced by Høedt-Rasmussen in 1967, rCBF is calculated from the slope of the initial part of the clearance curve regarded as monoexponential for the first one or two minutes of the recording. One then corrects for the λ of the grey matter only since it is assumed that during this early phase the bulk of the counts are coming from this compartment.

Despite understandable theoretical objections and a systematic difference between rCBF values obtained from the initial slope F (initial) and those calculated by the other types of analysis, as computed from 4 data-groups $-\Delta$ F(init) $-F_{10} = 17$ per cent, $p < 0.05$ (Table 5.1), the short duration of recording required and the rapid analysis of data possible without need of a computer has rendered the use of this simplified approach very popular for clinical purposes. Its results, however, should be regarded as a relative 'index' of cerebral perfusion rather than as an absolute flow value.

One major theoretical objection to the rCBF methods, whatever mode of calculation is used, involves recirculation and extracerebral contamination. In fact, the entire amount of gas washed out from the brain is not cleared completely in a single passage through the lungs; this is especially true in the case of patients with impaired ventilation:perfusion ratio. There will thus be during the course of the study a re-introduction of gas to the brain from the systemic circulation as well as contamination of the regional fields by radiations coming from the slowly perfused extracranial tissues (8–10 cc/min) by way of the external carotid artery. These two factors both act to blunt the initial slope of the clearance curves (Figs. 5.1A & B).

Normal values

We have collected the mean rCBF values obtained under local anaesthesia in control subjects by various authors (Table 5.1). In a few cases those measurements were done in healthy volunteers, but for the most part they were simultaneous with cerebral angiography in patients hospitalised for neurological investigation but in whom no overt organic brain pathology could be demonstrated.

Though one cannot strictly equate mean rCBF with hemispheric CBF measured by the Kety-Schmidt method or its variants, it is interesting to notice that the former is of the same order of magnitude as the latter for which we have reproduced some of the published results for healthy subjects (Table 5.2). No formal comparison has been attempted here in view of the differences in age, technique, and clinical conditions between the various data-groups involved.

Table 5.2 Mean global CBF (GCBF) values obtained in normal individuals with the Kety-Schmidt method or its variants.

Author	No. patients	Tracer	GCBF
Kety & Schmidt (1948)	14-Normal	N_2O	54
Lassen & Munck (1955)	20-Normal	Kr^{85}	52
Lassen, Feinberg and Lane (1960)	11-Normal	N_2O	50
Lewis et al. (1960)	9-Normal	N_2O	57
		Mean:	53

It can also be noticed that the bicompartmental analysis of rCBF has yielded, in man, a ratio of F_w to F_g close to that obtained in laboratory animals by autoradiographic technique—Freygang and Sokoloff (1959) in cats: 1/4.3; Reivich et al. (1969) in cats: 1/4.5. In the case of rCBF this ratio lies between 1/3.5 and 1/4, though the variation in the relative weight of the grey and white compartments puts emphasis on the functional nature of these 'compartments'.

Reproducibility and regional variations

In order to assess the clinical reliability and limitations of such a method, various authors (Agnoli et al., 1968; Ingvar & Lassen, 1965; Lassen et al., 1963; McHenry, Jaffe and Goldberg, 1969; Wilkinson et al., 1969) have studied its reproducibility and defined its 'measurement error', accounted for by methodological inaccuracies as well as normal physiological variations bound to occur during the procedure: these two factors cannot be separated experimentally. This measurement error is expressed as the coefficient of variation of the differences between two consecutive measurements done in the same subjects under similar conditions, and varies according to the author, from 4 to 9 per cent (Table 5.3).

The reproducibility of the rCBF method can thus be considered as good, provided enough time elapses between two consecutive injections of the tracer to permit its complete wash out from the tissues and a return of the counts to background level. Indeed, there exists no significant difference in mean hemispheric rCBF obtained from two subsequent measurements except in the case of Wilkinson et al. (1969) who found a 9 per cent lower value for the second study ($p<0.02$), a difference which cannot be explained by changes in P_{CO_2}, by variations in perfusion pressure or by too short a lag between tracer injections.

The normal distribution pattern and regional variation of rCBF constitute another important aspect of the method, though interpretation of the data in the literature on that subject remains open to discussion. Ingvar (1965) in seven normal volunteers found that the 'temporal' region had a significantly lower 'cortical flow' (Fg) than that of the three other regions studied, but, as he suggests, this could be due in part to recirculation 'which in this measuring field offers special problems'; the rCBF reported in his work, however, appears quite homogeneous. Wilkinson et al. (1969) in a carefully designed study of 16 regions in 10 control subjects without 'abnormal physical signs referable to the hemisphere' (though his series includes four epileptics, two pituitary tumours, and one

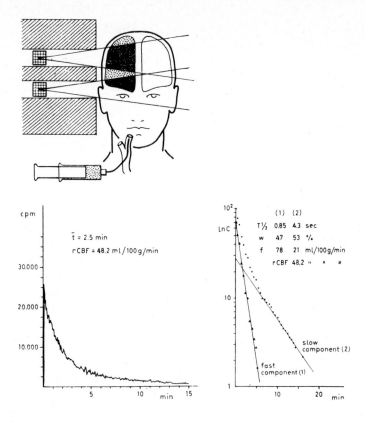

Fig. 5.1A (*Top*): Registration of the clearance curve of ^{85}Kr injected into the internal carotid artery. (*Bottom left*): Actual recording of a clearance curve. Regional blood flow can be calculated from the mean transit time $\bar{t}$ ($\bar{t}$ = area/height of the curve) on the basis of the equation:

$$\frac{1}{\bar{t}} = \frac{F}{V^{85}Kr} = \frac{F}{\lambda W} \times 100$$

where F = rCBF (ml/100 g/min); $V^{85}Kr$ = volume of distribution of ^{85}Kr; $\bar{\lambda}$ = mean partition coefficient of ^{85}Kr (1.09); W = unit weight of the brain (1 g). (*Bottom right*): Semilogarithmic plot of the clearance curve. Two exponential components are evident, showing the blood flow rates of the fast (f_1) and the slow (f_2) compartments and their relative weights (w_1 and $^1w_2$). Compartmental analysis is based on the following equations:

$$C(t) = I_1 e^{-k_1 t} + I_2 e^{-k_2 t}$$

where C = recorded radioactivity; I_1 and I_2 = intercepts with the y axis of the fast and the slow components; K_1 and K_2 = slopes of the fast and the slow components.

$$rCBF = \frac{I_1 \lambda_1 K_1 + I_2^* \lambda_2 K_2}{I_1 + I_2^*} \times 100 \ (ml/100 \ g/min)$$

where λ_1 (0.95) and λ_2 (1.30) = partition coefficients of ^{85}Kr for the fast and the slow components; I_2^* = intercept of the slow component corrected for the short injection time and partition coefficient

$$I_2^* = I_2 \frac{\lambda_1 K_2}{\lambda_2 K_2}$$

$$W_1\% = \frac{I_1}{I_1 + I_2^*} \times 100; \qquad W_2\% = \frac{I_2}{I_1 + I_2^*} \times 100$$

$$f_1 = K_1 \lambda_1 \times 100; \qquad f_2 = K_2 \lambda_2 \times 100 \ (ml/100 \ g/min)$$

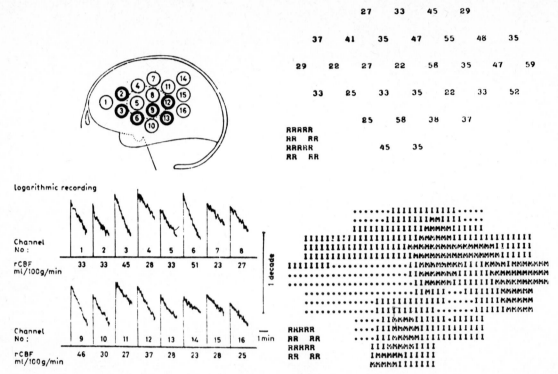

Fig. 5.1B (*Left*): rCBF measured with ^{133}Xe in 16 regions. The evaluation of the curves is limited to the initial two minutes. (*Right*): Further reduction of the size of probes allows rCBF to be measured in up to 35 regions. Use of a small digital computer on-line gives the rCBF values per unit time (numbers in the left upper part of the figure = rCBF in ml/100 g/min) along with a graphical representation of the regions with increased (MM) and decreased (...) blood flow. The symbol R indicates that the right hemisphere has been explored. (Courtesy of Dr N. A. Lassen.)

optic nerve glioma) reports a high rCBF in the insular and precentral regions, a Fg low in the temporal and high in the precentral areas, and a high Fw in the internal capsule area, all regions where values were significantly different from the mean values for the hemisphere. Lastly,

Risberg and Ingvar (1973), in 17 patients (16 alcoholics and one meningo-encephalitis in remission) studied with 35 probes, reports somewhat similar results in resting conditions.

It remains true that the regions explored by each probe do not correspond to circumscribed

Table 5.3 Measurement error of the rCBF method: coefficient of variation of the differences between two subsequent measurements done in similar conditions.

Author	Total no. of probes	Lag between meas. (min)	Tracer	Type of analysis	F_1	F_2	ΔF_{2-1} %	s.d. of differences	Meas. Error (coef. var.)	$P_a CO_2$ 1	2
Lassen *et al.* (1963)	19	20	85-Kr	Bicomp.	43	40	−7%, NS	2.6 pr[a]	6%		
Ingvar and Lassen (1965)	28	20	85-Kr	Stoc.-10'	50	49.5	−1%	4.4 pr[a]	9%	49.8–49.5	
Høedt-Rasmussen (1967)	8	15	85-Kr	Stoc.-10'	38	37	−3%, NS	1.8 pr[a]	5%	38.4–38.4	
Fieschi, *et al.* (1969)	70	>30	85-Kr	Bicomp	45.4	45.6	+0.5%	3.5 pr[a]	8%		
McHenry, Jaffe & Goldberg(1969)	80	25	133-Xe	Stoc.-10'	34	33.5	−1.5%, NS	1.25 pa[b]	4%	35–35	
Wilkinson *et al.* (1969)	80	30	133-Xe	Bicomp	53	48	−9%, p<0.02	1.75 pa[b]	4%	42.4–45.2	

[a]pr: Standard deviation obtained from differences for each individual probe.
[b]pr: Standard deviation obtained from mean hemispheric difference for each patient.

anatomical structures but represent more correctly cones of mixed tissues whose size will depend on the number of probes and type of collimation used, and in which the tissues nearer the surface will outweigh those more centrally situated. For that reason and because of rather inconclusive findings on the normal pattern of rCBF distribution, we believe that one should be content to obtain a randomised regional variability of rCBF values in a control series, sufficient to interpret the gross regional changes in flow and reactivity which are encountered in pathological cases.

Paulson (1970) has proposed that the mean of the coefficients of variation (CV) be determined individually in each subject of a control series studied under normal physiological conditions; accordingly, in any patient and in any region where the rCBF varies more than $CV + 2$ s.d. from the mean hemispheric rCBF, it may reasonably be assumed that there is a 'regional or focal disturbance in flow' at the <0.05 level of certainty. From the information available in the literature (Table 5.4), a limit of 20 per cent has been used in our analysis of the case records reported in the section on mathematical processing, above, to identify regions with focal flow disturbances, although some authors have accepted lesser changes when observed in a number of adjacent regions.

Reactivity of the cerebral vascular bed

For a better understanding of the results reported in the following sections we will summarise some of the inherent properties of the cerebral vascular bed: its capability for autoregulation and its sensitivity to CO_2. The former plays a protective role in that, within certain limits, it maintains the overall cerebral perfusion constant in the face of abrupt changes in perfusion pressure induced by alterations in arterial, venous, or intracranial pressure; the latter permits the fine adjustment of the local blood supply to the local metabolic needs and functional activity of the tissue. Reviews on the physiology of cerebral circulation such as those of Reivich (1969), Betz (1972), Fieschi, and Bozzao (1972a) and Purves (1972) discuss in detail the function of local myogenic reactivity and the role of the autonomic nervous system in the vasomotor responses of the cerebral vessels. These studies emphasise the predominant role of the local metabolic signals (CO_2, H^+, K^+, and to a lesser extent O_2) in modulating the tone of the smooth muscle of the cerebral arterioles, although neurogenic factors are probably also involved, especially when acute and marked changes in perfusion pressure are taking place.

These normal vasomotor responses can be

Table 5.4 Regional variability of rCBF as determined from the individual coefficients of variation obtained from a control series.

Author	No. of patients	No. of probes per patient	Tracer	Type of analysis	F ± s.d.	Mean coef. variation ± s.d.	Limit: C.V. ± 2 s.d.
Ingvar (1965)	7-Normal	4	133-Xe	Stoc.-10	49.8 ± 5.4	11%[a]	
Høedt-Rasmussen et al. (1967)	7-Hosp.	16	133-Xe	Stoc.-10		9.3%[b] ± 2.5	14%
Zingesser et al. (1968)	10-Normal	4	133-Xe	Bicomp.	53.4	11.1%[b] ± 3.4	18%
Agnoli et al. (1968)	15-Hosp.	4–5	85-Kr	Bicomp.	45.4 ± 7.3	16%[a]	
Jaffe, McHenry and Goldberg (1970)	5-Hosp.	8	133-Xe	Stoc.-10	54 ± 5.9	11%[a]	
Paulson (1970)	11-Hosp.	16	133-Xe	Stoc.-10		8.5%[b] ± 1.6	12%
				F(init.)		10.6%[b] ± 2.6	16%
Olesen, Paulson and Lassen (1971)	8-Hosp.	35	133-Xe	F(init.)	64 ± 9	8.2%[b] ± 1.2	11%

[a] Mean coefficient of variation obtained from pooled probe values.
[b] Mean coefficient of variation obtained from individual C.V. for each patient.

impaired to various degrees in pathological states, and this impairment may be the only local vascular disturbance which can be detected. Investigators have thus designed simple clinical tests to evaluate the reactivity of the cerebral vascular bed after induced changes in systemic arterial pressure (SAP) or P_aCO_2. To test the integrity of *autoregulation*, a controlled rise in SAP is induced with an intravenous drip-infusion of angiotensin II or a controlled hypotension with a short-acting ganglion blocking agent, such as tripmetaphon, while maintaining P_aCO_2 unchanged. The administration of these drugs must be adjusted to keep the SAP 25 to 30 mmHg above or below the patient's baseline pressure which will determine the choice of the drug to be used: the usual rates are approximately 1 γ/min for angiotensin and 5 mg/min for tripmetaphon. The entire duration of the test can be kept within 20 minutes if the initial slope analysis is used to calculate rCBF. Normally, rCBF should not be affected by these induced changes in SAP and should remain constant, within the experimental error of the method. But in interpreting this test, one must be aware that autoregulation operates within certain limits (60–160 mmHg) which may vary according to age, baseline SAP, and P_aCO_2 (Fig. 5.2). Below 60 mm and above 160 mm of Hg, brain perfusion will follow passively perfusion pressure; this may lead in the former case to cerebral ischaemia and in the latter to vasogenic oedema and hypertensive encephalopathy (the 'break-through phenomena') (Lassen and Agnoli, 1972; Strandgaard *et al.*, 1974).

To test the *CO_2 reactivity* it is usually easier, in most clinical circumstances, to induce hypercapnia by inhalation of 5 per cent CO_2 in air administered through a facial mask for 20 minutes (10 min to reach equilibrium and from 2 to 10 min to record the clearance curve). In young, co-operative subjects and in comatose patients passively ventilated, one can instead induce hypocapnia by resorting to hyperventilation. The response of the cerebral vascular bed to CO_2 is complex, but in physiological conditions and for a P_aCO_2 varying from 25 to 60 mm of Hg, brain perfusion is practically linear with P_aCO_2, with a positive slope in the normal

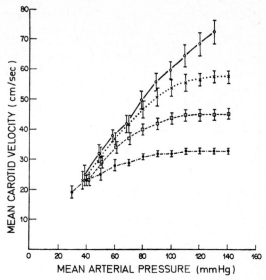

Fig. 5.2 Autoregulation: lowest curve was obtained on room air with the three succeeding ones obtained on 6, 9, and 12 per cent CO_2, respectively. (*From* Raichle and Stone (1971–1972) In *European Neurology*, p. 3, fig. 1.)

conscious man of 1.34 to 2.17 ml/100g/min per mm Hg of P_aCO_2 (Grubb, Raichle and Eichling, 1974). But since CO_2 also tends to influence SAP, the interpretation of this test can become rather difficult in cases where autoregulation is also impaired, for instance in ischaemic areas (Waltz, 1968) or at high levels of P_aCO_2 (Harper, 1965; Raichle and Stone, 1971), since the loss of autoregulation will also allow for an increase in CBF when SAP increases and may prevent in this case the differentiation of the specific effect of CO_2 on the vascular bed. To minimise the possible role of SAP, some investigators have used variation in cerebrovascular conductance (CVC = F/Δ SAP) to evaluate the alterations of the vasomotor reactivity to CO_2 (Ackerman *et al.*, 1973).

For practical purposes, in normal individuals breathing 5 per cent CO_2 in air, the rCBF is usually increased by 20 per cent or more. But in acute brain lesions such as trauma, intracerebral haemorrhage, ischaemia, or certain metabolic encephalopathies vessels can show variable degrees of 'vasoparalysis' to CO_2. Paradoxical reactions secondary to vasoparalysis may then take place in the damaged regions such as a regional reduction in flow during hypercapnia ('steal phenomenon') or a regional augmentation during hypocapnia ('counter-steal phenomenon') (Lassen and Palvölgyi, 1968).

Practical considerations for proper measurements

In closing this section on methodology, we would like to emphasise a few practical points we believe essential for a meaningful interpretation of the results. First, it is important that the patient remains immobile during the recording of the clearance curve and that the position of the external probes stays unchanged for a much longer period, if one wishes to perform repeated measurements to compare accurately the regional values, for instance, after infusion of a vasoactive drug. Ideally, the type of collimation used and the position of the probes on the scalp should be carefully standardised to facilitate comparison of the values obtained by different investigators using this technique.

It is also essential that haematocrit, SAP, and $P_a CO_2$ be monitored during the procedure since CBF may be affected by any of these three variables. Blood viscosity has been shown to influence brain perfusion in patients with long-standing polycythemia (Kety, 1950) or experimentally, in dogs, in which haematocrit was decreased by replacing blood with plasma or dextran (Haggendal and Norback, 1966).

We have already mentioned the importance of SAP and $P_a CO_2$; the ideal situation is one where both parameters remain fairly constant while spontaneous changes in rCBF are taking place or while rCBF changes are induced by drugs acting directly on the cerebrovascular bed. Only $P_a CO_2$ should change when reactivity to CO_2 is being tested, and only SAP when testing auto-regulation.

However precise the recording and analysis of the clearance curve and however numerous the probes, the complexity of the method makes us have reservations on the use of such a technique for clinical purposes, notwithstanding the valuable physiological, pharmacological, and pathophysiological information it has helped to gather. We might add that this technique is not entirely without risk, although the severity and frequency of its complications are lower than that reported for carotid angiography, provided that one follows the recommendations formulated by Ingvar and Lassen (1973) and by Mosmans (1974).

It follows that rCBF studies by direct puncture of the carotid artery or preferably by selective catheterisation of the vessel should always be performed in conjunction with an angiographic study, save in very specific instances (see p. 102) where it can be of direct potential benefit to the patient. We share the following view expressed by Mosmans (1974) in a recent review:

At the present stage the rCBF studies do not appear to contribute sufficiently to establish diagnosis and/or to localise cerebral lesions to justify introduction as a routine method of investigation in clinical neurology. This opinion is also motivated by the fact that the investigation involves catheterisation of the internal carotid artery, that a well trained multidisciplinary team and expensive sophisticated equipment are required.

RESULTS OBTAINED IN CEREBRO-VASCULAR DISEASES (CVD)

The following observations on rCBF in stroke and focal vascular diseases are derived from a comprehensive analysis of data published by four different groups of investigators: (1) Paulson (1970); Paulson, Lassen, and Skinhøj (1970); Skinhøj et al. (1970). (2) McHenry et al. (1972). (3) Fieschi et al. (1969); Agnoli et al. (1968). (4) Iliff et al. (1974); Ackerman et al. (1973).

rCBF measurements in brain softenings and haemorrhages

Global hemispheric changes. Following an ischaemic lesion in the territory of the internal carotid artery, the involved hemisphere, as might be expected, shows a lower mean rCBF than that of control subjects without organic brain disease. This is true for brain softening (BS) as well as brain haemorrhage (BH), and an analysis of variance has shown that the difference between the controls and the stroke patients is significant (Table 5.5). Indeed this reduction was noted in all case records for F(init) as well as for F_{10} and F_{BC}. Similar results had been found previously by Fieschi and Bozzao (1972b), who reported that the rCBF in 50 of their patients with cerebral ischaemic disease was significantly lower than that of controls, mainly due to a decrease in fast flow, in spite of a slightly higher $P_a CO_2$ (Table 5.6). These authors also showed that in cases where rCBF declined to levels of 20 ml/100g/min or less, the clearance curve tended to become mono-exponential: a true 'fast-phase' had practically disappeared. It seems from other observations (Høedt-Rasmussen and Skinhøj, 1964; Meyer, 1970) that this reduction in flow is not necessarily confined to the hemisphere ipsilateral to the lesion, but can also involve the contralateral undamaged hemisphere in what has been referred to as transneural diaschisis.

Moreover, one does not know if these diffuse alterations in rCBF are directly related to the stroke or can be partly accounted for by pre-existing vascular disease (Sokoloff, 1961). Our analysis indicates that in CVD there exists a correlation between the underlying vascular pathology and the magnitude of the rCBF reduction as demonstrated by the grouping of patients with stroke according to the presence or absence of an occlusion of the middle cerebral artery (MCA) or some of its major collaterals (Table 5.7). There is a significant difference in mean rCBF between these two groups of patients, though one must also be aware of other factors that may reduce perfusion after total occlusion of a major intracerebral vessel, such as secondary brain oedema or a decrease in brain

Table 5.5 Mean rCBF values in brain softenings, intracerebral haemorrhages, and transient ischaemic attacks as computed from data published by four groups of investigators.

	No. of cases	rCBF(init.)	No. of cases	$rCBF_{BC}^{10}$
Brain softenings	40	44.6 ± 16.8	85	37.8 ± 19.2
TIA	30	52.2 ± 12.7	29	46.0 ± 14.7
Brain haemorrhage			7	32.4 ± 11.3
Controls (see Table 5.1)		55–64		42–54

Table 5.7 Difference in mean hemispheric rCBF between cases with and without MCA occlusion[a]

	No. of cases	rCBF (init.)	$2\,CBF_{BC}^{10}$
MCA occlusion	38	30.2 ± 8.9	31.5 ± 6.9
No occlusion	68	47.3 ± 12.7	40.4 ± 10.1
Difference (%)		$+56.5^b$	$+28.0^b$

[a]Occlusion of main trunk or of some of its major branches as seen by angiography.
[b]$p < 0.01$.

The results summarised above are by no means specific for strokes since rCBF has been found similarly affected in other types of pathology such as tumours (Cronquist and Agee, 1968) or head injuries (Fieschi et al., 1972).

metabolism as shown by the marked impairment in the level of consciousness which may occasionally accompany a stroke. This correlation is also underlined by the significant difference in mean rCBF existing between patients with stroke and those with transient ischaemic attacks (TIA) studied at various times after the episode. It

Table 5.6 Mean rCBF in control subjects and in patients with cerebral ischaemic lesions. (From Fieschi and Bozzao, Progress in Brain Research. Vol. 35, p. 388, table 2.)

		Compartmental analysis				$P_a CO_2$ (Vol. %)
		f_1-Grey (ml/100 g/min)	f_2-White (ml/100 g/min)	$W_1 \%$	F	
Normals	$\bar{x}$	78.2	20.8	43.0	44.7	41.6
	s.d.	18.3	2.7	6.3	6.2	
Cerebral lesions	$\bar{x}$	51.4	15.8	40.8	30.2	44.8
	s.d.	14.4	4.3	9.0	8.4	
% reduction from controls		34.0^a	24.0^a	5.0	32.0^a	$(+3.2$ vol. %)

[a]$p < 0.01$.

appears that the cerebrovascular bed in TIAs is still capable of compensating for local reductions in perfusion (Table 5.5).

Lastly, the data of Prosenz *et al.* (1972) on hemisphere blood flow measured by 133 Xe clearance and a scintillation gamma camera can also be interpreted similarly. These authors report that among their 23 patients with ischaemic CVD studied in the subacute phase (two weeks to three months after the attack) who had no impairment of consciousness at the time of the measurement and who eventually survived, those with the greatest neurologic deficit had the lowest blood flow. It remains to be proven however that rCBF measurements can provide the clinician with as valuable prognostic information as these authors suggest.

Regional changes in flow. There are two types of circumscribed disturbance in brain perfusion that can be observed in stroke: regional ischaemia and regional hyperaemia, often called 'luxury perfusion'. The recognition of these alterations in flow is the major contribution of the rCBF method to the understanding of the physiopathology of cerebrovascular diseases.

The so-called 'luxury perfusion syndrome', an expression coined by Lassen (1966), corresponds to the angiographic findings of capillary blush and early filling of veins (Cronquist and Laroche, 1967) (Fig. 5.3) and to the venous congestion sometimes seen on the surface of the cortex by neurosurgeons, i.e. 'the red veins syndrome' of Feindell and Perot (1965). Localised reactive hyperaemia is not peculiar to CVD and has been noticed in post-traumatic (Reivitch, Marshall and Kassell, 1969) and post-epileptic states (Penfield, 1938). It is the consequence of lactic acidosis in or around hypoxic tissues provoking a localised dilatation of the arteriolar bed by a direct effect on the vessel walls (Michenfelder and Sundt, 1971). The significance to the brain of reactive hyperaemia is still unclear, but it probably indicates that the reactivity of the vessels to the chemical environment is still present. In fact, it appears to be in excess of the tissue metabolic activity inasmuch as O_2 extraction in such regions is frequently reduced below control levels (Symon, 1971). Therefore therapeutic measures aimed at a further increase in flow, such as administration

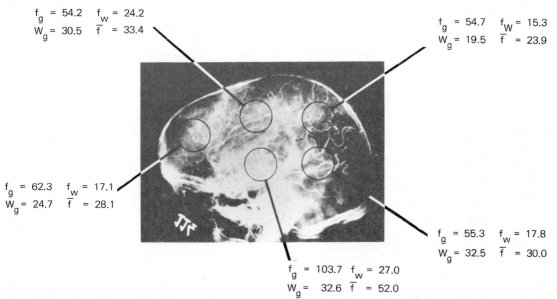

$f_g = 54.2 \quad f_w = 24.2$
$W_g = 30.5 \quad \bar{f} = 33.4$

$f_g = 54.7 \quad f_w = 15.3$
$W_g = 19.5 \quad \bar{f} = 23.9$

$f_g = 62.3 \quad f_w = 17.1$
$W_g = 24.7 \quad \bar{f} = 28.1$

$f_g = 55.3 \quad f_w = 17.8$
$W_g = 32.5 \quad \bar{f} = 30.0$

$f_g = 103.7 \quad f_w = 27.0$
$W_g = 32.6 \quad \bar{f} = 52.0$

Fig. 5.3 Reactive hyperemia: rCBF two days after an ischaemic softening. fg = flow rate of the fast component; fw = flow rate of the slow component; Wg = relative weight of fast compartment; $\bar{f}$ = mean regional flow. Reactive hyperemia ('luxury perfusion') is present in temporal region. Serio-angiography shows early filling of septal, thalamostriate and internal cerebral veins. (*From* Fieschi *et al., Neurology,* **18,** p. 1171, Fig. 2.)

of CO_2 or induced hypertension in cases with impaired autoregulation, would be of doubtful value to these regions at that stage.

Regional ischaemia and regional hyperemia are usually superimposed on a more diffuse hemispheric disturbance in flow and both may be present simultaneously in different areas of the same hemisphere, sometimes with hyperaemic foci of various sizes bordering a central nucleus of ischaemia. We remind the reader that we have adopted a variation in rCBF of ± 20 per cent from the hemispheric mean as an indication of the presence of a regional disturbance in perfusion. Data collected from the works quoted previously have been recalculated and reclassified accordingly. We are aware that these stringent criteria certainly lead to an underestimation of the number of regions with focal disturbances as determined by autoradiographic studies (Fig. 5.4). In spite of this, the proportion of patients with regional disturbances is seen to be high in the early phase of a stroke and tends to drop drastically after the first three days: this is especially true for focal hyperaemia (Fig. 5.5). Therefore it seems reasonable to conclude that these regional haemodynamic changes are directly related to the stroke.

Although it is impossible to predict in any given case the evolution of the disease from the regional perfusion pattern since this pattern is far from stable, the question arises whether the regional haemodynamic changes are topographically related to the causative pathological lesion. It has been impossible for us to answer this question from the information available in the various case records studied, although in a limited series of seven infarcts and seven haemorrhages not included in our analysis (Agnoli *et al.*, 1970) the correlation between disturbances in flow and pathological findings was significant. Marshall (1972) has also attempted to study this relationship in a group of completed strokes (Table 5.8), by comparing rCBF to clinical signs. He concluded that 'the agreement (between regional changes in perfusion and clinical localisation) for hemiparesis, hemisensory loss, and expressive dysphasia was high, while that for hemianopsia was less good, presumably because this sign may arise as a result of a lesion at a number of sites'.

Table 5.8 rCBF abnormalities coinciding with the site of the lesion as clinically determined in patients with completed stroke. (*From* Marshall (1972) Sixth Salzburg Conference, p. 71.)

Clinical defect	History		Physical examination	
	No. of cases	% coinciding	No. of cases	% coinciding
Paresis	22	73	20	85
Senory loss	9	78	11	82
Expressive dysphasia	11	82	6	83
Receptive dysphasia	2	0	2	0
Hemianopia	9	56	11	73

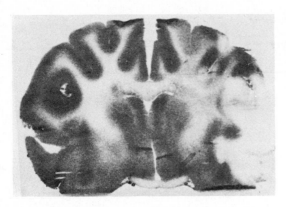

Fig. 5.4 ^{14}C autoradiography of cat brain four hours after ligation of the middle cerebral artery. $P_aCO_2 = 33$ mm Hg SAP = 150 mm Hg. During hypertension, there is a markedly irregular distribution of areas with low flow and high flow in the territory of the artery occluded.

Regional disturbances of vascular reactivity. As we have seen, the normal vasomotor responses of the cerebrovascular bed can be altered after a stroke; these alterations can be circumscribed or diffuse, simultaneous or dissociated, as for example when autoregulation is impaired while CO_2 reactivity is maintained. When the autoregulatory mechanisms are impaired, the brain is no longer protected against changes in perfusion pressure and CBF passively follows

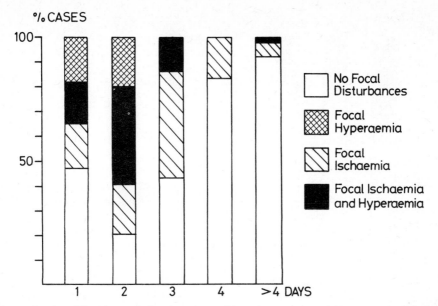

Fig. 5.5 Incidence of regional disturbances in flow in patients with stroke, as computed from case records included in Table 5.5.

SAP. At times, this impairment in autoregulation may lead to paradoxical reactions, i.e. a decrease in rCBF while SAP rises, or conversely an increase in rCBF during hypotension. This phenomenon could be the consequence of concomitant changes in the extravascular pressure in the same direction but of greater magnitude than the changes in SAP (Fieschi et al., 1972); the variation in extravascular pressure will thus neutralise or reverse the effect of SAP on perfusion pressure in these vascular beds where autoregulation is lost ('false' autoregulation).

When the reactivity to CO_2 is altered, the local circulation will no longer be regulated by the local metabolic needs of the tissues. Here also paradoxical responses can be encountered. Thus, during hypercarbia, rCBF may be decreased, rather than increased, in the diseased areas: this phenomenon is referred to as the 'intracerebral steal' (Lassen and Palvölgyi, 1968); or conversely, rCBF may be increased during hypocarbia in these same areas: this is known as the 'intracerebral counter-steal' (Pistolese et al., 1972). The 'intracerebral steal' would be accounted for by a redistribution of blood from the region with impaired reactivity to regions around the lesion which still react normally to CO_2 by vasodilation, thus creating a pressure gradient between non-reacting and reacting regions in favour of the latter. The 'countersteal' is explained by a similar mechanism operating in the opposite direction. These alterations in vasoreactivity can be brought out by the clinical tests already described.

As a threshold for impaired autoregulation, we have adopted the criterion of Fieschi et al. (1969), i.e. a variation in rCBF of ± 16 per cent from baseline after infusion of angiotensin or tripmetaphon. This value of 16 per cent corresponds to the mean difference in flow between the baseline and postinfusion measurements ± 2 s.d., over the mean rCBF for the baseline measurement, or twice the measurement error (Table 5.3). Impaired CO_2 reactivity has been defined as an increase in rCBF of less than 20 per cent during 5 per cent CO_2 inhalation, or decreases in rCBF of less than 20 per cent during a hyperventilation which lowers the P_aCO_2 by at least 5 mmHg. Our analysis has shown that CO_2 reactivity is impaired in approximately 45 per cent of cases after a stroke but that it is rapidly

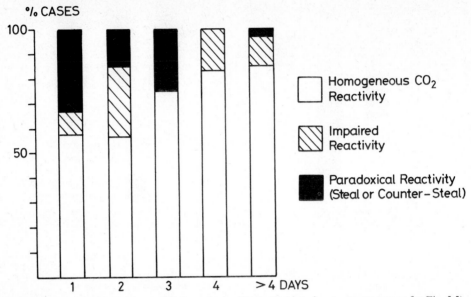

Fig. 5.6 Incidence of abnormal reactivity to CO_2 in patients with stroke (data from same sources as for Fig. 5.5).

regained after the first three days (Fig. 5.6). During this early phase, paradoxical responses are frequent. Autoregulation, on the other hand, is altered in 75 per cent of patients but here again it improves markedly three days after the stroke (Fig. 5.7). Therefore from a haemodynamic standpoint, the acute phase lasts usually no longer than three or four days.

These results, however, are to be interpreted cautiously because they are dependent to a large

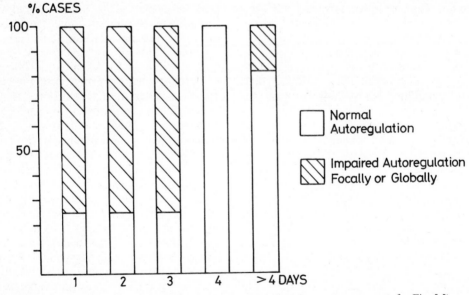

Fig. 5.7 Incidence of impaired autoregulation in patients with stroke (data from same sources as for Fig. 5.5).

extent on the ability of the regional method to depict localised and subtle alterations in flow. In that light, the recent findings by Symon and Brierly (1975) are worth mentioning. These authors measured cortical blood flow with hydrogen clearance in eight monkeys, three years after ligation of the MCA. They found that even if the mean regional flow in the infarcted zone was normal (48 ml/100 g/min), it was unevenly distributed: some regions of the infarct had as low a perfusion as 21 ml/100 g/min, others as high as 89 ml/100 g/min. Moreover even after three years, the CO_2 reactivity of the vascular bed remained impaired while autoregulation, preserved at the periphery of the infarct, was abolished in its centre; however, no paradoxical reactions were encountered.

rCBF and arterial occlusion

Frequently in stroke, no vascular abnormalities are seen on angiography; yet rCBF measurements will often indicate the presence of focal haemodynamic changes in the involved hemisphere. One would therefore expect to find more pronounced focal rCBF abnormalities in cases where an occlusion of the MCA or its branches can be demonstrated angiographically. In the case records we have analysed, 40 per cent of the patients with stroke showed such an occlusion. Although those with and without occlusion had a comparable proportion of focal abnormalities when studied in the acute phase (62 per cent and 55 per cent, respectively), in the group with occlusion there was a higher prevalence of ischaemic foci (56 per cent vs. 33 per cent), while hyperaemic foci were present in both groups in 43 per cent of the cases (Fig. 5.8). Moreover, as previously shown in Table 5.7, the mean hemispheric rCBF in cases without occlusion was 28 per cent higher than that for cases with occlusion; these differences in the mean hemispheric rCBF as well as in the pattern of the regional disturbances supports the view that there are two distinct types of haemodynamic disturbance.

Patients with and without occlusion showed a high proportion of impaired and/or paradoxical response to CO_2 as well as (though not always associated with) a frequent loss of autoregulation, the latter being found in 60 per cent of cases with occlusion and 86 per cent of cases without

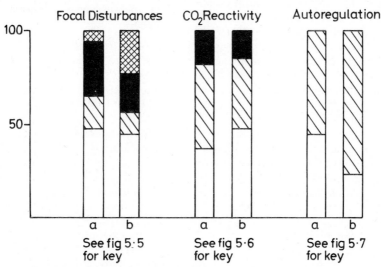

a. Patients with MCA occlusion

b. Patients without occlusion

Fig. 5.8 Incidence of foci of hyperaemia and ischaemia, and of disturbances of autoregulation and CO_2 reactivity in the acute phase (three days) of ischaemic strokes with and without MCA occlusion.

occlusion. Some patients without occlusion displayed a paradoxical or 'false' autoregulation in the involved region. The frequent loss of autoregulation stresses the fact that patients with acute stroke require careful monitoring of their blood pressure in the hours following the ictus: in those without demonstrable arterial occlusion, in which the perfusion pressure in the infarcted zones is less likely to be reduced, any rise in SAP should be prevented in order to forestall the development of vasogenic oedema, whereas in patients with occlusion, any fall in SAP should be corrected to avert further extension of ischaemia in or around the infarcted zones.

rCBF measurements in transient ischaemic attacks

In transient ischaemic attacks, clinical symptoms, although transient, usually last longer than the focal ischaemia since time must be allowed for recovery of tissue function. During the recovery phase, focal haemodynamic abnormalities such as various degrees of vasoparalysis may persist and continue after ischaemia has disappeared and neurological function been regained. The duration and degree of these focal disturbances are related to the severity of the insult, and the recording of such disturbances may help in establishing the period during which patients remain at risk after an episode of TIA.

In a study of 12 such patients, Skinhøj et al. (1970) were able to observe definite disturbances of the rCBF and of its regulation for up to one day following the attack, but not beyond; these disturbances were encountered for a somewhat longer period (up to four days) in 12 cases with 'minor apoplectic attacks' reported together with TIAs, though we feel these cases should rather be considered as completed strokes. In another work, Rees et al. (1971) observed focal disturbances in 7 out of 10 patients with TIA studied by compartmental analysis 8 to 90 days after the last clinical episode. These abnormalities consisted of changes in the fast phase flow (F_g), the slow phase flow (F_w), or the weight of the fast compartment (W_g) and were sometimes limited to a single region. These results, at variance with those of Skinhøj, are interpreted by the authors as an indication that following a TIA there remains a small 'silent' brain infarction. It may also indicate that the bicompartmental analysis is more suitable to depict subtle changes in regional perfusion. As far as the cerebral vasoreactivity is concerned, both authors agree on its integrity between attacks, a result which tends to discount the 'haemodynamic' hypothesis according to which TIA would occur most frequently in areas with marginal perfusion and where the local reactivity of the vascular bed is altered (Denny-Brown, 1960).

Because of these limited abnormalities, the mean rCBF measured after an episode of TIA remains in the normal range and is significantly higher ($+17$ ml/100 g/min—bicompartmental analysis—or $+48$ per cent; $p < 0.001$) than that found in completed strokes, as computed from 29 of the cases of TIA reported in the case records surveyed for which the F_{BC} was available (Table 5.5). It is probable that rCBF values in TIA would have been lower had they been obtained during the attack itself.

rCBF measurements in normal pressure hydrocephalus

Though this pathology is not related directly to CVD, we have thought it useful to mention here briefly some of the findings obtained with ^{133}Xe clearance in normal pressure hydrocephalus (NPH) since these results suggest that a haemodynamic derangement may be an important component of this syndrome.

According to Mathew et al. (1974), rCBF was focally reduced in 15 patients with NPH, particularly in the areas supplied by the anterior cerebral artery. When restudied after the operation, 'patients with higher preoperative rCBF and higher degrees of increase in rCBF after lowering CSF pressure (via a lumbar puncture) appeared to improve better with CSF shunting', while patients with low preoperative rCBF and lesser changes in perfusion after removal of CSF responded poorly to treatment.

The results obtained by Salmon and Timperman (1971) are somewhat different. In a limited

series of cases with post-traumatic encephalopathy these authors could find no correlation
between the value of the preoperative rCBF and
clinical improvement after the shunt. Their
results suggest, however, as in the previous case,
that the degree of clinical improvement could be
linked to the haemodynamic effects of the shunt,
since the only patients to benefit from the
operation were those who showed after the
procedure an increase in mean rCBF (especially
those with a marked increase in W_g). In the light
of these results, the pursuit of rCBF studies in
this condition may be of interest.

THERAPEUTIC APPLICATIONS

Effect of drugs on rCBF in CVD

Regional blood flow studies have shown that
the effect of most drugs on the normal cerebral
vascular tree is homogenous and have added
little to our knowledge of the pharmacology of
cerebral circulation since the comprehensive
review by Sokoloff (1959). We will thus only
comment briefly here on some of the results
obtained with the rCBF method in cerebrovascular diseases after administration of various
drugs.

Noradrenaline, angiotensin, and other hypertensive agents act on the cerebral circulation
through an increase in systemic blood pressure,
since their direct action on cerebral vessels is
negligible at concentrations sufficient to act
upon the peripheral vascular tree (Olesen, 1972).
These drugs do not induce cerebral vasoconstriction and can thus be safely used to increase
cerebral perfusion when SAP is reduced below
the threshold level for autoregulation or when
autoregulation is impaired. In spite of some
limited successes (Farhat and Schneider, 1967),
the beneficial effect of such a treatment in CVD
remains to be proven. In any case, it seems clear
that increases in perfusion pressure above the
upper threshold level are contraindicated for
they favour the development of brain oedema,
especially in infarcted areas (Lassen and Agnoli,
1972).

Similarly, many systemic vasodilators exert
no direct effect on the cerebral blood vessels

and act only on cerebral perfusion when autoregulation is abolished, through changes in
systemic pressure. This is true for ganglionic-
blocking agents and the majority of the peripheral vasodilators (Heiss, 1970).

A few drugs seem to have a direct effect on the
cerebral vessel wall; some, like serotonin (Deshmukh and Harper, 1973), prostaglandin F_{2A}
(Yamamoto et al., 1972), and the xanthine derivatives will constrict the normal cerebral vessel,
though prostaglandin F_{2A} may act on the cerebral oxygen consumption rather than on vascular smooth muscle (Pickard, 1973) and will
tend to trigger counter-steals in regions with
paralysed vessels. This underlies the use of
theophylline in the short-term treatment of
acute CVD (Skinhøj and Paulson, 1970) for the
same reason, of hypocapnia, though the results
of this form of therapy remain rather inconclusive (Christensen et al., 1973). Others, such as
hexobendine (McHenry et al., 1972), papaverine
(McHenry et al., 1970) acetazolamide and their
derivatives (Cotev, Lee and Severinghaus, 1968)
actively dilate the cerebrovascular bed. Their
clinical usefulness in CVD, however, remains
controversial since it has never been clearly
demonstrated that an increase in flow in infarcted
areas of the brain will modify the disease process.

More recently, interest has developed for the
use of intravenous infusions of hyperosmolar
agents, such as glycerol, during the acute phase
of a stroke (Ott, Mathew and Meyer, 1974). The
infusion is usually followed by a significant
increase in rCBF in infarcted areas; this increase
is presumed to be secondary to reduction in
local oedema in the early phase of an infarct and
to the subsequent reduction in capillary resistance. These agents thus act indirectly via perfusion pressure rather than directly on the vessel
wall. The increase in perfusion brought about
by hyperosmolar agents is not necessarily beneficial, since the lesions may already be irreversible and since blood flow in those areas may
already be higher than metabolic requirements.

rCBF measurements as a safeguard during carotid surgery

During internal carotid endarterectomy for
the prophylactic treatment of cerebral vascular

diseases, the artery may have to be temporarily occluded below the lesion. Since the use of an external shunt to protect the brain during the period of occlusion presents its own difficulty and cannot always be used efficiently, a reduction of cerebral blood flow during the period of carotid clamping is to be expected. The duration and degree of this reduction is obviously critical but cannot be predicted beforehand. Therefore a test has been devised in an attempt to evaluate the level to which rCBF will be reduced by clamping. If the level is too low, special procedures have to be employed during endarterectomy, or surgery avoided, because of the high risk of permanent ischaemic complications that may follow the operation.

One of the proposed tests, performed under anaesthesia immediately before the endarterectomy, consists in the total clamping, for two minutes, of the internal carotid artery above the stenosis. The ipsilateral rCBF F(init.) is measured before and during the test (Boysen, 1971). In a study conducted with one detector (Jennett, Harper, and Gillespie, 1966), it was reported that if the CBF of the homolateral hemisphere is reduced by more than 25 per cent from the pre-clamping value, the likelihood of neurological damage following the endarterectomy is high. Evidently, this threshold is likely to vary with the length of the carotid clamping since a given reduction in perfusion considered safe for a short period of clamping may become dangerous if the interruption of flow is prolonged. Because the time factor is difficult to assess in advance, a strict limit must be put on the critical rCBF level in order to avoid permanent cerebral ischaemia if the endarterectomy should last beyond the usual 10 to 20 minutes. This critical threshold is now put at 30 ml/100 g/min in normocapnic patients (Boysen, 1973). Below this level the incidence of ischaemic complications increases significantly. Thus if the rCBF should fall below 30 ml/100 g/min during the test, it is felt that the operation should not be attempted unless a better perfusion is achieved either by external shunts and/or by induced rises in the arterial pressure, a measure that should increase flow in regions where autoregulation is abolished. An elevation of arterial pressure by 20 to 30 mm of Hg with pressor amines has proved helpful in keeping blood flow above the safety limit in six out of eight cases reported by Pistolese *et al.* and has permitted the operation to be performed successfully. If that measure fails, only then should a shunt be attempted or other means to reduce complications be tried such as deep barbiturate anaesthesia, hypothermia, or hyperbaric oxygen (Jennett *et al.*, 1969), or the operation cancelled.

We would suggest, in concluding, that the best safeguard against complications produced by ischaemia due to carotid clamping consists in the monitoring of rCBF and arterial pressure above the stenosis (stump pressure) during an occlusion test of two minutes, to be repeated with moderate increments in SAP if flow in any region is below the critical threshold of 30 ml/100 g/min. This constitutes in our opinion one of the most valuable clinical applications of the rCBF method.

CONCLUSION

The Kety-Schmidt method for measurement of global CBF had led to a greater understanding of the physiological and pharmacological mechanisms acting upon the cerebral vasculature. More recently, rCBF determinations with radioactive inert gases have added to our knowledge by introducing newer concepts of pathophysiological and clinical importance such as the recognition that alterations in brain perfusion could be limited to circumscribed areas of brain, as illustrated by the 'luxury perfusion syndrome' and the local vasoparalysis of the post-hypoxic and ischaemic brain. Some of these new findings, such as the existence of the steal and counter-steal or the notion that a false autoregulation due to vasogenic oedema could take place during marked increases in SAP, have influenced our therapeutic approach to stroke. These observations have stressed the importance of SAP in the regulation of brain perfusion in the acutely damaged brain in which the vascular network will react passively to changes in transmural pressure. Therefore the control of blood pressure as well as the prevention of brain oedema seem of prime importance in any attempt to restore CBF in the acute phase of a stroke, or as a preventive measure during carotid surgery.

Yet, in spite of the impact these new notions have had on our understanding of brain infarction, the rCBF technique has not been widely used for patient care. It is in fact too complex to be employed routinely despite the specific information it can provide. This is why improvements to the method remain a main objective for the future in order to increase its usefulness. These objectives could be summarised as follows: the development, for clinical application, of *noninvasive* and reliable methods for measurement of rCBF and local or regional energy metabolism, and of techniques to assess the state of the microcirculation. These may help us understand the mechanisms leading to un-even distribution of flow in ischaemic brain and, in some regions, to the 'no reflow' phenomena, the immediate correction of which could possibly lead to more rapid resolution of ischaemia.

Until then and apart from its usefulness as a research tool in clinical physiology and pharmacology, the major practical applications of the rCBF method will remain confined to specific diagnostic problems such as those we have discussed: preoperative monitoring of patients undergoing carotid surgery or evaluation of the potential benefits to be expected of a ventriculo-atrial shunt in normal pressure hydrocephalus.

It is hoped that the methodological developments mentioned above will permit a reorientation of our efforts in this field towards more basic considerations and will further justify the interest already shown by many in the regional approach to cerebral blood flow.

REFERENCES

Ackerman, R. H., Zilkha, E., Bull, J. W. D., DuBoulay, G. H., Marshall, J., Ross Russell, R. W. & Symon, L. (1973) The relationship of the CO_2 reactivity of cerebral vessels to blood pressure and mean resting blood flow. *Neurology*, **23**, 21.

Agnoli, A., Fieschi, C., Bozzao, L., Battistini, N. & Prencipe, M. (1968) Autoregulation of cerebral blood flow. Studies during drug induced hypertension in normal subjects and in patients with cerebrovascular diseases. *Circulation*, **38**, 800

Agnoli, A., Prencipe, M., Priori, A. M., Bozzao, L. & Fieschi, C. (1969) Measurements of rCBF by intravenous injection of [133]Xe. A comparative study with the intra-arterial injection method. In *Cerebral Blood Flow*, (ed.) Brock, M. *et al.* Berlin: Springer-Verlag.

Agnoli, A., Fieschi, C., Prencipe, M., Battistini, N. & Bozzao, L. (1970) Relationships between regional haemodynamics in acute cerebrovascular lesions and clinico-pathological aspects. In *Research on the Cerebral Circulation. Fourth International Salzburg Conference*, ed. Meyer, J. S. *et al.* Springfield: Charles C. Thomas.

Battistini, N., Casacchia, M., Fieschi, C., Nardini, M. & Passero, S. (1971) Treatment of experimental cerebral infarction with passive hyperventilation. In *Brain and Blood Flow*. London: Pitman.

Betz, E. (1972) Cerebral blood flow: its measurement and regulation. *Physiological Reviews*, **52**, 595.

Blandino, G., Bonanno, N., Conforti, P. & Meduri, M. (1973) A comparison of standard carotidography, hemispheric scintigraphy (with MAAI-131) and regional blood flow measurements (with XE-133) in brain vascular patients. *Journal of Nuclear Biology and Medicine*, **17**, 58.

Boysen, G. (1971) Cerebral blood flow measurement as a safeguard during carotid endarterectomy. *Stroke*, **2**, 1.

Boysen, G. (1973) Cerebral haemodynamics in carotid surgery. *Acta Neurologica Scandinavica*, **49**, Suppl. 52.

Christensen, M. S., Paulson, O. B., Olesen, J., Alexander, S. C., Skinhøj, E., Dam, W. H. & Lassen, N. A. (1973) Cerebral apoplexy (stroke) treated with or without prolonged artificial hyperventilation: (1) cerebral circulation, clinical course, and cause of death. *Stroke*, **4**, 568.

Cotev, S., Lee, J. & Severinghaus, J. W. (1968) The effects of acetazolamide on cerebral blood flow and cerebral tissue Po_2. *Anesthesiology*, **29**, 471.

Cronquist, S., Laroche, F. (1967) Transitory hyperaemia in focal cerebral vascular lesions studied by angiography and regional cerebral blood flow measurements. *British Journal of Radiology*, **40**, 270.

Cronquist, S., Agee, F. (1968) Regional cerebral blood flow in intracranial tumours. *Acta Radiologica* (diagnosis), **7**, 393.

Denny-Brown, D. (1960) Recurrent cerebrovascular episodes. *Archives of Neurology*, **2**, 194.

Denton, I. C., White, R. P. & Robertson, J. T. (1972) The effects of prostaglandins E_1, A_1, and F_{2a} on the cerebral circulation of dogs and monkeys. *Journal of Neurosurgery*, **36**, 34.

Deshmukh, V. D. & Harper, A. M. (1973) The effect of serotonin on cerebral and extracerebral blood flow with possible implications in migraine. *Acta Neurologica Scandinavica*, **49**, 649.

Farhat, S. M. & Schneider, R. C. (1967) Observations on the effect of systemic blood pressure on intracranial circulation in patients with cerebrovascular insuffiency. *Journal of Neurosurgery*, **27**, 441.

Feindel, W. & Perot, P. (1965) Red cerebral veins: a report on arteriovenous shunts in tumours and cerebral scars. *Journal of Neurosurgery*, **22**, 315.

Fieschi, C., Agnoli, A., Battistini, N. & Bozzao, L. (1966) Regional cerebral blood flow in patients with brain infarcts. A study with the 85 K R clearance technique. *Archives of Neurology*, **15**, 653.

Fieschi, C., Agnoli, A., Battistini, N., Bozzao, L. & Prencipe, M. (1968) Derangement of regional cerebral blood flow and of its regulatory mechanisms in acute cerebrovascular lesions. *Neurology*, **18**, 1166.

Fieschi, C., Agnoli, A., Prencipe, M., Battistini, N., Bozzao, L. & Nardini, M. (1969) Impairment of the regional vasomotor response of cerebral vessels to hypercarbia in vascular diseases. *European Neurology*, **2**, 13.

Fieschi, C., Beduschi, A., Agnoli, A., Battistini, N., Collice, M., Prencipe, M. & Risso, M. (1972) Regional cerebral blood flow and intraventricular pressure in acute brain injuries. *European Neurology*, **8**, 192.

Fieschi, C. & Bozzao, L. (1972a) The physiology of cerebral circulation: Pharmacology of the cerebral circulation. In *International Encyclopedia of Pharmacology and Therapeutics*. London: Pergamon.

Fieschi, C. & Bozzao, L. (1972b) Clinical aspects of regional cerebral blood flow. In *Progress in Brain Research*, ed. Meyer, J. S. & Schade, J. P. Amsterdam, London, New York: Elsevier.

Freygang, W. H. & Sokoloff, L. (1959) Quantitative measurement of regional circulation in the central nervous system by the use of radioactive inert gas. In *Advances in Biological and Medical Physics*. London: Academic Press.

Grubb, R. L., Raichle, M. E., Eichling, J. O. & Ter-Pogossian, M. M. (1974) The effects of changes in P_aCO_2 on cerebral blood volume, blood flow, and vascular mean transit time. *Stroke*, **5**, 630.

Haggendal, E. & Norback, B. (1966) Effect of viscosity on cerebral blood flow. *Acta Chirurgica Scandinavica*, Suppl. 364, 13.

Harper, A. M. (1965) The inter-relationship between P_aCO_2 and blood pressure in the regulation of blood flow through the cerebral cortex. *Journal of Neurology, Neurosurgery and Psychiatry*, **28**, 449.

Heiss, W. D., Prosenz, P. & Roszuczky, A. (1972) Technical considerations in the use of a gamma camera 1600-channel analyser system for the measurement of regional cerebral blood flow. *Journal of Nuclear Medicine*, **13**, 534.

Heiss, W. D. (1973) Drug effects on regional cerebral blood flow. *Journal of the Neurological Sciences*, **19**, 461.

Høedt, Rasmussen, K. & Skinhøj, E. (1964) Transneural depression of the cerebral hemispheric metabolism in man. *Acta Neurologica Scandinavica*, **40**, 41.

Høedt-Rasmussen, K. (1967) Regional cerebral blood flow: the intra-arterial injection method. *Acta Neurologica Scandinavica*, **43**, Suppl. 27, 1.

Høedt-Rasmussen, K., Skinhøj, E., Paulson, O., Ewald, J., Bjerrum, J. K., Fahrenkrug, A. & Lassen, N. A. (1967) Regional cerebral blood flow in acute apoplexy. The luxury perfusion syndrome of the brain tissue. *Archives of Neurology*, **17**, 271.

Iliff, L. D., Zilkha, E., DuBoulay, G. H., Marshall, J., Ross Russell, R. W. & Symon, L. (1974) Cerebrovascular CO_2 reactivity of the fast and slow clearing compartments. *Stroke*, **5**, 607.

Ingvar, D. H. (1965) Normal values of rCBF in man, including flow and weight estimates of grey and white matter. *Acta Neurologica Scandinavica*, **41**, Suppl. 14, 72.

Ingvar, D. H. & Lassen, N. A. (1965) Methods for cerebral blood flow measurements in man. *British Journal of Anesthesia*, **37**, 216.

Ingvar, D. H. & Lassen, N. A. (1973) Cerebral complications following measurement of rCBF with intra-arterial 133-Xenon injection method. *Stroke*, **4**, 658.

Jaffe, M. E., McHenry, L. C. & Goldberg, H. I. (1970) Regional cerebral blood flow measurement with small probes. II. Application of the method. *Neurology*, **20**, 225.

Jennett, W. B., Harper, M. A. & Gillespie, F. C. (1966) Measurement of regional cerebral blood flow during carotid ligation. *Lancet*, ii, 1162.

Jennett, W. B., Ledingham, Mc. A., Harper, A. M., Smellie, G. D. & Miller, J. D. (1969) The effect of hyperbaric oxygen during carotid surgery. *Cerebral Blood Flow*, (ed.) Brock, M. *et al*. Berlin: Springer-Verlag.

Kety, S. S. & Schmidt, C. F. (1948) The nitrous oxide method for the quantitative determination of cerebral blood flow in man: theory, procedure and normal values. *Journal of Clinical Investigation*, **27**, 476.

Kety, S. S. (1950) Circulation and metabolism of the human brain in health and disease. *American Journal of Medicine*, **8**, 205.

Lassen, N. A. & Munck, O. (1955) The cerebral blood flow in man determined by the use of radioactive Krypton. *Acta Physiologica Scandinavica*, **33**, 30.

Lassen, N. A. (1959) Cerebral blood flow and oxygen consumption in man. *Physiological Reviews*, **39**, 183.

Lassen, N. A., Feinberg, I. & Lane, M. H. (1960) Bilateral studies of cerebral oxygen uptake in young and aged normal subjects and in patients with organic dementia. *Journal of Clinical Investigation*, **39**, 491.

Lassen, N. A. & Ingvar, D. H. (1961) The blood flow of the cerebral cortex determined by radioactive Krypton-85. *Experientia* (Basel), **17**, 42.

Lassen, N. A., Høedt-Rasmussen, K., Sorensen, S. C., Skinhøj, E., Cronquist, S., Bodforss, B. & Ingvar, D. H. (1963) Regional cerebral blood flow in man determined by Krypton-85. *Neurology*, **13**, 719.

Lassen, N. A. (1966) The luxury perfusion syndrome and its possible relation to acute metabolic acidosis localised within the brain, *Lancet*, ii, 1113.

Lassen, N. A. & Palvölgyi, R. (1968) Cerebral steal during hypercapnea and the inverse reaction during hypocapnea observed by the 133-Xenon technique in man. *Scandinavian Journal of Clinical and Laboratory Investigation*, **22**, Suppl. 102.

Lassen, N. A. & Agnoli, A. (1972) The upper limit of autoregulation of cerebral blood flow. On the pathogenesis of hypertensive encephalopathy. *Scandinavian Journal of Clinical and Laboratory Investigation*, **30**, 113.

Leech, P. J., Miller, J. D., Fitch, W. & Barker, J. (1974) Cerebral blood flow, internal carotid artery pressure, and the EEG as a guide to the safety of carotid ligation. *Journal of Neurology, Neurosurgery and Psychiatry*, **37**, 854.

Lewis, B. M. Sokoloff, L., Wechsler, R. L. Wentz, W. B. & Kety, S. S. (1960) A method for the continuous measurement of cerebral blood flow in man by means of radioactive Krypton (KR79). *Journal of Clinical Investigation*, **39**, 707.

Marshall, J. (1972) The evaluation and prognosis of acute cerebrovascular insufficiency as determined by rCBF analysis. In *Sixth Salzburg Conference on Cerebrovascular Diseases*, ed. Meyer, J. S. *et al.*, Stuttgart: Thieme.

Mathew, N. T. (1974) The importance of CSF pressure-regional CBF dysautoregulation in the pathogenesis of normal pressure hydrocephalus. Intracranial pressure II. In *Proceedings of the Second International Symposium on Intracranial Pressure*, ed. Lundberg, N. *et al.*, Berlin: Springer Verlag.

McHenry, L. C., Jaffe, M. E. & Goldberg, H. I. (1969) Regional cerebral blood flow measurements with small probes. I. Evaluation of the method. *Neurology*, **19**, 1198.

McHenry, L. C., Jaffe, M. E., Kawamura, J. & Goldberg, H. I. (1970) Effect of papaverine in regional blood flow in focal vascular disease of the brain. *New England Journal of Medicine*, **282**, 1167.

McHenry, L. C., Goldberg, H. I., Jaffe, M. E., Kenton, E. J., West, J. W. & Cooper, E. S. (1972) Regional cerebral blood flow: response to carbon dioxide in cerebrovascular disease. *Archives of Neurology*, **27**, 403.

McHenry, L. C., Jaffe, M. E., West, J. W., Cooper, E. S., Kenton, E. J., Kawamura, J., Oshiro, T. & Goldberg, H. I. (1972) Regional cerebral blood flow and cardiovascular effects of hexobendine in stroke patients. *Neurology*, **22**, 217.

Meyer, J. S. (1970) Diaschisis resulting from acute unilateral cerebral infarction. *Archives of Neurology*, **23**, 241.

Michenfelder, J. D. & Sundt, T. M. (1971) Cerebral ATP and lactate levels in the squirrel monkey following occlusion of the middle cerebral cortex. *Stroke*, **2**, 319.

Mosmans, P. C. M. (1974) *Regional Cerebral Blood Flow in Neurological Patients: Clinical Significance and Correlation with EEG*. Van Gorcum: Assen.

Obrist, W. D., Thompson, H. K., Herschel King, C. & Shan Wang, H. (1967) Determination of regional cerebral blood flow by inhalation of 133-Xenon. *Circulation Research*, **20**, 124.

Olesen, J. & Paulson, O. B. (1971) The effect of intra-arterial papaverine on the regional cerebral blood flow in patients with stroke or intracranial tumour. *Stroke*, **2**, 148.

Olesen, J., Paulson, O. B. & Lassen, N. A. (1971) Regional cerebral blood flow in man determined by the initial slope of the clearance of intra-arterially injected ^{133}Xe. *Stroke*, **2**, 519.

Olesen, J. (1972) The effect of intracarotid epinephrine, nor-epinephrine, and angiotensin on the regional cerebral blood flow in man. *Neurology*, **22**, 978.

Olesen, J. (1974) *Cerebral Blood Flow: Methods for Measurement, Regulation, Effects of Drugs and Changes in Disease*. Copenhagen: Fadls Forlag.

Ott, E. O., Mathew, N. T. & Meyer, J. S. (1974) Redistribution of regional blood flow after glycerol infusion in acute cerebral infarction. *Neurology*, **24**, 1117.

Palvölgyi, R. (1969) Regional cerebral blood flow in patients with intracranial tumours. *Journal of Neurosurgery*, **31**, 149.

Paulson, O. B. (1970) Regional cerebral blood flow in apoplexy due to occlusion of the middle cerebral artery. *Neurology*, **20**, 63.

Paulson, O. B., Lassen, N. A. & Skinhøj, E. (1970) Regional cerebral blood flow in apoplexy without arterial cerebral occlusion. *Neurology*, **20**, 125.

Penfield, W. (1938) The circulation of the epileptic brain. *Research publication of the Association for Research in Nervous and Mental Diseases*, **18**, 605.

Pickard, J. D. (1973) The mechanism of action of prostaglandin F2a on cerebral blood flow in the baboon. *Journal of Physiology*, **234**, 46.

Pistolese, R., Faraglia, V., Agnoli, A., Prencipe, M., Pastore, E., Spartera, C. & Fiorani, P. (1972) Cerebral hemispheric 'counter-steal' phenomenon during hyperventilation in cerebrovascular diseases. *Stroke*, **3**, 456.

Planiol, T., Floyrac, R., Itti, R., Rouzaud, M., Degiovanni, E. & Gories, P. (1971) La gamma-angio-encephalographie dans l'insuffisance circulatoire cerebrale. *Revue Neurologique*, **125**, 56.

Posner, J. B. (1973) Newer techniques of cerebral blood flow measurements. *Sixth Conference on Cerebro-Vascular Diseases, Princeton, January 1972*. New York: Grune and Stratton.

Prosenz, P., Chimani, N., Heiss, W. D., Kothbauer, P., Tschabitscher, H. & Sollner, E. (1972) Prognosis of brain infarction based on blood flow measurements by means of the Xenon clearance method. *European Neurology*, **8**, 124.

Prosenz, P., Heiss, W. D., Tschabitscher, H. & Ehrmann, L. (1974) The value of regional cerebral blood flow measurements compared to angiography in the assessment of obstructive neck vessel disease. *Stroke*, **5**, 19.

Purves, M. J. (1972) The physiology of the cerebral circulation. *Monographs of the Physiological Society*, No. 28. Cambridge University Press.

Raichle, M. E. & Stone, H. L. (1971) Cerebral blood flow autoregulation and graded hypercapnia. *European Neurology*, **6**, 1.

Rees, J. E., DuBoulay, E. P. G. H., Bull, J. W. D., Marshall, J., Russell, R. W. R. & Symon, L. (1971) Persistence of disturbance of regional cerebral blood flow after transient ischaemic attacks. In *Brain and Blood Flow*, London: Pitman.

Reivich, M. (1969) Regulation of the cerebral circulation. In *Clinical Neurosurgery*. Baltimore: William and Wilkins.

Reivich, J., Jehle, J., Sokoloff, L. & Kety, S. S. (1969) Measurement of regional cerebral blood flow with antipyrine-^{14}C in awake cats. *Journal of Applied Physiology*, **27**, 296.

Reivich, M., Marshall, W. J. S. & Kassell, N. (1969) Loss of autoregulation produced by cerebral trauma. *Cerebral Blood Flow*, (ed.) Brock, M. *et al.* Berlin: Springer-Verlag.

Risberg, J. & Ingvar, D. H. (1973) Patterns of activation in the grey matter of the dominant hemisphere during memorizing and reasoning: A study of rCBF changes during psychological testing in a group of neurologically normal patients. *Brain*, **96**, 737.

Shah, S., Bull, J. W. D., DuBoulay, G. H. Marshall, J., Russell, R. W. R. & Symon, L. (1972) A comparison of rapid serial angiography and isotope clearance measurements in cerebrovascular disease. *British Journal of Radiology*, **45**, 294.

Skinhøj, E. & Paulson, O. B. (1970) The mechanism of action of aminophylline upon cerebral vascular disorders. *Acta Neurologica Scandinavica*, **46**, 129.

Skinhøj, J. E., Høedt-Rasmussen, K., Paulson, O. B. & Lassen, N. A. (1970) Regional cerebral blood flow and its autoregulation in patients with transient local cerebral ischaemic attacks. *Neurology*, **20**, 485.

Sokoloff, L. (1959) The action of drugs on the cerebral circulation. *Pharmacological Reviews*, **11**, 1.

Sokoloff, L. (1961) Aspects of cerebral circulatory physiology of relevance to cerebrovascular disease. *Neurology*, **11**, 34.

Salmon, J. H. & Timperman, A. L. (1971) Cerebral blood flow in post-traumatic encephalopathy. The effect of ventriculo-atrial shunt. *Neurology*, **21**, 33.

Strandgaard, S., MacKenzie, E. T., Sengupta, D., Rowan, J. O., Lassen, N. A. & Harper, M. (1974) Upper limit of autoregulation of cerebral blood flow in the baboon. *Circulation Research*, **18**, 435.

Sveinsdottir, E., Torlof, P., Risberg, J., Ingvar, D. H. & Lassen, N. A. (1971) Monitoring regional cerebral blood flow in normal man with a computer-controlled 32-detector system. *European Neurology*, **6**, 228.

Symon, L. (1968) Experimental evidence for 'intra-cerebral steal' following CO_2 inhalation. *Scandinavian Journal of Clinical and Laboratory Investigation*, **22**, Suppl. 102.

Symon, L. (1971) Hyperemia in the cerebral circulation. In *Brain and Blood Flow*. London: Pitman.

Symon, L. & Brierly, J. B. (1975) Morphological changes in cerebral blood vessels in chronic ischaemic infarction; functional changes obtained by hydrogen clearance. *Stroke* (in press).

Waltz, A. G. (1968) Experimental cerebral ischaemia: effects on cortical microvasculature and blood flow. *Scandinavian Journal of Clinical and Laboratory Investigation*, **22**, Suppl. 102.

Wilkinson, I. M. S., Bull, J. W. D., DuBoulay, G. H., Marshall, J., Russell, R. W. R. & Symon, L. (1969) Regional cerebral blood flow in the normal cerebral hemisphere. *Journal of Neurology, Neurosurgery and Psychiatry*, **32**, 367.

Wilkinson, I. M. S. & Browne, D. R. G. (1970) The influence of anesthesia and of arterial hypocapnia on regional blood flow in the normal human cerebral hemisphere. *British Journal of Anesthesiology*, **42**, 472.

Yamamoto, Y. L., Feindel, W., Wolfe, L. S., Katoh, H. & Hodge, C. P. (1972) Experimental vasoconstriction of cerebral arteries by prostaglandins. *Journal of Neurosurgery*, **37**, 385.

Zierler, K. L. (1965) Equations for measuring blood flow by external monitoring of radioisotopes. *Circulation Research*, **16**, 309.

Zingesser, L. H., Schechter, M. M., Dexter, J., Katzman, R. & Scheinberg, L. C. (1968) On the significance of spasm associated with rupture of a cerebral aneurysm. *Archives of Neurology*, **18**, 520.

6. The Investigation of Strokes

M. J. G. Harrison

The investigation of patients suffering from cerebrovascular disease seeks to answer a series of questions:

1. Is the patient's neurological problem in fact due to vascular disease, or is some totally different pathology responsible—e.g., tumour, subdural haematoma, epilepsy, multiple sclerosis, etc.?

2. Is the pathological lesion in the brain an infarct or a haematoma?

3. What is the anatomy of the vascular lesion? Is the occlusion intracranial or extracranial? Is the source of embolism cardiac or in neck vessels? Is the haematoma accessible or deep?

4. What stage has the dynamic process reached? Is the haematoma extending? Is embolism likely to recur?

5. Can preventative vascular surgery be considered, e.g., carotid artery stenosis, the subclavian steal syndrome?

Investigation	Main role

A CSF
  EEG
  Echo-encephalography
  Radioisotope brain scan
  EMI scan
	Determination of pathology
	Infarct/haematoma/tumour

B Ophthalmodynamometry
  Doppler studies
	Indirect measurement of
	  flow in internal carotid
	  artery

Thermography
  Intravenous radioisotope
  Angiography
	Detection of occlusion or
	  severe stenosis of extra-
	  cranial vessels

C EMI scan Angiography	Site and size of haematoma Vascular pathology

All these questions are important in the management of individual patients, and the investigations supplement the information to be gained about site, pathology, and time course from history and physical examination (Ross Russell and Harrison, 1973).

Non-invasive techniques will be considered before angiography, and the role of measurements of rCBF will be dealt with elsewhere. The investigations can be grouped according to the type of information they provide.

Cerebrospinal fluid

The examination of the cerebrospinal fluid (CSF) may be of value in the differential diagnosis of cerebral haemorrhage and cerebral infarction.

Pressure

Elevation of cerebrospinal fluid pressure at lumbar puncture is more frequent in intracranial haemorrhage than in cerebral infarction. Thus Aring and Merritt (1935) found that the CSF pressure was normal in 78 per cent of cases with cerebral infarction while pressures of over 300 mm of water were found in 38 per cent of cerebral haemorrhage (Table 6.1). In the case of cerebral infarction with presumed oedema the pressure may be slightly elevated (Plum, 1971). Patients having a pressure over 200 mm tended to have a worse prognosis.

Table 6.1 Findings in the CSF in fatal cases of cerebral thrombosis and cerebral haemorrhage. (*After* Aring and Merritt, 1935.)

	Thrombosis	Haemorrhage
Pressure > 400 mm H_2O	0%	18%
> 300 mm H_2O	4%	38%
Bloody sample	1.5% (1 case)	73%

Appearance

Xanthochromia or blood staining of the CSF is indicative of cerebral haemorrhage and can be expected in 80 per cent of cases (McKissock, Richardson, and Walsh, 1959). A few cases of cerebral infarction are associated with mild xanthochromia (Merritt and Fremont Smith, 1937), and blood staining may occur with embolic haemorrhagic infarction. Xanthochromia appears four to six hours after the onset of bleeding and may persist for three to four weeks (Merritt and Fremont Smith, 1937).

Cell content

A red cell content of 100 to 1 000 000 per mm^3 may be found with cerebral haemorrhage. A few cells are to be found in some cases with cerebral infarction. Sornas, Ostlund, and Muller (1972) found it impossible to distinguish haemorrhagic and non-haemorrhagic infarction by reference to the erythrocyte content.

In 66 per cent of cases of infarction Sornas found the white cell content of the CSF to be normal (Sornas et al., 1972). A pleocytosis was commoner in cerebral haematoma. A transitory rise in polymorphonuclear neutrophilic leukocytes occurred in up to 60 per cent of cases of haemorrhage. Individual patients may show white cell counts of up to 20 000 per mm^3. Occasional cases of cerebral infarction may show 6 to 50 white cells. Septic emboli often produce infarction with pleocytosis in the CSF of 100 to 4000 cells.

Protein content

Merritt (1974) reported a mild elevation of protein in approximately one in three cases of acute brain infarction.

Enzymes

Certain enzymes are increased in the CSF in the presence of cerebral infarction or cerebral haemorrhage, e.g. creatine phosphokinase, aldolase, and lactic dehydrogenase (Wolintz et al., 1969). The changes do not appear to be sufficiently specific to be helpful in differential diagnosis.

EEG

Acute cerebrovascular lesions are usually accompanied by an abnormality of the surface recorded electroencephalogram. A variety of changes may be seen.

Local delta activity

The presence of a slow wave focus is usually indicative of cortical involvement (Cohn, et al., 1948). This develops within a few hours of an infarct and if there is associated oedema the abnormality may increase for 3 to 10 days (Cobb, 1963). As the majority of acute cerebrovascular lesions involve the territory of the middle cerebral artery, such focal change is found mainly over the temporal lobe. The local abnormality often resolves in weeks (Roseman, Schmidt and Foltz, 1952) providing valuable information in the differential diagnosis from tumour, especially when combined with brain scanning (Murphy, et al., 1967). However, the focal EEG abnormality may persist for months and occasionally years, especially if epilepsy develops. Eventually there is a tendency for the abnormality to decline even in these cases.

Local reduction in voltage

Ipsilateral diminution of the frequency or amplitude of the alpha rhythm is common after cerebral infarction and may co-exist with a delta focus (Fig. 6.1).

Spikes and sharp waves

Focal spikes may appear early in the development of a cortical infarct and be associated with focal seizures.

Normal record

In a series recorded within two weeks of the onset Cohn (1949) found 25 per cent to have a normal record, or to show only mild changes. Normal records are common with brain stem vascular lesions.

It is not usually possible to distinguish between cerebral haemorrhage and cerebral infarction, since the slow wave pattern with flattening or asymmetry of the alpha rhythm may occur in either case. As haematomas less often involve the cortex, they are less likely to cause a focal abnormality.

The site of the vascular lesion within the brain may be indicated. As already noted a focus of delta activity suggests a cortical lesion. By contrast discordance between the EEG signs and the severity of the hemiplegia is common with an internal capsular lesion. In these latter

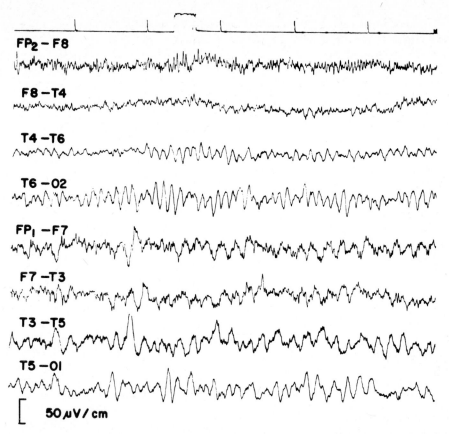

Fig. 6.1   EEG delta activity and reduction in normal activity on side of cerebral infarct affecting the cortex. Lower four channels anteroposterior chain of electrodes on side of lesion. Upper four channels from unaffected contralateral side.

situations delta or theta waves may occur, although rarely. A local absence of sleep spindles or altered K complexes may be demonstrable. Thalamic lesions may cause synchronous bilateral bursts of delta and theta activity.

Normal records are common with small brain stem vascular lesions but generalised slow wave patterns, intermittent generalised runs of theta activity, frontal intermittent delta activity (FIRDA), and bitemporal changes (Phillips, 1964) may all be seen on occasion. Akinetic mutism or coma associated with a normal EEG may be seen in the case of brain stem lesions below the pons.

Subdural haematomas may frequently be detected by electroencephalography. An area of reduced local activity together with local or frontal delta or FIRDA is suggestive. EEG flattening on the wrong side, i.e. over the hemisphere ipsilateral to affected limbs, is particularly suggestive. (Turrell, Levy and Roseman, 1956). Rarely triphasic waves occur over a haematoma. Although 90 per cent of chronic subdural haematomas are associated with EEG changes these are rarely sufficiently specific for a confident interpretation to be made.

Echoencephalography

Detection of the mid-line through the intact skull was first reported in the English literature by Leksell in 1955. The technique depends on the reflection of ultrasound transmitted into the skull by a piezo-electrical crystal. The same crystal mounted in the head of a mobile probe detects the reflections. After conversion to electrical currents these are displayed on an oscilloscope. Polaroid exposures are taken for record purposes and measurement. The technique is simple but requires considerable experience if reliable identification of echoes is to be made. As with many of the non-invasive techniques it has the advantage of enabling serial studies to be carried out in the individual patient.

The occurrence of bleeding into the substance of the brain will usually cause an immediate displacement. If the haematoma develops in the cerebral hemisphere, the mid-line echo may be displaced. In practice shift of the mid-line of more than 3 mm can be detected in up to 86 per cent of cases of cerebral haemorrhage (Table 6.2). Serial studies may show increasing shift in the deteriorating patient.

Table 6.2. Incidence of mid-line shift in hemisphere lesions.

Author	Cerebral haemorrhage	Infarction
Achar, Coe and Marshall, (1966)	77%	3.9%
Widen (1967)	86%	6%
deVlieger and Krull (1968)	66%	17%

By contrast cerebral infarction only produces shift of the mid-line when massive hemisphere oedema develops. A shift of the mid-line echo may be found in approximately 10 per cent of cases (Table 6.2). Since extensive oedema does not develop in the first few hours following infarction, mid-line shift detected within a short interval of the occurrence of a stroke is very good evidence that haemorrhage has occurred. The appearance of shift on days three to five would be equally in keeping with the development of oedema around an infarct, and Widen (1967) found an increased incidence of shift in patients with infarction studied between days two and seven. This phenomenon was rare, however. No case of infarction in Widen's series still had a mid-line shift after seven days, whilst many of the cases of cerebral haematoma did.

With increasing skill in the recognition of abnormal echoes, further help may be obtained in the distinction between cerebral haemorrhage and other lesions. Kanaya et al., 1968) showed

that 94 per cent of a series of 52 cases of supratentorial haemorrhage, confirmed at surgery or autopsy, showed abnormal, multiple, spike-like echoes associated with the haematoma.

Brain scans

During recent years brain scanning (cerebral scintigraphy, isotope encephalography) has become a standard method of investigation of intracranial disease. The method is simple, repeatable, and free from complications.

In 1948 Moore demonstrated that it was possible to detect abnormal areas of brain tissue (metastases) by external counting after administration of intravenous radioactive fluorescein derivative. The advent of rectilinear scanners and the Anger gamma camera have shortened the time involved, and better resolution has followed the development of new isotopes. Currently 197 Hg-chlormerodrin, 99 m Tc-pertechnecate, and 113 m INDTPA are favoured. The last two isotopes can be 'milked' from a generator source in the local laboratory and therefore enable emergency scanning to be carried out.

The increased uptake of isotopes and their delayed clearance from areas of pathological cerebral tissue are probably due to alterations in the blood brain barrier, increased vascular permeability, and to surrounding oedema.

With currently used rectilinear scanning and the use of high doses of isotopes of short half life, e.g. 99 m TC, areas of abnormality can be detected if they are greater than approximately 10 ml in volume. Thus Boller, Patten and Howes (1973) found 84 per cent of such lesions to have a positive scan, whilst smaller lesions of all types were only detectable in 10 per cent of cases.

CEREBRAL INFARCTION

The potential usefulness of brain scanning after cerebral infarction was noted in 1964 by Rhotan, Carlsson, and Ter Pogossian, and subsequent series (e.g., Rhotan et al., 1966; Glasgow et al., 1965) have confirmed this.

Although tumour and infarct may both present areas of increased isotope concentration, a distinction can sometimes be made. The appearance of an abnormal tumour scan is often

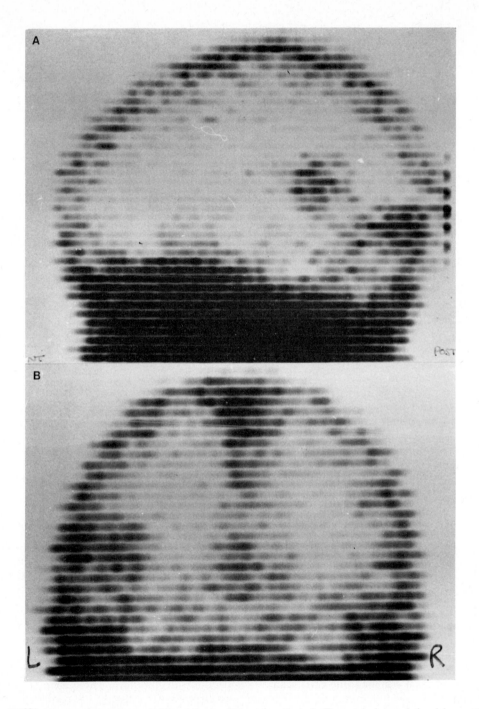

Fig. 6.2   TC^{99} brain scan after acute onset of fluent dysphasia due to a metastasis. The uptake is rounded and does not involve the periphery. (Fig. 6.2A: left lateral view; Fig. 6.2B: posterior view.)

well defined and rounded and does not extend to the cortex (Fig. 6.2). Infarct scans often extend to the cortex, and may be wedge-shaped (Fig. 6.3). Their outline is less clear cut and is irregular. The siting of the lesion may also be helpful: the scan uptake may for example coincide with the middle cerebral territory (Deland, 1971). These features cannot always be relied upon in individual cases, however (Heiser and Quinn, 1966).

Serial scanning is of great help in distinguishing between a tumour and an infarct. Scans performed within a week of the onset of a non-haemorrhagic stroke are usually negative (only 25 per cent are positive). By the third week a positive scan may be expected in 75 per cent. By six weeks many such scans will have faded or reverted to normal (Tow *et al.*, 1969).

When the scan is positive in the first week, it may well show a characteristic increase in density and reduction in area by the third week. Patients with an abnormal scan after a non-haemorrhagic stroke are more likely to have a residual clinical deficit (Gutterman and Shenkin, 1969; Usher and Quinn, 1969). The scan may remain positive for many months, particularly in those with persistent deficit. Brain stem infarction cannot usually be detected by isotope scanning, and a negative scan is the rule after transient ischaemic attacks in which little or no infarction has occurred.

CEREBRAL HAEMORRHAGE

Intracerebral haematomas may also produce a positive scan. The pattern of uptake is unlikely to include the cortex and it is frequently impossible to distinguish from that due to abscess or tumour.

SUBDURAL HAEMATOMA

While a crescentic peripheral area of uptake may be due to other causes, in the context of the differential diagnosis of a stroke it would strongly suggest a chronic subdural haematoma (Heiser, Quinn and Mollihan, 1966).

Computerised axial scanning (the EMI scan)

Computerised axial scanning is an exciting new non-invasive radiological technique which has added an entirely new dimension to neuro-

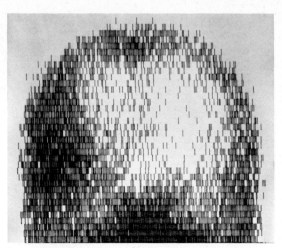

Fig. 6.3 TC^{99m} brain scan after cerebral infarction in the right hemisphere. The uptake is wedge-shaped and extends to the periphery. (Anterior view.)

logical investigation. A narrow X-ray beam scans the head linearly. Two sodium iodide crystal detectors take readings of photon transmission. The unit is then rotated 1 degree around the head and the process is repeated. After 180 scans some 28 000 readings have been obtained and these are processed by the computer to give a visual display of the absorption coefficients at each point in a series of adjacent slices of cranial tissue. Effectively a soft tissue tomographic view of the brain is obtained in the transverse axial plane (Hounsfield, 1973).

CEREBRAL INFARCTION

Infarction can be detected by an area of low density including both cortex and white matter (Fig. 6.4). The change due initially to oedema may be detectable within 24 hours. The boundaries tend to be irregular. By the second week the area of low density is better demarcated. The differential diagnosis from tumour is further helped by the absence of mid-line shift in most cases despite the large size of the abnormal area

CEREBRAL HAEMORRHAGE

As blood breaks down in a haematoma blood products accumulate. These have a high X-ray absorption value due to the content of calcium ions and haemoglobin. The EMI scan shows an area of high density (Fig. 6.5). Extension of the haematoma into the ventricular system can be readily identified by the association of a high density area within the brain substance and an outline of part of the ventricular system by a similar high density shadow (Ambrose, 1974).

One of the most useful roles for this unique development will be its ability, without danger to the patient, to distinguish between cerebral infarction and cerebral haemorrhage in the early days after a stroke. The location of the cerebral haematoma can also be defined when surgery is contemplated. Infarction and haemorrhage into the brain stem cannot always be identified. Subdural haematomas and brain tumours can be identified with a high degree of reliability (Uttley, 1974), though there are technical difficulties in demonstrating bilateral subdural haematomas which have caused no shift of the mid-line.

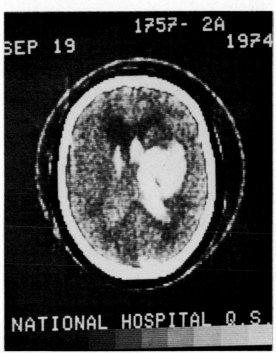

Fig. 6.5 EMI scan: Coronal view shows an area of high density (white) due to an intracerebral haematoma in right capsular region. The ventricular system is partly outlined by a high density shadow indicating the presence of blood in the ventricle. (Both EMI scans made available by kind permission of Dr. G. Gawler, National Hospital, Queen Square.)

Ophthalmodynamometry

Normally the pressure in the trunk of the ophthalmic artery is approximately 75 per cent of that in the carotid syphon. The pressure in the central retinal artery is a little lower. In the presence of occlusion or a tight stenosis of the internal carotid artery there is a drop in ophthalmic artery pressure, the extent of the drop depending on the adequacy of the collateral circulation.

A method of estimating blood pressure in the ophthalmic-retinal artery was introduced by Bailliart in 1917. The pulsations of retinal vessels are observed ophthalmoscopically, while a measured compressive force is applied to the globe. The pressure is applied progressively until retinal arteriole pulsation becomes obvious

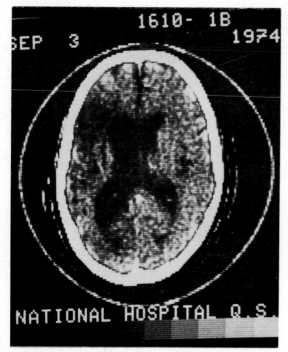

Fig. 6.4 EMI scan: Coronal view shows area of reduced density (blacker) on the left due to an infarct, six weeks previously. The mildly dilated ventricular system is also shown.

at the margins of the optic disk (diastolic end point) and then until blanching occurs (systolic end point). Difficulties are encountered in the presence of cardiac arythmias, and the techniques should not be used in the presence of a history of retinal detachment. High myopia impairs accurate assessment as does glaucoma, and patients with these conditions are not usually examined.

Normally the ophthalmic artery pressures, as assessed in this way, are symmetrical. A difference of 20 to 25 G is highly suggestive of carotid artery occlusion of recent occurrence (Ross Russell and Cranston, 1961). The technique may be combined with ophthalmo-dynamography to improve its reliability (Bettelheim, 1967).

Doppler studies

The percutaneous measurement of arterial blood flow using the Doppler principle was introduced by Franklin et al. in 1961. A flow-meter was devised which depends on the shift in frequency of continuous wave ultrasonic energy if it is back scattered off moving blood. The difference in frequency between transmitted and reflected sound is a mixed spectrum due to the different velocities of different blood components. The mean frequency, however, is proportional to the mean blood flow. It falls within the audible range (Stegell, Rushmer, and Baker, 1966). Modern instruments enable the direction of flow to be determined (Muller, 1973).

Direct measurements of flow in the internal carotid artery are difficult due to the superimposition of the internal and external carotid artery in the neck. Flow in the common carotid artery can be measured, however (Brisman, Grossman and Correll, 1970). Also, the diameter of the carotid artery low in the neck can be calculated from B mode scans or echotomography (Planiol, et al., 1972). The technique that has been most successful in clinical use has, however, been that proposed by Goldberg (Spencer et al., 1974) and reported by Muller (1973). The direction of flow in the trunk of the supratrochlear and nasal arteries is assessed at the inner canthus of the eye by a directional Doppler device or by noting whether flow is arrested by digital compression of the superficial temporal artery. In the presence of severe stenosis of occlusion of the internal carotid artery, the ophthalmic artery and its supratrochlear and nasal branches fill by retrograde flow from the external carotid circulation. Muller found reversed flow in these orbital branches in 31 of 37 cases of angiographically confirmed carotid occlusion, and in 9 of 27 cases of stenosis. Planiol has pointed out that increased accuracy is achieved if Doppler studies are combined with thermography (Planiol et al., 1972). Supraorbital Doppler studies appear to be more accurate than ophthalmodynamometry (Wise et al., 1971).

Reversal of flow in the vertebral artery in the neck due to stenosis of the proximal subclavian vessel (subclavian steal syndrome) may also be detectable by the directional Doppler instrument (Grossman, Brisman, and Wood, 1970; Yao, 1972). Increasing retrograde flow in the vertebral artery during exercise hyperemia of the arm can also be demonstrated.

Further advances in technique can be expected to increase the usefulness of Doppler angiography. Thus B scanning can outline the carotid bifurcation and provide a profile of the diseased vessel lumen (Planiol et al., 1972), and Korpel et al. (1974) have reported preliminary studies in which they were able to produce in vitro ultrasonic images of arteriosclerotic plaques.

Thermography

Infra-red photography of the face detects the pattern of heat emitted from the skin. Since the latter depends on cutaneous blood flow, the method provides an indirect but simple measure of the cutaneous blood flow. Although the face is mainly perfused by branches of the external carotid artery, an area in the supraorbital region is supplied by a terminal branch of the ophthalmic artery. An obstructive lesion of the internal carotid artery between its origin and the origin of the ophthalmic artery may thus impair cutaneous blood flow and heat emission from the supraorbital area (Fig. 6.6).

The method is, of course, completely atraumatic to the patient. Although the infra-red pictures can be obtained within a minute or two, a period of equilibration in a cool room is required before the photograph is taken.

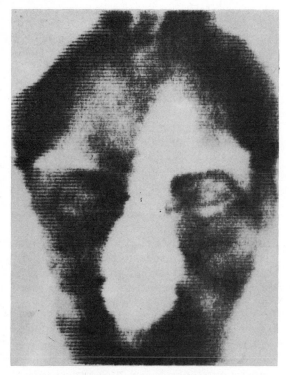

Fig. 6.6 Thermography frontal view of face. The naturally cool areas (eyebrows, nose, cheeks, and sclerae) are white. The periorbital areas are warmer (darker). On the left side the supraorbital area is much cooler than on the opposite side. This is due to poor flow in the supraorbital branch of the left ophthalmic artery following occlusion of the left internal carotid artery. (Illustration kindly supplied by Dr M. Gross, and with the permission of the Editors of *Traité de Radio Diagnostic*.)

The results of this method have been compared with angiography in a series of publications. In the presence of severe stenosis or occlusion of one internal carotid artery, abnormal thermograms are found in over 80 per cent of cases (Wood, 1965: 88 per cent; Mawdsley *et al.*, 1968: 82 per cent). Gross and Popham (1969) found an abnormal thermogram in 87 per cent of cases of carotid occlusion and in 12 out of 12 examples of severe carotid stenosis. Bilateral carotid artery narrowing or occlusion is less

reliably detected. Vertebrobasilar ischaemia is not regularly associated with thermal changes in the face.

Intravenous radioisotope angiography

The delayed arrival of intravenously injected isotope (e.g., Tc^{99m}) on one side of the head may be used to identify occlusion or severe stenosis of the internal carotid artery (Burke and Halko, 1968). Rapid sequence gamma camera scans of the head and neck are obtained in the anteroposterior view during the first half minute after injection. Evidence of unilateral extracranial carotid artery obstruction is seen as an asymmetry of radioactivity in the region of the carotid vessels in the first six seconds. Rarely asymmetrical radioactivity in the cranial portion of the scan reflects intracranial vascular obstruction (Wise *et al.*, 1971).

The presence of ulcerated lesions in the internal carotid artery, which may be the source of embolic material but which have little or no effect on blood flow, will not be detected by thermography, ophthalmodynamometry, isotope angiography or by Doppler flow studies, and this is the major drawback of these methods.

Angiography

The atraumatic techniques described so far will often be sufficient to detect the occasional apparent 'stroke' that is due not to vascular disease but to a cerebral tumour or other cause (Silverstein, 1965). They can also in most cases discriminate between cerebral haemorrhage and cerebral infarction. In the case of cerebral haemorrhage, the EMI scanner can provide the additional information on localisation of the haematoma needed for possible neurosurgical intervention. In the absence of an EMI scanner only angiography can provide this information, and this therefore represents a primary role for angiography in the investigation of stroke.

Thermography, ophthalmodynamometry isotope angiography, and Doppler studies may be able to detect recent occlusion of the internal carotid artery, or severe stenosis causing reduced flow in this vessel. They are not applicable to the vertebral artery, and provide no information about intracranial vessels. Also abnormalities of the vessel wall, which may well be important as sources of emboli, cannot be detected by these methods. At present only angiography is capable of providing detailed information on abnormalities of the cerebral vasculature and of the extent of extracranial atheromatous disease in carotid and vertebral arteries. Limitations of resolution and superimposition restrict the possibilities of detecting small vessel changes, for example, in cortical branches and in the vascular bed in the basal ganglia. Magnification techniques and angiotomography go some way to overcome these problems and can be expected to improve as high resolution equipment is developed further (Goldberg and McHenry, 1973). Colour subtraction is also useful in identifying small vessel occlusion (du Boulay, 1973).

Some information on rates of blood flow can be obtained by the use of rapid serial angiography. The time of arrival of dye is compared in the arterial, capillary, and venous phases in different parts of the vascular bed. This modern development compares quite well with measurements of regional blood flow by isotope clearance techniques (Shah et al., 1972). The maximum data can best be obtained by combining angiography with rapid serial films of the intracranial circulation, and a rCBF measurement.

The choice of angiographic technique will depend on the type of information required in the individual case. Arch angiography has the advantage of giving an overall view of the extent, severity, and localisation of atheromatous disease in the extracranial vessels. Since clinical localisation of the vascular territory that is affected may often be faulty, the ability of arch angiography to identify disease in 'other' vessels is important (Sutton and Davies, 1966). The correspondence of clinical and angiographic abnormality is greatest with disease in the carotid territory, but only reaches 65 per cent (Alter et al., 1972). There are disadvantages to using arch angiography alone. Thus the intracranial vessels may be inadequately visualised. Also minor vessel wall changes, in the cervical part of the carotid artery particularly, are underestimated (Cronquist, 1966). In many centres arch angiography is combined with selective catheterisation or puncture of those vessels which are identified clinically or by the arch angiograms as containing possible abnormalities. The choice of catheterisation or direct puncture is usually decided by the experience of the radiologist. Biplanar views should be taken of the origin of the internal carotid artery or ulceration of the wall may be missed. Slow 'trickle' injections may help to identify an ulcer crater (du Boulay, 1973).

The complications of angiography have been assessed in the co-operative study group in 4000 patients with transient cerebral ischaemia, some with a permanent deficit before angiography (Hass et al., 1968). There was an overall mortality of 0.7 per cent, and 0.5 per cent developed a severe hemiplegia. Grave complications in direct carotid arteriography appeared to be related to advanced disease of the artery close to the puncture site or in intracranial arteries. On the other hand complications of retrograde procedures were related to the number of injections, the total amount of contrast, and to the presence of brain stem abnormality. In a number of cases complications occurred in spite of the absence of any occluding arterial lesions. Minor complications occurred in 5.3 per cent of direct carotid punctures and consisted of local haematoma formation and extravasation of contrast into the arterial wall. Such mishaps can be minimised by employing a small preliminary test injection. The most important minor complication of the retrograde technique is occlusion of the peripheral artery used for the injection with loss of the pulse distally (7.1 per cent brachial; 14 per cent femoral). In general the best results are obtained by avoiding high risk patients and by combining direct puncture with retrograde techniques.

TRANSIENT ISCHAEMIC ATTACKS (CAROTID TERRITORY)

The possibility of finding an operable stenosis or source of emboli in the internal carotid artery is the principal rationale for angiographic study of patients with transient ischaemic attacks in the carotid territory. If cases with an obvious cardiac source for embolism or other cause of TIAs are excluded, an example of the

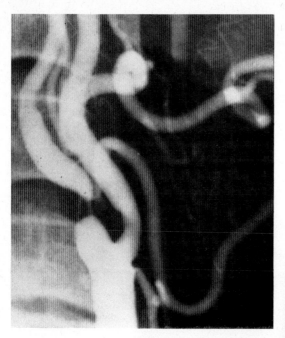

Fig. 6.7 Carotid angiogram: tight stenosis of the internal carotid artery.

yield of selective angiography of the carotid artery on the side of the symptoms is shown in Table 6.3 (Harrison and Marshall, 1975a). Approximately one in four cases in this series had stenosis of the cervical part of the carotid artery (Figs. 6.7 and 6.8) and a similar number had lesser degrees of atheromatous change in the carotid either in the neck or siphon (Fig. 6.9). Approximately 1 in 10 proved to have an occlusion of the carotid. Views of the intracranial circulation may occasionally reveal evidence of small vessel occlusions. Rapid serial angio-

Table 6.3 Results of angiography of carotid artery ipsilateral to a hemisphere transient ischaemic attack (Harrison and Marshall, 1975a).

Angiographic finding	Number	Per cent
Normal	91	43
Stenosis	48	22.5
Atheroma	48	22.5
Occlusion	18	9
Branch occlusion	6	3
Total	211	

graphy may also show areas of low flow after TIAs (Shah *et al.*, 1972).

The finding of carotid stenosis is more common in the presence of a localised bruit over the bifurcation (Harrison and Marshall, 1975a). Combined hemisphere and retinal involvement, with a history of amaurosis fugax, increases the chances of finding a total occlusion of the carotid artery. Operable lesions were found in one in three of those patients in which there was either a bruit or retinal involvement on the side of the symptoms of hemisphere ischaemia in the series described by Harrison and Marshall.

There are many instances in which four-vessel (arch) angiography and selective angiography of the carotid artery fail to show any abnormality.

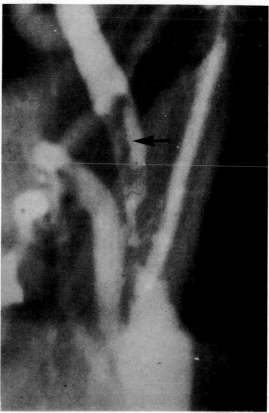

Fig. 6.8 Carotid angiogram. There is a tight stenosis of the internal carotid artery. A filling defect in the vessel above the stenosis reveals the presence of a thrombus (*arrowed*) within the arterial lumen.

There are a number of possible reasons for this. Some of the cases may be due to emboli from the heart which have been undetected by clinical examination. Others may have been due to emboli from the aorta, or from minor irregularities in the vessel wall too small to be detected. Yet others may have had TIAs due to temporary cardiac arrythmias (Walter *et al.*, 1970, McAllen and Marshall, 1973), hypotension and hypertension (Marshall 1968), etc. It has already been noted that the clinical localisation of the symptoms may be faulty, and if only a carotid angio-gram is performed it may fail to disclose a significant extracranial lesion in another artery.

TRANSIENT ISCHAEMIC ATTACKS (VERTEBRO-BASILAR TERRITORY)

The more benign clinical outcome from TIAs in the basilar circulation (Marshall, 1964) tends to mean that angiographic study is less often pursued. Persistent attacks, doubt about the diagnosis, relationship of the attacks to head turning or use of the arm may all prompt angiography, as may the finding of a bruit or

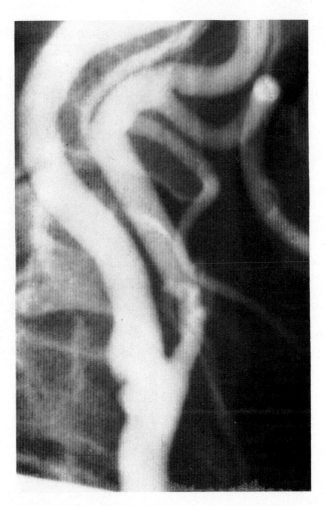

Fig. 6.9 Carotid angiogram. There is no stenosis of the internal carotid artery, but atheromatous ulcers are seen in the wall of the internal and external carotid arteries.

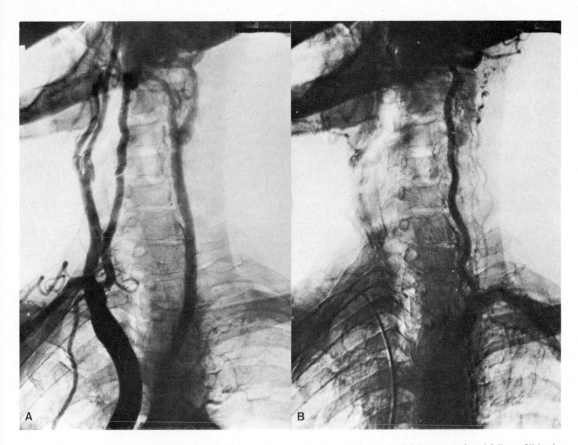

Fig. 6.10 Arch angiogram (subtraction films). The proximal subclavian artery on the left is stenosed and fails to fill in the early films (Fig. 6.10A). Later films (Fig. 6.10B) shows its filling by retrograde flow in the left vertebral artery. Subclavian steal syndrome.

absent or delayed pulses. In this context arch angiography is usually employed. Operable stenosis of the vertebral artery is rare (Gortvai, 1964), but narrowing of the vertebral vessels by osteophytes on head turning may be demonstrable (Toole and Tucker, 1960).

The subclavian steal syndrome (Reivich et al., 1961; Fields and Lemak, 1972) is diagnosed by the angiographic demonstration of subclavian artery stenosis and delayed filling of the distal subclavian artery by retrograde flow in the vertebral artery (Fig. 6.10). In a patient with vertebrobasilar TIA exercise hyperemia in the arm may increase the distal run off. The size and involvement by atheroma of the other neck vessels may determine whether the subclavian steal provokes symptoms. In a series of patients with cerebrovascular disease, Chase and Kricheff (1966) found the haemodynamic features of a subclavian steal to be present on angiography in approximately 5 per cent. When subclavian stenosis is the only angiographic abnormality, the prognosis is good, a completed stroke being rare in one study with a follow-up period of up to eight years (Fields and Lemak, 1972).

CEREBRAL HAEMORRHAGE

The value of angiography in cases of cerebral haemorrhage lies principally in the localisation of the haematoma. Haematomas in the cerebral hemispheres are either deep in the putamen or thalamus, or lie in the subcortical white matter in the region of the external capsule. The lateral or medial displacement of lenticulostriate vessels on PA projections of the carotid angiogram will demonstrate the deep or superficial siting of the haematoma which appears as an avascular mass (Fig. 6.11). Rarely leakage of dye may be seen.

Haemorrhage into a cerebellar hemisphere may be confirmed by angiography. Carotid arteriograms reveal the acute hydrocephalus, and ventriculography or vertebral angiography is needed to define the situation further prior to neurosurgical intervention.

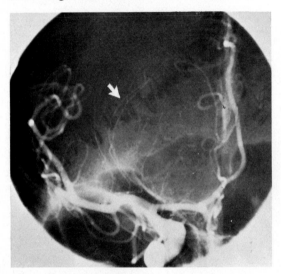

Fig. 6.11 Carotid angiogram (AP view). The anterior cerebral artery is bowed slightly across the mid-line, and lenticulo-striate vessels are bowed laterally (arrowed). The appearances are those due to deep (thalamic) haemorrhage.

CEREBRAL INFARCTION

In the investigation of cerebral infarction angiography serves firstly to distinguish cerebral infarction from cerebral haemorrhage, and from tumour and subdural haematoma. An infarct may be revealed as an avascular area with or without displacement of peripheral vessels due to the development of oedema. Delayed filling or emptying of an artery, local stasis of contrast material, or the absence of the normal capillary blush in a particular area may be seen (Waddington and Ring, 1968). Colour subtraction and angiotomography or magnification techniques may be needed to reveal these features, particularly when they affect the basal ganglia or small cortical territories. Early filling veins may reflect

the hyperaemia surrounding an infarct due to the vasodilating effect of accumulated tissue metabolites. Areas of low flow (delayed filling or emptying of an artery) are encountered more often than areas of rapid flow (early filling or 'shunt' veins), but are more difficult to identify (Shah *et al.*, 1972).

Occlusion of vessels is found in the majority of cases of recent cerebral infarction, perhaps in as many as 90 per cent of cases (Ring, 1971). The commonest clinical situation is infarction in the middle cerebral territory, and this will be used to illustrate the findings of angiography following an ischaemic stroke (Table 6.4). Occlusion of the internal carotid artery in its cervical segment is found in up to 20 per cent (Bull *et al.*, 1960; Harrison and Marshall, 1975b) (Fig. 6.12).

Table 6.4 Results of angiography of carotid artery ipsilateral to a hemisphere infarct (Harrison and Marshall, 1975b).

Angiographic finding	Number	Per cent
Normal	127	42
Occluded carotid	61	20
Atheroma in the neck or siphon	85	28
Intracranial branch occlusion alone	31	10
Total	304	

The frequency with which intracranial occlusion is found depends on both the techniques employed (Ring, 1971) and the timing of the study. The effect of the timing of the angiogram appears to depend on the spontaneous disobliteration of intracranial occlusions. Serial angiograms may show patency of a vessel previously obstructed. This may be due in part to thrombolysis (Dalal *et al.*, 1965), but haemodynamic factors also play a role since repeat angiography may show the obstruction to have moved more distally. The earlier that angiography is carried out after the onset of an infarct the higher the prevalence of occlusions. Feischi and Bozzao (1969) found 49 of 86 cases studied within 24 hours had occlusions of the carotid or its branches. Middle cerebral artery occlusion was found in one in three cases studied early (Feischi, 1965) but only in 5 to 10 per cent studied late (Bauer *et al.*, 1962; Harrison and

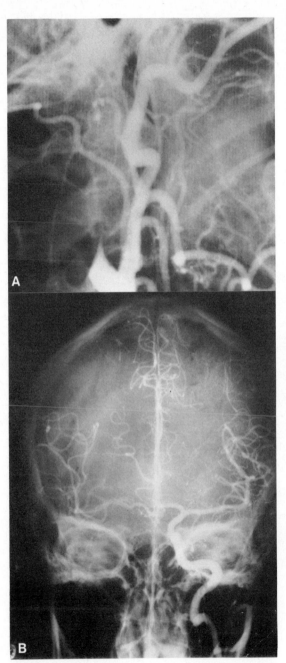

Marshall 1975b; Fig. 6.13). Feischi and Bozzao found that repeat angiography never revealed recanalisation of an occlusion of the cervical part of the carotid artery. The published series, in which angiography performed at various intervals after onset revealed a prevalence of carotid occlusions of 20 per cent, are probably reliable. Occlusions of the carotid artery in the siphon and of the middle cerebral artery often did show disobliteration; it follows that late angiography will seriously underestimate such occlusions and many normal angiograms after stroke may be due to this phenomenon. Furthermore without specialised techniques many small cortical arterial occlusions will be missed (Waddington and Ring, 1968; Ring, 1971).

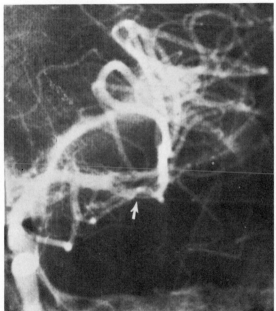

Fig. 6.13 Carotid angiogram. Detailed view of the AP projection. There is a filling defect at the bifurcation of the middle cerebral artery due to the presence of an embolus (arrowed).

Fig. 6.12 Carotid angiogram. The right internal carotid artery fails to fill more than 1 cm above its origin (Fig. 6.12A) An injection of contrast medium in the left carotid artery (Fig. 6.12B) spontaneously fills the middle and anterior cerebral vessels of both sides.

While there is no doubt about the pathological relevance of angiographically demonstrated vessel occlusions, the role of carotid atheroma without occlusion is more difficult to clarify. Angiograms show atheromatous changes in asymptomatic individuals (Faris *et al.*, 1963) as frequently as in patients with cerebrovascular disease. The severity of the changes appears greater in the patients with cerebrovascular symptoms, however, with more vessels affected (Poser et al., 1964).

The prognosis for patients with normal angiograms is better than that for those with arterial lesions (Shenkin, Haft, and Somach, 1966). Whether an internal carotid artery occlusion leads to ischaemia in several intracranial territories with a large infarct or to more re-stricted damage depends partly on whether the occlusion extends beyond the bifurcation of the internal carotid artery (Castaigne et al., 1970). Further factors influencing the severity of the effects of such an occlusion are the degree of involvement of intracranial vessels in athero-matous disease (Stein et al., 1962) and the anatomical normality of the Circle of Willis (Barry and Alpers, 1959; Battacharji, Hutchinson, and McCall, 1967) both of which may be assessed angiographically to some extent.

REFERENCES

Achar, V. S., Coe, R. P. K. & Marshall, J. (1966) Echo encephalography in the differential diagnosis of cerebral haemorrhage and infarction. *Lancet*, i, 161

Alter, M., Kieffer, S., Resch, J. & Ansari, K. (1972) Cerebral infarction. Clinical and angiographic correlations. *Neurology*, **22**, 590.

Ambrose, J. (1974) Computerised X-ray scanning of the brain. *Journal of Neurosurgery*, **40**, 679.

Aring, C. D. & Merritt, H. H. (1935) Differential diagnosis between cerebral haemorrhage and cerebral thrombosis. *Archives of Internal Medicine*, **56**, 435.

Battacharji, S. K., Hutchinson, E. C. & McCall, A. J. (1967) The Circle of Willis —the incidence of developmental abnormalities in normal and infarcted brains. *Brain*, **90**, 747.

Bauer, R. B., Sheehan, S., Wechsler, N. & Meyer, J. S. (1962) Arteriographic study of sites incidence and treatment of arteriosclerotic cerebrovascular lesions. *Neurology*, **12**, 689.

Berry, R. G. & Alpers, B. J. (1959) Anatomical studies of the Circle of Willis II. Vascular disorders of the brain. *Transactions of the American Neurological Association*, **84**, 12.

Bettelheim, H. C. (1967) Experiences with ophthalmodynamography in the diagnosis of carotid occlusion. *American Journal of Ophthalmology*, **64**, 689.

Boller, F., Patten, D. H. & Howes, D. (1973) Correlation of brain-scan results with neuropathological findings. *Lancet*, i, 1143.

Brisman, R., Grossman, B. L. & Correll, J. W. (1970) Accuracy of transcutaneous Doppler ultrasonics in evaluating extra-cranial vascular disease. *Journal of Neurology*, **32**, 529.

Bull, J. W. D., Marshall, J. & Shaw, D. A. (1960) Cerebral angiography in the diagnosis of the acute stroke. *Lancet*, i, 562.

du Boulay, G. H. (1973) Radiological investigation of stroke. *British Journal of Hospital Medicine*, **10**, 258.

Burke, G. & Halko, A. (1968) Cerebral blood flow studies with sodium pertechnecate Tc 99M and the scintillation camera. *Journal of the American Medical Association*, **204**, 109.

Castaigne, P., Lhermitte, F., Gautier, J. C., Escourelle, R. & De Rouesne, C. (1970) Internal carotid artery occlusion. *Brain*, **93**, 231.

Chase, N. E. & Kricheff, I. I. (1966) Cerebral angiography in the evaluation of the patients with cerebrovascular disease. *Radiological Clinics of North America*, **4**, 131.

Cobb, W. A. (1963) In *Electroencephalography*, ed. Hill, D., & Parr, G. London: Macdonald.

Cohn, R. (1949) *Clinical Electroencephalography*. New York: McGraw Hill.

Cohn, R., Raines, G. N., Mulder, D. W. & Neumann, M. M. (1948) Cerebral vascular lesions: electroencephalographic and neuropathological correlations. *Archives of Neurology and Psychiatry* (Chicago), **60**, 163.

Cronquist, S. (1966) Total angiography in evaluation of cerebrovascular disease. *British Journal of Radiology*, **39**, 805.

Dalal, P. M., Shah, P. M., Sheth, S. C. & Deshpande, C. K. (1965) Cerebral embolism. Angiographic observations on spontaneous clot lysis. *Lancet*, i, 61.

Deland, F. H. (1971) Scanning in cerebral vascular diseases. *Seminars in Nuclear Medicine*, **1**, 31.

Faris, A. A., Poser, C. M., Wilmore, D. W. & Agnew, C. H. (1963) Radiologic visualisations of neck vessels in healthy men. *Neurology*, **13**, 386.

Fields, W. S. & Lemak, N. A. (1972) Joint study of extracranial arterial occlusion VII. Subclavian steal —a review of 168 cases *Journal of the American Medical Association*, **222**, 1139.

Fieschi, C. (1965) Considerazioni sulla patogenesi dei rammollimenti cerebrali derivati dall studio di casi acuti. *Archivio di Psicologia, Neurologia e Psichiatria*, **26**, 143.

Fieschi, C. & Bozzao, L. (1969) Transient embolic occlusion of the middle cerebral and internal carotid arteries in cerebral apoplexy. *Journal of Neurology, Neurosurgery and Psychiatry*, **32**, 236.

Franklin, D. L., Schegal, E. & Rushmer, R. F. (1961) Blood flow measured by Doppler frequency shift of back scattered ultrasound. *Science*, **134**, 564.

Glasgow, J. L., Currier, R. D., Goodrich, J. K. & Tutor, F. T. (1965) Brain scans at varied intervals following C.V.A. *Journal of Nuclear Medicine*, **6**, 902.

Goldberg, H. I. & McHenry, L. C. (1973) Cerebral magnification angiography and angiotomography in stroke. In 8th *Conference Cerebral Vascular Diseases*, ed., McDowell, F. H. & Brennan, R. W. New York: Grune & Stratton.

Gortvai, P. (1964) Insufficiency of vertebral artery. Treated by decompression of its cervical part. *British Medical Journal*, ii, 233.

Gross, M. & Popham, M. (1969) Thermography in vascular disorders affecting the brain. *Journal of Neurology, Neurosurgery and Psychiatry*, **32**, 484.

Grossman, B. I., Brisman, R. & Wood, E. H. (1970) Ultrasound and the subclavian steal syndrome. *Radiology*, **94**, 1.

Gunning, A. J., Pickering, G. W., Robb Smith, A. H. T. & Ross Russell, R. W. (1964) Mural thrombosis of the internal carotid artery and subsequent embolism. *Quarterly Journal of Medicine*, **33**, 155.

Gutterman, P. & Shenkin, H. A. (1969) Cerebral scans in completed strokes. Value in prognosis of clinical course. *Journal of the American Medical Association*, **207**, 145.

Harrison, M. J. G. (1974) Transient ischaemic attacks. In *10th Symposium on Advanced Medicine*, ed. Ledingham, J. G. G. London: Pitman.

Harrison, M. J. G. & Marshall, J. (1975a) Indications for angiography and surgery in carotid artery disease. *British Medical Journal*, i, 616.

Harrison, M. J. G. & Marshall, J. (1975b) The results of carotid angiography in cerebral infarction in normotensive and hypertensive subjects. *Journal of Neurological Science*, **24**, 243.

Hass, W. K., Fields, W. S., North, R. R., Krecheff, I. I., Chase, N. E. & Bauer, R. B. (1968) Joint study on extracranial arterial occlusion II. Arteriography, techniques, sites and complications. *Journal of the American Medical Association*, **203**, 159.

Heiser, W. J. & Quinn, J. L. (1966) Analysis of brain scan patterns in cerebral ischaemia and astrocytoma. *Archives of Neurology*, **15**, 125.

Heiser, W. J., Quinn, J. L. & Mollihan, W. V. (1966) The crescent pattern of increased radioactivity in brain scanning. *Radiology*, **87**, 483.

Hounsfield, G. N. (1973) Computerised transverse axial scanning (tomography). I. Description of system. *British Journal of Radiology*, **46**, 1016.

Kanaya, H., Yamasaki, H., Saiki, I. & Furukaura, K. (1968) The use of echo-encephalography to differentiate intracerebral haemorrhage and brain softening. *Journal of Neurosurgery*, **28**, 539.

Korpel, A., Whitman, R. L., Ahmed, M., Davies, H., Steele, P. & Barnes, F. S. (1974) An ultrasonic image of arteriosclerotic deposits. I. EEE *Transactions on Biomedical Engineering*, **21**, 171.

Leksell, L. (1955–1956) Detection of intracranial complications following head injury. *Acta Chirurgica Scandinavica*, **110**, 301.

McAllen, P. M. & Marshall, J. (1973) Cardiac dysrhythmia and transient cerebral ischaemic attacks. *Lancet*, ii, 1212.

McKissock, W., Richardson, A. & Walsh, L. (1959) Primary intracerebral haemorrhage. *Lancet*, ii, 683.

Marshall, J. (1964) The natural history of transient ischaemic cerebrovascular attacks. *Quarterly Journal of Medicine*, **33**, 309.

Marshall, J. (1968) The differential diagnosis of little strokes. *Postgraduate Medical Journal*, **44**, 543.

Mawdsley, C., Samuel, E., Sumerling, M. D. & Young, G. B. (1968) Thermography in occlusive cerebrovascular diseases. *British Medical Journal*, iii, 521.

Merritt, H. H. (1974) *A Textbook of Neurology*. Philadelphia: Lea and Febiger.

Merritt, H. H. & Fremont Smith, F. (1937) *The Cerebrospinal Fluid*. Philadelphia: Saunders.

Moore, G. E. (1948) Use of radioactive diiodo fluorescein in the diagnosis and location of brain tumours. *Science*, **107**, 569.

Muller, H. R. (1973) Directional Doppler sonography. A new technique to demonstrate flow reversal in the ophthalmic artery. *Neuroradiology*, **5**, 91.

Murphy, J. T., Gloor, P., Yamamoto, Y. L. & Feindel, W. (1967) A comparison of electroencephalography and brain scan in supratentorial tumours. *New England Journal of Medicine*, **276**, 309.

Phillips, B. M. (1964) Temporal lobe changes associated with the syndromes of basilar-vertebral insufficiency: an electro-encephalographic study. *British Medical Journal*, ii, 1104.

Planiol, T. H., Pourcelot, L., Pottier, J. M. & De Giovanni, E. (1972) Etude de la circulation carotidienne par les methodes ultrasoniques et la thermographie. *Revue Neurologique*, **126**, 127.

Plum, F. (1971) Edema in cerebral infarction. In *Cerebral Vascular Diseases*, ed., Moossy, J. & Janeway, R. New York: Grune & Stratton.

Poser, C. M., Zosa, A. M., Gomez, A. J. & Hardin, C. A. (1964) Cervicocephalic angiography for cerebrovascular insufficiency. *Acta Neurologica Scandinavica*, **40**, 321.

Reivich, M., Holling, H., Roberts, B. & Toole, J. F. (1961) Reversal of blood flow through the vertebral artery and its effect on cerebral circulation. *New England Journal of Medicine*, **265**, 878.

Rhotan, A. L., Carlsson, A. M. & Ter Pogossian, M. M. (1964) Brain scanning with chlomerodrin Hg[197] and chlormerodrin Hg[203] *Archives of Neurology*, **10**, 369.

Rhotan, A. L., Klinkerfuss, G. H., Lilly, D. R. & Ter Pogossian, M. M. (1966) Brain scanning in ischaemic cerebrovascular disease. *Archives of Neurology*, **14**, 506.

Ring, A. (1971) Detection of small-vessel intracranial occlusions by angiography. In *Cerebral Vascular Diseases*, ed. Moossy, J. & Janeway, R., New York: Grune & Stratton.

Roseman, E., Schmidt, R. P. & Foltz, E. L. (1952) Serial electroencephalography in vascular lesions of the brain. *Neurology*, **2**, 311.

Ross Russell, R. W. & Harrison, M. J. G. (1973) The completed stroke. *British Journal of Hospital Medicine*, **10**, 244.

Ross Russell, R. W. & Cranston, W. I. (1961) Ophthalmodynamometry in carotid artery disease. *Journal of Neurology Neurosurgery, and Psychiatry*, **24**, 281.

Shah, S., Bull, J. W. D., duBoulay, G. H., Marshall, J., Ross Russell, R. W. & Symon, L. (1972) A comparison of rapid serial angiography and isotope clearance measurements in cerebrovascular disease. *British Journal of Radiology*, **45**, 294.

Shenkin, H. A., Haft, H. & Somach, F. M. (1966) Prognostic significance of arteriography in non-haemorrhagic strokes. *Journal of the American Medical Association*, **194**, 612.

Silverstein, A. (1965) Arteriography of stroke. I Incidence of mass lesions in patients with clinical diagnosis of occlusive cerebrovascular disease. *Archives of Neurology*, **12**, 387.

Skinhøj, E., Høedt-Rasmussen, K. & Paulson, O. B. (1970) Regional cerebral blood flow and its autoregulation in patients with transient focal ischaemic attacks. *Neurology*, **20**, 485.

Sörnäs, R., Östlund, H. & Müller, R. (1972) Cerebrospinal fluid cytology after stroke. *Archives of Neurology*, **26**, 489.

Spencer, M. P., Reid, J. M., Davis, D. L. & Paulson, P. S. (1974) Cervical carotid imaging with a continuous-wave Doppler flowmeter. *Stroke*, **5**, 145.

Stegell, H. F., Rushmer, R. F. & Baker, D. W. (1966) A transcutaneous ultrasonic blood velocity meter. *Journal of Applied Physiology*, **21**, 707.

Stein, B. M., McCormick, W. F., Rodriguez, J. N. & Taveras, J. M. (1962) Radiography of atheromatous disease involving the extracranial arteries as seen at post mortem. *Archives of Neurology*, **7**, 545.

Sutton, D. & Davies, E. R. (1966) Arch aortography and cerebrovascular insufficiency. *Clinical Radiology*, **17**, 330.

Thompson, J. F. (1973) Discussion with De Weese, J. A., Robb, C. G., Satran, R., Marsh, D. O., Joynt, R. J., Sumner, S. D. & Nichol, S. C. *Annals of Surgery*, **178**, 263.

Toole, J. F. & Tucker, S. H. (1960) Influence of head position upon cerebral circulation. *Archives of Neurology*, **2**, 616.

Tow, D. E., Wagner, H. N., Deland, F. H. & North, W. A. (1969) Brain scanning in cerebral vascular disease. *Journal of the American Medical Association*, **207**, 105.

Turrell, R. C., Levy, L. L. & Roseman, E. (1956) The value of the electroencephalogram in selected cases of subdural haematoma. *Journal of Neurosurgery*, **13**, 449.

Usher, M. S. & Quinn, J. L. (1969) Serial brain scanning with technetium 99 m pertechnetate in cerebral infarction. *American Journal of Roentgenology*, **105**, 728.

Uttley, D. (1974) Computerised axial scanning. In *10th Symposium on Advanced Medicine*, ed. Ledingham, J. G. G. London: Pitman.

de Vlieger, M. & Krull, G. H. (1968) Echo-encephalography in the diagnosis of cerebral vascular diseases. In *Cerebral Vascular Diseases*. New York: Grune & Stratton.

Waddington, M. M. & Ring, B. A. (1968) Syndrome of occlusions of middle cerebral artery branches. *Brain*, **91**, 685.

Walter, P. F., Reid, S. D. & Wenger, N. K. (1970) Transient cerebral ischaemia due to arrythmia. *Annals of Internal Medicine*, **72**, 471.

Widen, L. (1967) Echo-encephalography in the differential diagnosis between intracranial haemorrhage and cerebral infarction. In *Thule International Symposium*, ed. Engel, A. & Larson, T. Stockholm: Nordiska Bokhandelns Forlag.

Wise, G., Brockenbrough, E. C., Marty, R. & Griep, R. (1971) The detection of carotid artery obstruction: a correlation with arteriography. *Stroke*, **2**, 105.

Wolintz, A. M., Jacobs, L. D., Christoff, N., Solomon, M. & Chernik, N. (1969) Serum and cerebrospinal fluid enzymes in cerebrovascular disease. *Archives of Neurology*, **20**, 54.

Wood, E. H. (1965) Thermography in the diagnosis of cerebrovascular disease. *Radiology*, **85**, 270.

Yao, S. T. (1972) Ultrasound in the transcutaneous assessment of blood flow. *British Journal of Hospital Medicine*, **8**, 521.

7. Transient Cerebral Ischaemia

R. W. Ross Russell

A transient ischaemic attack (TIA) is a focal disturbance of the cerebral circulation, often repetitive, which results in a period of impaired function lasting a short time and recovering without residual disability. The briefest last only a few seconds, most last 10 to 20 minutes, and some do not clear for some hours. The duration allowed within the definition is arbitrary, but most authors accept a maximum period of 24 hours.

Transient cerebral ischaemia is a common symptom having a yearly incidence of two per 1000 at ages 65 to 74 (Whisnant, 1974). Men with TIA outnumber women except in the over 80 age group. In the U.S.A. negroes are more commonly affected than whites. The chief importance of a TIA is as a forerunner of a permanent stroke; estimates of the risk of subsequent infarction differ widely according to the definition used for TIA and for stroke, from 13 per cent (Fields *et al.*, 1970) to 50 per cent (Acheson and Hutchinson, 1964). The consensus of opinion puts the chance of developing infarction within five years of a TIA at approximately 30 per cent (Toole *et al.*, 1975). The risk of subsequent stroke increases with age and is slightly greater in women than men; it appears to be less in the vertebrobasilar territory than in the carotid territory (Ziegler and Hassanein, 1973). The number of attacks suffered by individual patients is also variable (Table 7.1). One-third of patients suffer only a single attack; most have 2 to 10 attacks; only 12 per cent have a total of more than 10 (Friedman *et al.*, 1969).

There are also differences in the recurrence rate between the two main territories; vertebrobasilar ischaemic attacks are more than twice as frequent as carotid and tend to recur over a longer period (Ziegler and Hassanein, 1973). In those patients who subsequently develop a

Table 7.1 Clinical characteristics of transient ischaemic attacks. (Friedman *et al.*, 1969).[a]

	Number of patients	Per cent
Number of attacks		
1	22	37
2	7	12
3	7	12
5	2	3
10	1	2
uncertain < 10	14	23
uncertain > 10	6	10
unknown	1	2
Duration of typical attack		
< 10 min	9	15
10 min–1 hour	21	35
1–24 hours	24	40
Unknown	6	10
Vascular territory involved		
Carotid	47	78
Vertebrobasilar	11	18
Unknown, probably both	2	3
Previous cardiovascular disease		
Hypertension	29	48
Coronary artery disease	27	45
Abnormal ECG	29	48
Enlarged heart on X-ray	9	15
Cardiac failure	9	15
Atrial fibrillation	5	8

[a]Friedman *et al.* studied the occurrence of TIA in a retirement community. Eighteen per cent developed a stroke during 29 months of observation. The following features were correlated with stroke: female sex, age over 70, carotid location, brief TIA. Number of TIAs, blood pressure, and cardiac status showed no correlation.

permanent deficit, 50 per cent of strokes develop within one year, and 21 per cent during the first month (Whisnant, 1974). Although after a TIA the expectation of developing a stroke is considerably higher than in a control population the expectation of life is comparatively little altered since at this age both groups have a high incidence of death from heart disease and other causes. Mortality is 23 per cent at four years, more than half the deaths being attributable to myocardial infarction (Toole *et al.*, 1975).

Carotid ischaemic attacks

The symptomatology of carotid TIA is very variable and many minor attacks probably escape recognition. Although in an individual patient the attacks tend to conform to a single type there may be differences in severity, duration, and distribution. The onset is abrupt and unexpected and affects the patient in the course of everyday activity; the time of day most favoured for attacks is within two hours of rising. In individual patients attacks may be provoked by sudden standing, exertion, coughing, laughing, smoking, or anger; most attacks are unprovoked and unpredictable. The disability reaches a maximum within a few seconds or minutes and wears off more slowly over minutes or hours. The commonest variety affects the territory of the middle cerebral artery and consists of weakness, numbness, or heaviness of the contralateral arm and leg. The patient may exhibit slowness and clumsiness of movement out of proportion to weakness or sensory loss. In the usual type of attack facial paresis also occurs but may pass unnoticed by the patient. Other types of attack affect the arm alone, the leg alone, the face and arm, and arm and leg, in that order of frequency (Fisher, 1962). Positive sensory features such as paraesthesiae frequently affect the distal parts of the limbs spreading to one side of the face and mouth and to half the tongue. Visual scintillations in the homonymous field do not occur in carotid attacks. A true focal convulsive seizure is most unusual although the patient may experience irregular jerking or trembling of the affected side.

Examination of the patient during an attack may reveal flaccid weakness of the arm and leg affecting especially abduction of the shoulder, intrinsic muscles of the hand, flexors of the hip, and dorsiflexors of the ankle. Sensation may be quite normal, or there may be sensory loss of a cortical type. The reflexes may be somewhat brisker on the affected side, the plantar response extensor even in the presence of good power in the leg. Speech disturbance of a dysphasic type may accompany ischaemia of the dominant hemisphere and may be the only symptom. A true dysarthria with preservation of full comprehension and verbal content should raise the suspicion of a brain stem or subcortical lesion. In patients seen some hours after an attack there may be no deficit, but asymmetry of the reflexes or an extensor plantar response may persist. Amaurosis fugax or transient visual uniocular loss in the eye contralateral to the hemiparesis has been calculated to occur in 40 per cent of patients with carotid TIA (Fisher, 1962). Only very exceptionally does it occur at the same time as the hemiparesis. It is a reliable index of carotid disease and is discussed more fully on page 141.

Transient vertebrobasilar ischaemia

Transient vertebrobasilar ischaemia or vertebrobasilar insufficiency (VBI) produces symptoms of disturbed function in the brain stem or the posterior parts of the hemisphere either individually or in groups. In a single patient the attacks tend to conform to one type although the intensity may vary. The commonest symptom, vertigo, occurs in two-thirds of patients and is the most difficult to interpret as it cannot easily be distinguished from that originating in disordered labyrinthine function. It is a good general rule that VBI cannot be diagnosed with certainty when recurrent vertigo is the only symptom, but occasionally the labyrinth itself may suffer a temporary reduction in its blood supply via the internal auditory artery. Vertigo is severe, sometimes with vomiting, often related to changes in posture or to rotation or extension of the neck. Very rarely it is accompanied by a fluctuating bilateral deafness, or by tinnitus. Ataxia on walking is often found in association with vertigo, and there may be subjective movement of the field of vision. Sometimes there is distortion and apparent tilting of the visual field or oscillopsia. Brief attacks of diplopia or rarely polyopia may accompany vertigo and are an important point of distinction from purely labyrinthine disorder. The diplopia may be horizontal or vertical and relates to a disturbance of conjugate gaze rather than to an individual nerve palsy. It usually lasts for 5 to 10 minutes, occasionally for as long as half an hour (Hoyt, 1970). Slurring dysarthria may also be experienced with vertigo and the patients may notice paraesthesiae and numbness around the mouth and tongue on one or both sides.

Visual disturbances are second in importance only to vertigo and occur in 50 per cent of patients. They consist of abrupt attacks of dimness or loss of focus, often with positive scotomas such as black and white lines or patterns with shimmering scotomas. These may be bilateral, confined to one homonymous half-field or to both upper fields. On other occasions vision may be retained but distorted as though looking through water or a moving veil. Complex visual hallucinations, often elaborate and pleasing, are a feature of some attacks (Williams and Wilson, 1962). Total loss of vision or the coloured scotomas of migraine are rare in transient vertebrobasilar attacks. Headache is present during an attack to some degree in the majority of patients. It is usually occipital, has a throbbing, bursting quality, and may be intense (Denny-Brown, 1951).

The syndrome of transient global amnesia in which the patient loses orientation of time and place and memory of past events for a period of some hours, yet remains capable of speech and with no physical deficit, is usually described as an isolated event occurring in elderly male patients. Exactly similar attacks may, however, be encountered in patients with vertebrobasilar insufficiency when the amnesia may be combined with a right homonymous hemianopia. Recurrent attacks may leave a permanent amnesic defect (Benson, Marsden, and Meadows, 1973).

Disturbance of consciousness affects only a small minority of patients with vertebrobasilar insufficiency, and a true epileptic seizure rarely if ever occurs. More commonly there are short periods of confusion or loss of awareness without loss of consciousness (Mathew and Meyer, 1974). At other times there may be decorticate posturing, periodic stupor, or akinetic mutism. These symptoms may last some hours and may

be followed by complete and rapid recovery. Leg weakness, sudden unexpected falling (drop attacks) without loss of consciousness or headache, is a symptom of vertebrobasilar insufficiency in about 15 per cent of patients. The symptom is commoner in women, usually occurs unexpectedly while walking or standing, and may be provoked by movements of the head or neck (Kremer, 1958). This particular symptom has a number of other causes and vertebrobasilar ischaemia should not be diagnosed when drop attacks are the only feature. Attacks of weakness or sensory disturbance localised to one side of the body happen in about 10 per cent of patients. In this type of attack it may be impossible to differentiate carotid from vertebrobasilar TIA. Alternating attacks involving the right and left side on different occasions, or marked dysarthria with left sided attacks are suggestive of brain stem localisation. Simultaneous involvement of all four limbs does not occur, although a common feature of basilar occlusion. There is some evidence that patients who experience alternating hemiparesis as a symptom of vertebrobasilar insufficiency are more likely to develop a permanent stroke than those with other symptoms (Marshall, 1964). Abnormal visceral sensations such as distortion of taste, feelings of fear or unreality may in rare instances be experienced at the same time as other symptoms of vertebrobasilar insufficiency. They probably relate to ischaemia in the temporal lobes (Williams and Wilson, 1962).

Differential diagnosis

Focal epilepsy may cause attacks of localised limb weakness or positive sensory symptoms, but there is usually additional evidence of an irritative motor lesion in the form of repeated jerking or involuntary movements which tend to begin distally and spread up the limb and may on occasion culminate in a generalised seizure. Electroencephalography may indicate a focus of abnormal electrical activity and there may be other evidence of a local cerebral lesion such as a cerebral tumour. The EEG is almost always normal after a TIA.

Focal cerebral symptoms, possibly also due to

ischaemia, are also a feature of many attacks of **migraine**. These are easy to differentiate from TIA when they conform to a classical type with a visual prodrome, unilateral headache, and vomiting. However, many migrainous patients suffer incomplete attacks where the prodromal symptoms occur without headache and in which the symptomatology may be identical with TIA, either in the carotid or basilar territory. In these cases the diagnosis must rely on the age or sex of the patient, on the past history of previous attacks affecting one or other side of the body, and on the family history. Vertebrobasilar migraine is commonly found only in young women.

In **diabetic patients** under treatment, some of whom may have latent cerebrovascular disease, focal symptoms exactly similar to those of transient cerebral ischaemia may occur during hypoglycaemia (Meyer and Portnoy, 1958).

Vertebrobasilar insufficiency may be confused with **peripheral labyrinthine disorders** such as Meniere's syndrome and positional vertigo. The diagnosis of a vascular aetiology depends on the history of a group of symptoms, the commonest of which are vertigo, visual blurring, ataxia, and diplopia, occurring in a patient with negative nervous system findings and in a setting of arterial degenerative disease. Vascular disease can seldom be diagnosed with confidence on the basis of a single symptom.

Acute hypertension by causing local regions of cerebral oedema may present with symptoms resembling a transient ischaemic attack (Kendall and Marshall, 1963). There are usually other symptoms of a more generalised kind such as headache, seizures, clouding of consciousness, and the onset is seldom as rapid as in TIA.

In any patient with transient hemiparesis suspected of being ischaemic in origin specific enquiry should be made for attacks of fugitive visual loss affecting the contralateral eye. These may not be mentioned spontaneously by the patient but when present are conclusive evidence of a vascular disorder involving the carotid artery.

It is important and sometimes difficult to differentiate focal transient ischaemia from attacks of more **generalised cerebral ischaemia** (syncope) such as that which results from a sudden reduction in cardiac output. Most types of syncope occur only when the patient is upright and the onset may be preceded by feelings of lightheadedness, nausea, sweating, pallor, palpitations, and heaviness in the limbs. Visual symptoms are also constantly present in syncope and consist of concentric contraction or altitudinal defects of the fields of vision, loss of colour vision, spots before the eyes, and sometimes complete blindness. Loss of consciousness in the vasovagal type of syncope is rapid and accompanied by bradycardia.

PATHOGENESIS OF TRANSIENT ISCHAEMIC ATTACKS

Much of the past disagreement over the aetiology of TIA is due to attempts to identify a single factor accounting for all attacks when there are certainly numbers of possible causes. Furthermore, patients with single attacks of transient ischaemia may be distinct from those with multiple repetitive attacks. If an attack recovers completely it is assumed that no structural damage has been sustained, but this assumption is not always justified. Pathological study of the brain of a patient who suffered a single episode of transient ischaemia in life may reveal an unexpected small softening or even haemorrhage (Van der Drift and Kok, 1973), and minor alterations in regional blood flow can be detected six months after TIA in some cases (Rees et al., 1970). It has to be accepted that the clinical definition of TIA includes a number of patients who have sustained a minor infarction or haemorrhage. When there are repetitive attacks then a true TIA without infarction becomes much more likely.

In considering the various causes of transient ischaemia without infarction the first major category, which may be termed occlusive, is due to a temporary arterial blockage during the attack as by an embolus or by external compression of an artery. In the second major category there is no such occlusion and the attack is due to a temporary defect in the homeostatic mechanisms regulating cerebral blood flow.

Embolism

Embolism has become accepted as an important cause of transient ischaemia, especially in the carotid circulation, as a result of both clinical and pathological evidence. Firstly, many attacks develop abruptly on a background of a normal circulation and are unrelated to changes of posture, cardiac irregularity, or symptoms of systemic hypotension; this sequence of events is more consistent with a sudden vascular occlusion than with a reduction of blood flow from disordered homeostasis.

Secondly, separate attacks may affect different parts of the same carotid territory, e.g. hemisphere and retina. If they were due to a reduction in blood flow through the carotid artery the attacks would be more stereotyped and would consistently tend to affect the same region.

Thirdly, evidence is frequently found of a source of embolism in the heart or major extra-cranial artery (Symonds, 1927; Gunning et al., 1964). Furthermore in a patient with carotid stenosis transient attacks cease when the artery becomes completely blocked (Fisher, 1962).

Fourthly, emboli may be visible in retinal arteries, sometimes passing rapidly through the circulation in the course of an attack (Fisher, 1959). Fibrin-platelet or cholesterol containing material derived from large arteries may also be identified pathologically in the small vessels of brain and retina (David et al., 1963; Russell, 1961).

The main objection to embolism as a cause of transient ischaemia is the difficulty of explaining repeated attacks. Research on the composition and behaviour of emboli in the circulation has shown that freshly formed thrombus composed of platelets and fibrin may break up after causing temporary arrest in the circulation and pass into smaller arteries. Finally they may disappear completely as a result of lysis or fragmentation. Subsequent emboli tend to take a similar path and may then cause repetitive symptoms.

Haemodynamic crisis

This term was introduced by Denny-Brown to signify a temporary breakdown in circulatory homeostasis of the brain. The concept was derived from experimental work showing the importance of systemic blood pressure in maintaining blood flow via collateral vessels to an area of brain after occlusion of one of the main cerebral arteries. (Meyer and Denny-Brown, 1957).

In practice, systemic hypotension appears to be a relatively rare cause of cerebral ischaemia since blood pressure measured during attacks is usually normal. Attempts to reproduce attacks by reduction of blood pressure are either ineffective or if the reduction is severe, loss of consciousness occurs due to generalised cerebral ischaemia (Kendell and Marshall, 1963). This is understandable since cerebral autoregulation remains effective even in the presence of arterial disease and the precise range of blood pressure which will reduce blood flow in one region of the brain while maintaining an adequate flow to other regions is a narrow one. Nevertheless, well authenticated cases are recorded where hypotension, usually due to abrupt reduction in cardiac output, has resulted in a focal cerebral deficit (Shanbrom and Levy, 1957). Homeostatic mechanisms quickly tend to restore systemic blood pressure and bring the attack to an end. Attacks of this type more often affect the vertebrobasilar circulation, and this may account for the less serious prognosis of TIA in the vertebral as compared to the carotid territory. In clinical diagnosis haemodynamic crisis should be suspected when the attacks are related to the upright posture, are accompanied by features of generalised cerebral ischaemia, or by other evidence of reduced cerebral blood flow, such as pallor, palpitations or brady-cardia or anginal pain. The onset of attacks is less abrupt than in the case of embolism.

Compression of arteries

The lumen of an extracranial artery, especially the vertebral (Toole and Tucker, 1960) and to a lesser extent the carotid arteries (Boldrey, Maass and Miller, 1956), may be reduced during movement of the neck and the resistance to blood flow may be increased. This is more likely to occur in the presence of arterial disease, cervical spondylosis, or congenital abnormality (Janeway *et al.*, 1966). Because the resistance of neck arteries is only a part of the total cerebral vascular resistance and because there are alternative routes of blood supply available, notably the other extracranial arteries and the Circle of Willis, neck movements are seldom the cause of transient cerebral ischaemia except in the presence of extensive extracranial occlusive disease, e.g. in bilateral carotid occlusion. Indentation of the vertebral arteries is produced by lateral protrusion of intervertebral discs and osteophytes and is commonly present at a number of levels (Payne and Spillane, 1957). Occasionally the removal of single disc protrusions has led to cessation of attacks (Gortvai, 1964).

Stealing and redistribution of blood

Reversal of blood flow in the vertebral artery may occur when there is a localised proximal occlusion or severe stenosis of one subclavian artery, usually on the left side. The blood passes up one vertebral artery, down the other, and into the arm. It was originally proposed that vasodilatation in the arm during exercise might increase temporarily the amount of diverted blood and lead to cerebral ischaemia (Reivich *et al.*, 1961). Although reversal of vertebral blood flow is a relatively common finding in the case of extensive proximal extracranial disease it is unusual to obtain a history of cerebral attacks related to arm exercise as regularly as earlier reports suggest (North *et al.*, 1962). Held, Jipp, and Schreier (1973) showed that arm blood flow on the side of a subclavian occlusion is usually normal although the normal increase in flow during exercise of the arm may be impaired.

Complex patterns of collateral flow with reversal of blood flow in some arteries are a feature of arterial occlusive disease in many sites and do not always imply 'stealing' of blood. In carotid occlusion, for instance, reversal of blood

flow in the ophthalmic artery is a frequent angiographic finding. The term 'steal' should be reserved for the situation in which an increase in flow to one part of a vascular territory is accompanied by clinical symptoms of ischaemia in another. An alteration in the cerebrovascular resistance in one vascular territory should not have any effect on the blood flow through other territories provided blood pressure remains unaltered. However, if it happens that a fall in systemic blood pressure occurs and one vascular bed or its supplying artery is incapable of further dilatation, then the effective blood pressure for the tissue is reduced with a consequent fall in flow in that region. In the case of subclavian steal, hind brain ischaemia presumably occurs because of the large vasodilatory potential of the arm and the impaired vasodilatation of atherosclerotic cerebral arteries.

The symptomatology of patients with subclavian steal syndrome is little different from other forms of vertebrobasilar insufficiency and consists of recurring occipital headache, dysarthria, vertigo, visual blurring, or limb weakness. Tinnitus and loss of consciousness may also occur, and the only distinctive symptom is weakness or pain in the arm on the side of the occluded artery (Toole, 1964).

Other examples of reversed flow and steal may be seen in the extracranial circulation. Blood may flow from the Circle of Willis down the right carotid and into the right subclavian artery in patients with occlusion of the brachiocephalic trunk: extensive anastomoses may develop between the two carotid arteries via thyroid branches, or between the external carotid artery and the vertebral artery via occipital branches. In all these situations the possibility of reduction of cerebral blood flow is present should the effective cerebral blood pressure be reduced by diversion of a large quantity of blood to extracerebral tissues.

A similar haemodynamic situation may obtain in arteriovenous fistula between the carotid artery and vein in the cavernous sinus, or between vertebral artery and vein. In both these cases large volumes of arterial blood may be diverted into low pressure venous pool, and in some circumstances intermittent focal ischaemia may occur in the territory of the vessels affected (Russell and Green, 1971).

Temporary failure of homeostasis may also occur as a result of variation in the cerebrovascular resistance. In polycythaemia, leukaemia, or dysproteinaemic states alterations in the relative amounts of plasma and cells or in the physical characteristics of plasma may lead to changes in blood viscosity. The resultant increase in peripheral resistance may be offset to some extent by vasodilatation but may be sufficient to impair the regulatory efficiency of the cerebral circulation during periods of minor circulatory stress. Vasoconstriction caused by hypocapnia may account for the temporary increase in ischaemic deficit noticed by some patients on overbreathing. Pathological degrees of vasoconstriction (arterial spasm) undoubtedly occur after subarachnoid haemorrhage and possibly in migraine, and following intra-arterial injection of contrast media, and may account for the temporary focal cerebral symptoms which may occur in these conditions.

The concept of 'stealing' has also been extended to the intracerebral circulation. An unstable situation in which different areas of brain receive a variable blood supply depending on fluctuations in blood pressure, gas tensions, and intracranial pressure undoubtedly occurs after acute vascular occlusion (intracerebral steal) (Symon, 1969) and is relevant to the management of cerebral infarction. The evidence that such a mechanism may cause repeated transient ischaemic attacks without infarction is, however, not convincing.

Carotid artery disease in TIA: further evidence for embolism

Since the pioneer observations of Fisher (1954) transient ischaemic attacks in the middle cerebral territory and in the retina have come to be linked to disease of the internal carotid artery. How the attacks are produced is still a matter for debate.

Thrombosis of the internal carotid artery has been recognised for many years as a cause of cerebral infarction (Hunt, 1914) but was commonly thought to be less important than thrombosis of intracranial vessels. There were good reasons for this view since it was known that surgical ligation of the internal carotid artery in the neck was not usually followed by brain damage, a fact used by Willis to deduce the function of the circular anastomosis at the base of the brain. Even in patients with atherosclerosis, complete carotid occlusion may be asymptomatic and has been demonstrated angiographically in approximately 1 to 2 per cent of patients undergoing angiography for brain tumour. On the other hand angiography in patients with clinical cerebrovascular disease has shown occlusion to be much more prevalent than in patients without vascular disease. A prevalence rate of 17.5 per cent (Bull, Marshall, and Shaw, 1960) agrees closely with that found by Schwartz and Mitchell (1961) in an unselected autopsy series of patients with stroke.

There is thus good reason to incriminate carotid *occlusion* as a factor in cerebral infarction. It may be deduced that in those patients who escape infarction a collateral blood supply is established via the Circle of Willis from the contralateral internal carotid and from the basilar system as well as by way of external-internal carotid anastomoses such as the ophthalmic artery.

A link between cerebral ischaemia and *stenosis* of the carotid artery is less clear. Fisher (1954) showed the presence of unsuspected lesions of the carotid artery in 10 per cent of routine autopsies (including patients with cerebral infarction). Hutchinson and Yates (1957), who examined at autopsy the entire extracranial vasculature of 83 patients who had cerebrovascular symptoms during life, found occlusive changes in 40 per cent although they did not separate complete occlusion from severe stenosis. On the other hand Schwartz and Mitchell (1961), looking at an unselected autopsy population, also found 40 per cent to have severe stenosis of one or more extracranial arteries. Less than half of these patients had a history of cerebral symptoms in life (Fig. 7.1A).

Since caroticovertebral stenosis seems to be no more frequent at autopsy in cases of stroke than in a random population it has been questioned whether stenosis plays any part in the causation of ischaemic symptoms. Further doubts arise from measurements of pressure in the carotid artery and pial vessels, which show that the major part of cerebrovascular resistance is in the smaller pial arteries and intracerebral arterioles and that a comparatively small proportion is due to the neck vessels. The calibre of the neck vessels can thus be substantially reduced before having a controlling influence on cerebrovascular resistance. Russell and Cranston (1961) showed that in patients with mild or moderate stenosis of the internal carotid artery the ophthalmic artery pressure was normal and only when stenosis was almost complete was there a reduction in pressure. Similar conclusions were reached by Brice, Dowsett, and Lowe (1964) who measured flow in the carotid artery during progressive clamping of the vessel. From these observations it may be deduced that mild or moderate narrowing of a single carotid artery is haemodynamically insignificant and unlikely to cause transient cerebral ischaemia by interference with blood flow. Even after surgical ligation of the carotid artery (in the treatment of aneurysm) transient attacks very rarely occur (Fisher, 1962), demonstrating the functional reserves of the collateral circulation. If multiple lesions are present in extracranial arteries, however, haemodynamic factors such as blood pressure may become critical.

In spite of these theoretical objections there is a strong clinical and angiographic body of evidence linking cerebral ischaemic attacks with all grades of stenosis of the carotid artery and even with atheromatous ulceration of the artery without narrowing (Fisher, 1954) (Figs. 7.1A, 7.1B, and 7.1C). For instance in patients with unilateral carotid stenosis the symptoms are significantly more frequent on the side of the stenosis than on the other side (Drake and Drake, 1968).

It seems that the likeliest mechanism of transient ischaemia in patients with mild stenosis or ulceration of the carotid artery is not a haemodynamic effect but the formation of mural thrombus and embolism to the brain of fragments of thrombus (Figs. 7.1D and 7.1E). Examination of resected specimens of carotid artery from patients with transient ischaemic attacks has confirmed the frequent presence of mural thrombus on the surface of the atheromatous lesions especially in those patients experiencing recent attacks (Gunning et al., 1964). It is known that some atherosclerotic lesions may enlarge progressively by the accumulation of thrombus over months and years while others remain stationary (Gurdjian, Darmody, and Thomas, 1969). The final effect of successive layering of mural thrombus is to occlude the lumen of the vessel (Fig. 7.1B).

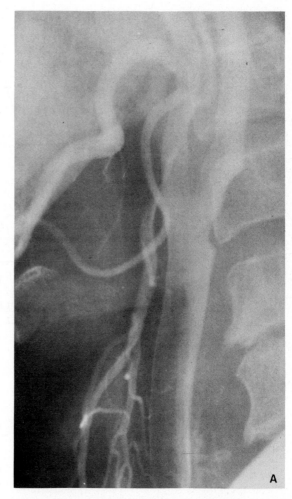

Fig. 7.1A Carotid atheroma. Atheromatous plaque at carotid bifurcation producing minor stenosis.

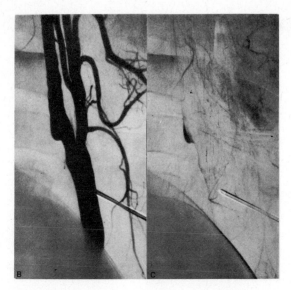

Fig. 7.1B Carotid atheroma. Shallow ulcer of the carotid artery near its origin.

Fig. 7.1C Stasis of contrast material in ulcer.

Angiography in transient ischaemic attacks

The sites of arterial narrowing and occlusion found on four vessel angiography in patients with transient ischaemia are shown in Figures 7.2A and B taken from the Co-operative Study (Hass *et al.*, 1968). The frequency of stenotic lesions at the origin of the internal carotid (33.8 per cent) and the vertebral artery (20 per cent) is emphasised; 19.4 per cent of patients showed no occlusion, 6.1 per cent showed

intracranial vascular lesions. In patients with carotid occlusion propagation of thrombus takes place throughout the artery so that it is not possible to determine the original site of occlusion. The high proportion of multiple lesions (67.3 per cent) is important and has a bearing both on pathogenesis and treatment.

On the basis of history and clinical examination it is possible to predict which patients are most likely to show an angiographic abnormality (Table 7.2). Harrison and Marshall (1975) have shown that the prevalence of carotid lesions is greatest in those patients having attacks in both retina and hemisphere and in those with a carotid bruit. Carotid stenosis of a type suitable for surgery was found in 33 per cent and 61 per cent, respectively. This compares with a figure of 13 per cent in those patients having hemisphere attacks without a carotid bruit.

The height of the blood pressure is another factor influencing the yield of positive findings on angiography. Prineas and Marshall (1966), examining patients with completed stroke, showed that extracranial arterial lesions were more frequent in patients having a normal blood pressure whereas hypertensive patients had fewer large vessel extracranial occlusions but more intracranial small vessel disease.

SURGICAL TREATMENT

The first successful carotid endarterectomy for transient cerebral ischaemia was published

Table 7.2 Angiographic findings (*from* Harrison and Marshall, 1975).

	Retinal	Retinal and hemisphere	Hemisphere only With ipsilat bruit	Without bruit	Total
Normal	6 (32%)	8 (27%)	6 (21%)	71 (52%)	91 (43%)
Stenosis	4 (21%)	10 (33%)	17 (61%)	17 (13%)	48 (22%)
Atheroma	6 (32%)	4 (13%)	4 (14%)	34 (25%)	48 (24%)
Occlusion	3 (15%)	8 (27%)	1 (4%)	6 (5%)	18 (9%)
Branch occlusion	—	—	—	6 (5%)	6 (3%)
Total	19 (100%)	30 (100%)	28 (100%)	134 (100%)	211 (100%)

Note: 211 patients with carotid TIAs were investigated by carotid angiography.

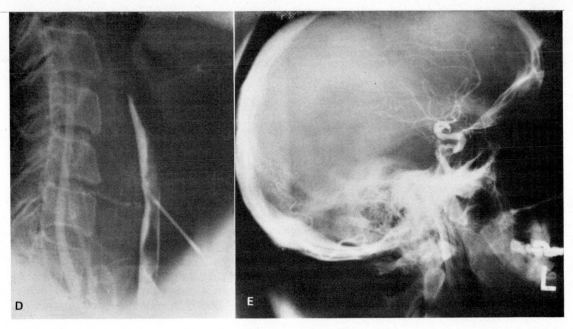

Fig. 7.1D Carotid atheroma. Distal carotid occlusion with retrograde propagation of thrombus in the internal carotid artery shown as a filling defect.

Fig. 7.1E Carotid thrombosis. Thrombus producing a filling defect in cavernous portion of internal carotid artery.

by Eastcott, Pickering, and Rob in 1954 and the subsequent 20 years have seen reports of many hundreds of patients treated by a variety of surgical techniques.

The results of extracranial vascular surgery for transient cerebral ischaemia were carefully assessed by the Cooperative Study group (Fields, et al., 1970). There were a total of 316 patients randomly allocated to surgical and non-surgical categories; some of the non-surgical group received anticoagulants. All patients had a history of transient cerebral ischaemia in any vascular territory but no fixed neurological deficit.

In patients with **unilateral carotid stenosis** with no lesion on the opposite side followed for an average period of three and a half years, 43 per cent of the surgical group continued to experience transient attacks compared to 44 per cent of control group. These were mostly vertebrobasilar ischaemia. In only 4 to 5 per cent of the surgical group were there continuing

attacks in the carotid circulation compared with 8.3 per cent in the non-surgical group; 36.3 per cent of the operated cases were asymptomatic compared with 37.5 per cent in the non-surgical group. Completed stroke, both fatal and non-fatal, occurred in two surgical patients and five non-surgical patients. There was thus no significant difference between the two groups.

In patients with **bilateral carotid stenosis** the surgical group underwent single or multiple endarterectomy and 45.5 per cent were asymptomatic on follow-up as compared with 25.4 per cent of the non-surgical group, this difference being significant. Three strokes occurred in the surgical group.

In patients with **carotid stenosis and a contralateral occlusion**, most of whom underwent endarterectomy on the stenosed carotid, 85 per cent of surgical patients became asymptomatic; in the non-surgical group 48 per cent were asymptomatic. One permanent stroke occurred in the follow-up period in the surgical group and

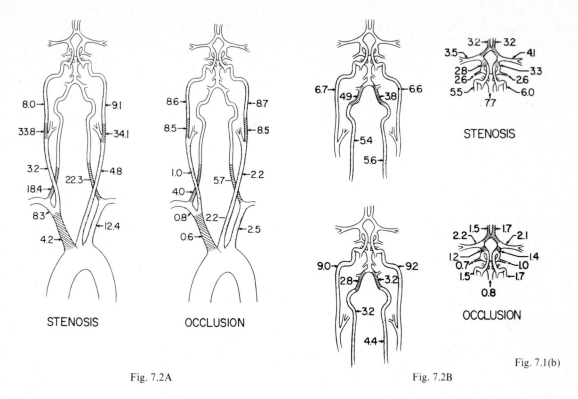

STENOSIS

OCCLUSION

STENOSIS

OCCLUSION

Fig. 7.2A

Fig. 7.2B

Fig. 7.1(b)

Figs. 7.2A and 7.2B Frequency of stenosis and occlusion found at four vessel angiography on patients with transient cerebral ischaemic attacks. (Reproduced from the joint study of extracranial arterial occlusion by courtesy of Dr W. K. Hass and the editor of the *Journal of the American Medical Association*.)

four in the non-surgical group. In the whole series the percentage of asymptomatic surviving patients was significantly greater in the surgical group, though in the sub group with unilateral carotid stenosis no significant difference emerged. **Over the whole group** transient ischaemic attacks continued in 36 per cent of cases in the surgically treated group as against 47 per cent in the non surgical group; the percentage differed in all three sub groups but was always lower in surgically treated cases. Furthermore when transient ischaemic attacks occurred in the surgical group they were usually referred to the territory of the cerebral artery other than the one operated on. New strokes occurred in 4 per cent of the operated group and 12.4 per cent of the non surgical group. The mortality in both groups was due primarily to factors other than cerebrovascular disease.

A number of criticisms can be made of the Cooperative Study, the most serious of which is that the mortality of the surgical procedure itself was not taken into account when comparing the two groups. There was, however, evidence that the surgical mortality declined during the period of study from 5 to 1.5 per cent. A second criticism is that the non-surgical group had a variety of medical treatments. All patients also underwent angiography before inclusion in the trial, which leads to difficulty in applying the results of the study since angiography is a necessary preliminary for surgery but not for non-surgical management. In spite of these difficulties the Cooperative trial remains the most authoritative guide to surgical management so far available.

Many other reports have appeared of series of patients treated surgically. None of these has included a control group treated by non-surgical means but in general they support the claims for the efficacy of this form of treatment. Wylie and Ehrenfeld (1970) reported 91 patients with unilateral carotid stenosis having transient symptoms; 85 were symptom-free during an average followup period of four years, three patients were unchanged. Operative mortality in patients with transient symptoms improved from 1.7 per cent to 0.5 per cent over the 10 years of the study. In bilateral carotid stenosis of 135 patients 95 per cent were rendered symptom free after an operation on both arteries. In carotid stenosis and contralateral occlusion there were 21 patients of whom 15 had no symptoms on follow-up.

The great majority of surgical reports refer to stenotic lesions of the internal carotid artery (De Weese *et al.*, 1971). Reconstructive procedures have been applied at various other extracranial sites, notably to stenosis of the vertebral artery at its origin or in the bony canal, occlusions or stenoses of the brachiocephalic trunk and subclavian arteries. The procedure used is most commonly endarterectomy, and the arterial lumen may be widened by insertion of a homograft or patch graft. Extensive proximal disease of the extracranial arteries can be treated by bypassing procedures originating directly from the aorta or from remaining healthy arteries (De Bakey *et al.*, 1965). Complete occlusion of the internal carotid artery is not operable except in its very early stages since propagation of thrombus occurs throughout the vessel and no back flow can be obtained.

ANTICOAGULANT TREATMENT

After the initial reports from the Mayo Clinic on the effectiveness of anticoagulant drugs in the control of attacks of transient cerebral ischaemia this form of treatment was widely used for a time (Millikan, Siekert, and Schick, 1955). However it soon became apparent that there was wide variation in the natural history both in the number of attacks and in the risks of subsequent stroke. Doubts were cast on the effective-ness of anticoagulants, and it became necessary to subject them to critical evaluation.

One report of this kind was a cooperative study involving seven American hospitals (Baker *et al.*, 1962). Twenty control patients were compared with 24 treated with anticoagulants of the coumarin group. Completed stroke occurred in 4 out of 20 control patients and in 1 out of 24 treated patients. Two control patients and five treated patients died during the period of observation, which averaged 20 months. In two patients receiving anticoagulants the cause of death was cerebral haemorrhage. Similar results were reached in a second study (Baker, Schwartz, and Rose, 1966) from a Veterans hospital which included only male patients and excluded seriously ill and aged patients. Pearce, Gubbay, and Walton (1965) compared 17 treated patients with 20 controls. Two of the controls and one of the treated patients developed a stroke in the subsequent 11 months; three control patients died. This report can be criticised on the grounds of small numbers and short follow-up and cannot be considered conclusive evidence against anticoagulants. The largest single study is by Siekert, Whisnant, and Millikan (1963). One hundred and seventy-five treated patients were followed for 60 months during which time seven (4 per cent) developed a stroke. Forty (23 per cent) died, and of 160 control patients, 51 (32 per cent) developed a stroke and 44 (28 per cent) died. There were considerable differences between the control study populations, and some of the controls received anticoagulants for a brief period. A recent retrospective community study looked at the problem from a different angle (Whisnant, Metsumoto, and Elveback, 1973), comparing the prognosis of 80 elderly patients who received long-term anticoagulants for transient cerebral ischaemia with 118 untreated patients using a life table method over a five year period. The two groups had comparable blood pressures, but the number of transient attacks before diagnosis may have been greater in the treated groups.

There was no difference in the death rate between the two groups, probably because the primary cause of death in patients with vascular disease was cardiac rather than cerebral. However, the probability of developing a stroke was significantly greater in the untreated group throughout the period from one to five years. At one year the probabilities were 12 per cent for the treated and 23 per cent for the untreated. After five years the probabilities were 24 per cent for the treated and 45 per cent for the untreated. Both groups develop more strokes than a control population of equivalent age and sex. Five per cent of patients on anticoagulants develop intracranial haemorrhage compared with 4 per cent among untreated patients. Most of the difference between the two groups appeared during the first two months after the onset of transient ischaemia. After that time the stroke rates were not significant. Whisnant *et al.*, suggest that mural thrombosis releases microemboli for a limited period during which time anticoagulants may exert an effect.

Frank (1971) has attempted to bring together the results of a number of comparable control studies. Of a total treated population of 246 patients drawn from four studies, 13 (5 per cent) developed a stroke within 40 months and 43 (18 per cent) died. Of the control population of 230 patients the equivalent figures were 54 (23 per cent) strokes and 50 (22 per cent) deaths (Table 7.3).

Table 7.3 Comparison of natural history, anticoagulants, and surgical therapy. Pooled results to 40 month follow-up (*from* Frank, 1971).

	Natural history (no treatment)	Anticoagulant treatment	Surgical treatment including postoperative complications
Cases	230	246	169
Strokes	54 (23%)	13 (5%)	18 (11%)
Deaths	50 (22%)	43 (18%)	28 (17%)

They also compared these results with the co-operative trial of surgically treated patients adjusted to include postoperative complications, to show that the surgically treated group, although developing fewer strokes than the controls, did not fare as well as those treated with anticoagulants. These figures should not be taken too literally since the surgical group contained only patients with extracranial arterial stenosis whereas in the other two groups the state of the extracranial arteries was unknown.

Even after reviewing the results of the above trials, it is permissible to have some reservations about the effectiveness of anticoagulant treatment. Very few of the published trials satisfy all the rigid criteria for a controlled study; some were retrospective rather than prospective; in some the treated and control groups were not comparable with respect to important factors such as age, sex, blood pressure and other risk factors; in some patients were not randomly allocated or their progress followed with equal care by an impartial observer. In many instances the patients received more than one treatment at the same time.

It also has to be borne in mind that positive results of a trial are more likely to be published than negative results and that the criteria for assessment (subsequent transient ischaemic attacks) are subjective and not subject to pathological confirmation.

It is also strange that anticoagulants have not been shown to influence the prognosis of completed stroke or of myocardial infarction, two conditions also due to arterial thromboembolic disease.

The explanation for the apparent marginal benefit conferred by anticoagulants is probably that they act only in some types of transient ischaemia—possibly only on that due to embolism from cardiac or mural thrombus—and that all other varieties are unaffected.

SURGERY AND ANTICOAGULANTS COMPARED

It is often necessary to make general recommendation for treatment of TIA as a group since the exact mechanism may be obscure. There is moderately good evidence that anticoagulant treatment reduces the incidence of completed strokes during the first three years after onset. Surgery seems rather less effective but preferable to no treatment. One patient in five on no treatment can be expected to develop a completed stroke within three years and one in three within five years (Table 7.3). Mortality seems unaffected by either medical or surgical treatment suggesting either that death is due to unrelated causes unaffected by anticoagulants or else that the benefits of treatment are evenly counterbalanced by the increased risks of therapy.

For patients with carotid stenosis and TIA, although there is no clear evidence that either medical or surgical treatment is superior, surgery is preferred at the present time. This is because internal carotid stenosis offers a simple and safe site for endarterectomy and because surgery avoids the risks and inconvenience associated with long-term anticoagulant therapy.

Platelets in cerebral vascular disease

The initial event in arterial thrombosis is adhesion of platelets to a region of damaged vessel possibly under the influence of collagen. This is followed by a rapid growth of a platelet thrombus due to aggregation of further platelets induced by adenosine diphosphate released from the platelets themselves. Soon after its formation the platelet thrombus becomes stabilised by the incorporation of fibrin. At any stage portions of thrombus can become detached and carried downstream to impact in smaller vessels. It is thought that successive embolisation of the cerebral and retinal circulations with fragments of mural thrombus may be responsible for attacks of transient ischaemia (McBrien, Bradley, and Ashton, 1963).

The behaviour of platelets can be studied in platelet-rich plasma *in vitro* and measurements made of the speed and reversibility of aggregation and of the effects of agents added to the plasma (Born and Cross, 1963). Aggregation can be induced by ADP, thrombin, collagen, or adrenaline. Dipyridamole inhibits primary ADP-induced aggregation while aspirin and other non-steroid, anti-inflammatory agents inhibit the 'secondary stage' of aggregation caused by the release of ADP from the platelets themselves (Mitchell, 1968).

Platelet behaviour can also be studied by estimation of the proportion of platelets which adhere to glass or other surfaces under standard conditions. Increased adhesiveness has been demonstrated in patients after cerebral infarction and also with other neurological diseases such as multiple sclerosis and may be a secondary rather than a primary event.

Finally direct observations of the effects of agents on platelet thrombus in the arteries of experimental animals may be made. Both dipyridamole and aspirin have been shown to prevent growth and embolisation of thrombus, a property shared by protaglandin E_1 and adenosine (Mitchell, 1968).

These laboratory findings have led to the clinical evaluation of agents acting on platelets. Acheson, Danta, and Hutchinson (1969), using dipyridamole, failed to detect any change in the natural history of platelets with established cerebral vascular disease including a group with TIA.

However, Sullivan, Harken, and Gorlin (1968) showed that following insertion of an artificial cardiac valve the incidence of cerebral embolism was reduced by a combination of dipyridamole and dicoumerol when compared with dicoumerol alone.

Aspirin has been reported to reduce the number of attacks in patients with amaurosis fugax (Evans, 1973) and is currently under evaluation in prevention of cerebral TIA.

Since aspirin and dipyridamole appear to act in different ways it is possible that combination of the two agents may prove to have a synergistic action.

MANAGEMENT OF TRANSIENT CEREBRAL ISCHAEMIA

Guidelines for management of transient cerebral ischaemia can be laid down in the light of natural history and the results of available trials of medical and surgical treatment. The following scheme is orientated towards the detection of extracranial vascular disease on the premise that surgery is the most satisfactory treatment for those patients with accessible lesions of the internal carotid artery. General recommendations can be made, but in each individual patient there are other variables which must be taken into account, such as the availability and quality of angiography and vascular surgery, the age and cardiac status of the patient, the mental state of the patient and his relatives, and the facilities for anticoagulant control.

The first step in the management of recent transient ischaemic attacks is the detection of the small number of patients suffering from cerebral ischaemia as the result of systemic blood disease such as polycythaemia or severe anaemia, since in this case the attacks may respond to treatment of the underlying abnormality (Table 7.4). The next step is to select out those patients whose transient attacks are secondary to cardiovascular disease other than atheroma and bearing in mind pathological studies which suggest that embolism from the heart is frequently undetected (Torvik and Jörgensen, 1964). Examples of these are TIA with valvular heart disease, severe hypertension, postural hypotension (spontaneous or drug-induced) or those with attacks related to vertebral artery narrowing during neck movements.

Diagnosis of this group is helped by attention to the circumstances of onset of the attacks and any relationship to posture or neck turning. These patients require treatment of the underlying abnormality.

Selection of this kind leaves a large residuum of patients with no clear underlying abnormality, either systemic or cardiovascular, whose presumptive diagnosis is atherosclerotic cerebrovascular disease and who are potential candidates for medical or surgical treatment (Table 7.4). The height of the blood pressure is an important consideration since in hypertensive patients not only is arteriography more hazardous but the yield of potentially treatable extracranial lesions is relatively small, because of the frequency of intracerebral, small-vessel disease (Prineas and Marshall, 1966). It is also necessary at this stage to decide whether the patient is fit or unfit to undergo vascular surgery, since it is unjustifiable to submit a patient in the latter category to the possible hazards of arteriography. Patients unfit for surgery are assigned at once to the medical treatment group. Patients

Table 7.4 Initial clinical screening of patients with transient cerebral ischaemia.

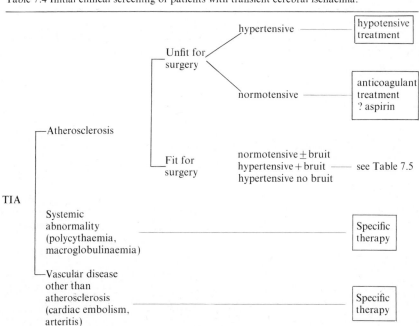

passed fit for surgery are examined for signs of extracranial vascular disease or for hypertension. On this basis they may be assigned to one of three groups:

1. **Normotensive patients with or without signs of extracranial disease** are subjected to arteriography. If operable extracranial stenosis is discovered, surgical treatment is advised (see below). The remainder are treated with anticoagulants.

2. **Hypertensive patients (diastolic pressure above 110 mm Hg) with no signs of extracranial arterial disease** (normal carotid, superficial temporal and radial pulses with no bruits) are treated medically with hypotensive drugs designed to reduce the diastolic pressure to the range 90 to 100 mmHg. If the attacks continue despite adequate control of blood pressure, aspirin or dipyridamole may be used.

3. **Hypertensive patients with signs of extracranial vascular disease** are also recommended for arteriography. If carotid stenosis is found and provided that the lesion is localised, surgery is advised. If extensive atheroma or complete carotid occlusion is found no surgery is possible and medical treatment should be undertaken only with extreme caution. Patients in this group tend to suffer an increased number of attacks on hypotensive treatment and the administration of anticoagulants to patients with uncontrolled hypertension is also hazardous. On the whole this category is best left untreated.

The type of arteriography depends on the experience and the facilities available. When unilateral carotid disease is suspected or when hypertension is present there is much to be said for a single common carotid angiogram to visualise both extracranial and intracranial portions of the artery. However before surgery is undertaken it is generally advisable to perform a second carotid angiogram on the other side or an arch aortogram to assess the state of the collateral circulation.

Surgical treatment is recommended for patients with internal carotid artery stenosis and for the smaller number of patients with common carotid or innominate stenosis or for subclavian stenosis with retrograde vertebral flow. Multiple lesions are not a contraindication to operation. In general carotid lesions are operated on before vertebral, and proximal lesions before distal. Surgical treatment is not carried out for complete carotid occlusion, and vertebral stenosis is not regarded as an indication for operation unless there is occlusion of other vessels. Common carotid, subclavian, or innominate occlusions may be treated with bypass operations in patients with multiple lesions.

Where anticoagulant treatment is proposed patients should first be screened for any bleed-

Table 7.5

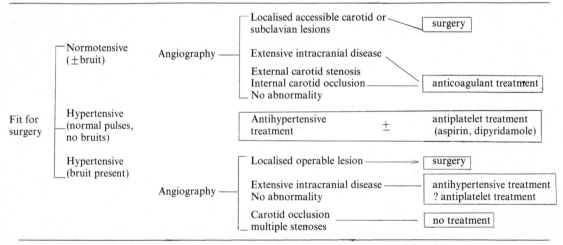

ing disorder, peptic ulceration, or other contra-indication to anticoagulants. If suitable they are placed on coumarin anticoagulants (Warfarin) in a dose sufficient to prolong the prothrombin time by a factor of 2 to $2\frac{1}{2}$. The prothrombin time is checked daily for the first 10 days and less frequently thereafter. Anticoagulation is continued for two to three years. It should be discontinued slowly since there is some evidence of a rebound period of increased risk of thrombosis if the drug is stopped abruptly (Marshall and Reynolds, 1965).

If aspirin is used the therapeutic dose is 600 to 1000 mg/day in divided doses. It regularly causes gastric erosion and some gastric bleeding and should not be given to patients with past or present symptoms of peptic ulceration. Patients taking aspirin and dicoumerol together require particularly careful assessment. The therapeutic dose of dipyridamole is 300 mg/day in divided doses. Many patients notice some headache whilst taking the drug.

TRANSIENT OCULAR ISCHAEMIA

The retina derives blood from two sources, the outer layers being nourished by the short ciliary arteries, two or more in number, which also supply the optic disc and the major part of the optic nerve. The inner retina, including nerve fibre layer and ganglion cells, receives blood from the central retinal artery. Both central retinal artery and ciliary arteries arise from the ophthalmic artery.

Temporary reduction of ocular blood supply in either the retinal or choroidal system may produce transient uniocular loss of vision (amaurosis fugax). This symptom should be distinguished from transient loss of the homonymous half field due to ischaemia in the posterior cerebral territory.

As in the brain there are a number of possible mechanisms which may sometimes be separated by attention to the circumstances of onset of attack and the type of visual field loss. The number of attacks varies widely: some patients suffer only a single attack; in others the symptom may occur many times a day.

Retinal embolism

Embolism is probably the commonest single cause of amaurosis fugax. Emboli may originate in the heart or from the walls of arteries at any point from the aorta to the ophthalmic artery. The commonest source is mural thrombus in the carotid artery, either near its origin or in its cavernous portion. Thrombus forms on the surface of an atheromatous plaque or ulcer. The artery is usually but not necessarily narrowed at the point of thrombus formation. The composition of emboli also varies: those which are derived from mural thrombus are composed of platelets, fibrin and red cells in various proportions; those from other sources may contain fragments of heart valve or atheromatous material including cholesterol esters (Russell, 1968). Rarely fat, tumour cells or air may be encountered.

The degree and duration of retinal ischaemia depends on the number and composition of the emboli.

Fibrin-platelet emboli most commonly derive from thrombus in the carotid artery or from vegetations on cardiac valves. It should be noted that these patients do not necessarily have bacterial endocarditis; they usually have chronic rheumatic valvular disease (Swash and Earl, 1970). Emboli commonly arrest in the retinal circulation at the onset of an attack, but in the course of the attack they fragment and pass through the capillary circulation allowing the normal circulation to be restored. The patient experiences an abrupt, painless loss of vision in one eye. Visual field loss may be total, or altitudinal from occlusion of the upper or lower retinal branch artery. Duration of visual loss is usually 30 seconds to 10 minutes and recovery is gradual. The attacks are often repetitive and may be very frequent (50 or more a day). Very similar symptoms probably occur with embolic obstruction of ciliary arteries, but field loss is not complete; in this case there may be a vertical type of hemianopia.

Cholesterol emboli also originate from ulcerating atheromatous lesions in the proximal arteries. They are multiple and may be symptomless since they can lodge in retinal arteries without causing obstruction. At other times a transient amaurosis may occur which is relieved as the embolus is displaced distally. Occasionally total occlusion of a retinal branch occurs with a permanent altitudinal or sector loss. Cholesterol emboli have a characteristic yellow refractile appearance and are usually found at points of branching. They usually disappear from the retinal vessels within a few weeks, leaving behind a short segment of arterial sheathing.

Retinal insufficiency from other causes

Bilateral visual loss with contraction of the fields of vision, spots before the eyes, and loss of colour perception is a frequent early symptom of syncope or systemic hypotension. It is unusual for visual loss in only one eye to be due to this cause except in patients with carotid occlusion when the perfusion pressure in the retinal circulation on one side is already reduced, and when a further fall may exceed the regulatory reserve of the retinal circulation. In this case uniocular visual loss may be provoked by cardiac dysrhythmia, or by orthostatic or drug-induced hypotension. Amaurosis fugax may also be a symptom in patients with high retinal vascular resistance either to narrowed arteries, as in malignant hypertension or arteritis, or to an increased blood viscosity, as in macroglobulinaemia, sickle cell disease, thrombocythaemia, or polycythaemia vera. Retinal arterial spasm is a possible cause and may occur in some patients with Raynaud's disease or in migraine. Sometimes amaurosis fugax is a symptom of ocular disease; in glaucoma, for instance, raised intraocular tension may produce intermittent reduction in blood flow in the early stages, and by a similar mechanism unilateral papilloedema may present with transient visual loss, usually related to posture, and due in this case to venous obstruction.

Management

When blood disorders, migraine, and local ocular disease have been excluded the great majority of patients with amaurosis fugax are found to have widespread atherosclerosis. There is a predominance of men and a high incidence of hypertension, diabetes, heart disease, and intermittent claudication. About one-third of patients presenting with amaurosis fugax will be found to have evidence of carotid stenosis and a localised bruit over the bifurcation of the artery or a history of transient cerebral ischaemia. The prevalence of carotid artery disease as shown by arteriography has been estimated at 78 per cent (Morax, Aron-Rosa, and Gautier, 1970) and 50 per cent (Marshall and Meadows, 1968). The carotid abnormality may be complete occlusion, stenosis, or atheromatous ulceration (Table 7.2).

Doubts still exist on the management of transient retinal ischaemia and on the natural history of untreated patients. The risk of subsequent blindness in patients presenting with transient loss of vision is small (7 to 11 per cent), but the risk of permanent cerebral infarction has been variously estimated at 6 per cent to 60 per cent (Morax *et al.*, 1970; Hollenhorst, 1962; Marshall and Meadows, 1968). These differences are due to great variation in the selection of patients. In the majority of cases cerebral ischaemia occurs within three months of the onset of amaurosis fugax. Patients who are fit for surgery and who have either a carotid bruit or a history of cerebral ischaemia should have a common carotid angiogram. If localised stenosis or an area of atheromatous ulceration is found in an accessible part of the internal carotid artery, an arch angiogram or contralateral carotid angiogram is performed to determine the state of the other arteries supplying the brain. Carotid endarterectomy is then undertaken as the treatment of choice in this group. Complete carotid occlusion cannot be treated surgically.

Opinion is divided on the correct management of patients with amaurosis fugax who do not have a carotid bruit or symptoms of cerebral ischaemia. The yield of positive findings on carotid arteriography in this group is low (20 per cent have carotid stenosis as compared to 75 per cent in those with both the above features) (Harrison and Marshall, 1975), but small numbers of potentially operable lesions may be discovered. In transient cerebral ischaemia the presence of hypertension further reduces the likelihood of finding a lesion in the extracranial arteries.

Patients unfit for surgery or with no carotid abnormality may be treated with aspirin (600 mg per day). This appears to arrest transient retinal ischaemia in some cases by its action on platelet aggregation (Evans, 1973; Mundall *et al.*, 1972).

There are no adequate controlled trials on the treatment of amaurosis fugax with coumarin anticoagulants.

Table 7.1 is reprinted from the *Journal of the American Medical Association*, November 24, 1969, volume 210. Copyright 1969, American Medical Association. Figs. 7.2A and B are reprinted from the *Journal of the American Medical Association*, March 11, 1968, volume 203. Copyright 1968, American Medical Association.

REFERENCES

Acheson, J., Danta, G. & Hutchinson, E. C. (1969) Controlled trial of dipyridamole in cerebral vascular disease. *British Medical Journal*, i, 614.

Acheson, J. & Hutchinson, E. C. (1964) Observations on the natural history of transient cerebral ischaemia. *Lancet*, ii, 871.

Baker, R. N., Broward, J. A., Fang, H. C., Fisher, C. M., Groch, S. N., Heyman, A., Karp, H. R., McDevitt, E., Scheinberg, P., Schwartz, W. & Toole, J. F. (1962) Anticoagulant therapy in cerebral infarction. Report of Cooperative Study. *Neurology* (Minneapolis), **12**, 823.

Baker, R. N., Schwartz, W. S. & Rose, A. S. (1966) Transient ischaemic strokes. A report of a study of anticoagulant treatment. *Neurology* (Minneapolis), **16**, 84.

Benson, D. F., Marsden, C. D. & Meadows, J. C. (1973) The amnesic stroke. *Neurology* (Minneapolis), **23**, 400.

Boldrey, E., Maas, L. & Miller, E. R. (1956) The role of atlantoid compression in the aetiology of internal carotid thrombosis. *Journal of Neurosurgery*, **13**, 127.

Born, G. V. R. and Cross, J. (1963) The aggregation of blood platelets. *Journal of Physiology*, **168**, 178.

Brice, J. G., Dowsett, D. J. & Lowe, R. D. (1964) The effect of constriction on carotid blood flow and pressure gradient. *Lancet*, i, 84.

Bull, J. W. D., Marshall, J. & Shaw, D. A. (1960) Cerebral angiography in the diagnosis of the acute stroke. *Lancet*, i, 562.

De Bakey, M. E., Crawford, E. S., Cooley, D. A., Morris, G. C., Garrett, H. E. & Fields, W. S. (1965) Cerebral arterial insufficiency: one to 11-year results following arterial reconstruction. *Annals of Surgery*, **161**, 921.

David, N. J., Klintworth, G. K., Friedberg, S. J. & Dillon, M. (1963) Fatal atheromatous cerebral embolism associated with bright plaques in the retinal arterioles. Report of a case. *Neurology* (Minneapolis), **13**, 708.

De Weese, J. A., Rob, C. G., Satran, R., Marsh, D. O., Joynt, R. J., Lipchik, E. O. & Zehe, D. N. (1971) Endarterectomy for atherosclerotic lesions of the carotid artery. *Journal of Cardiovascular Surgery*, **112**, 299.

Denny-Brown, D. E. (1951) The treatment of recurrent cerebrovascular symptoms and the question of vasospasm. *Medical Clinics of North America*, **35**, 1457.

Drake, W. E. & Drake, M. L. (1968) Clinical and angiographic correlates of cerebrovascular insufficiency. *American Journal of Medicine*, **45**, 253.

Eastcott, H. H. G., Pickering, G. W. & Rob, C. G. (1954) Reconstruction of internal carotid artery in a patient with intermittent attacks of hemiplegia. *Lancet*, ii, 994.

Evans, G. (1973) Effect of platelet suppressive agents on the incidence of amaurosis fugax and transient cerebral ischaemia. In *Cerebrovascular Disease 8th Conference*, ed. McDowell, F. H. & Brennan, R. W. New York: Grune & Stratton.

Fields, W. S., Maslenikov, V., Meyer, J. S., Hass, W. K., Remington, R. D. & Macdonald, M. (1970) Joint study of extracranial arterial occlusion. Progress report of prognosis following surgery or nonsurgical treatment for transient cerebral ischaemic attacks and cerebral carotid artery lesions. *Journal of American Medical Association*, **211**, 1993.

Fisher, C. M. (1954) Occlusion of the carotid arteries. *Archives of Neurology and Psychiatry*, **72**, 187.

Fisher, C. M. (1959) Observations of the fundus oculi in transient monocular blindness. *Neurology* (Minneapolis), **9**, 333.

Fisher, C. M. (1962) Concerning recurrent transient cerebral ischaemic attacks. *The Canadian Medical Association Journal*, **86**, 1091.

Frank, G. (1971) Comparison of anticoagulation and surgical treatment of transient ischaemic attacks; a review and consolidation of recent natural history and treatment studies. *Stroke*, **2**, 369.

Friedman, G. D., Wilson, W. S., Mosier, J. M., Calandrea, M. A. & Nichaman, M. Z. (1969) Transient ischaemic attacks in a community. *Journal of the American Medical Association*, **210**, 1428.

Gunning, A. J., Pickering, G. W., Robb-Smith, A. H. T. & Ross Russell, R. (1964) Mural thrombosis of the internal carotid artery and subsequent embolism. *Quarterly Journal of Medicine*, **33**, 155.

Gurdjian, E. S., Darmody, W. R. & Thomas, L. M. (1969) Recurrent stroke due to occlusive disease of extracranial vessels. *Archives of Neurology* (Chicago), **21**, 447.

Gortvai, P. (1964) Insufficiency of the vertebral artery treated by decompression of the cervical part. *British Medical Journal*, ii, 233.

Harrison, M. J. G. & Marshall, J. (1975) Indications for angiography and surgery in carotid artery disease. *British Medical Journal*, i, 616.

Hass, W. K., Fields, W. S., North, R. R., Kricheff, I. I., Chase, N. E. & Bauer, R. B. (1968) Joint study of extracranial arterial occlusion II. Arteriography, techniques sites and complications. *Journal of the American Medical Association*, **203**, 961.

Held, K., Jipp, P. & Schreier, A. (1973) Natural history and muscle blood flow of patients with occlusion of the subclavian arteries and aortic arch syndrome. In *Cerebrovascular Disease 6th International Conference, Salzburg 1972*, ed. Meyer, J. S., Lechner, H., Reivich, M. & Eichhorn, O. Stuttgart: Thieme.

Hollenhorst, R. W. (1962) Carotid and vertebrobasilar arterial stenosis and occlusion: Neuro-ophthalmologic considerations. *Transactions of American Academy of Ophthalmology and Otolaryngology*, **66**, 166.

Hoyt, W. F. (1970) In *Extracranial occlusive cerebrovascular disease diagnosis and management*, ed. Wylie, E. J. & Ehrenfeld, W. K. Philadelphia: Saunders.

Hunt, J. R. (1914) The role of the carotid arteries in the causation of vascular lesions of the brain with remarks on certain special features of the symptomatology. *American Journal of Medical Science*, **147**, 704.

Hutchinson, E. C. & Yates, P. O. (1957) Carotico-vertebral stenosis. *Lancet*, i, 2.

Janeway, R., Toole, J. F., Leinbach, L. B. & Miller, H. S. (1966) Vertebral artery obstruction with basilar impression. *Archives of Neurology*, **15**, 211.

Kendall, R. E. & Marshall, J. (1963) Role of hypotension in the genesis of transient focal cerebral ischaemic attacks. *British Medical Journal*, ii, 344.

Kremer, M. (1958) Sitting, standing and walking. *British Medical Journal*, ii, 63.

Marshall, J. (1964) The natural history of transient ischaemic cerebrovascular attacks. *Quarterly Journal of Medicine*, **33**, 309.

Marshall, J. & Meadows, S. P. (1968) The natural history of amaurosis fugax. *Brain*, **91**, 419.

Marshall, J. & Reynolds, E. H. (1965) Withdrawal of anticoagulants from patients with transient ischaemic cerebrovascular attacks. *Lancet*, i, 5.

Mathew, N. T. & Meyer, J. S. (1974) Pathogenesis and natural history of transient global amnesia. *Stroke*, **5**, 303.

McBrien, D. J., Bradley, R. D. & Ashton, N. (1963) The nature of retinal emboli in stenosis of the internal carotid artery. *Lancet*, i, 697.

Millikan, C. H., Siekert, R. G. & Shick, R. M. (1955) Studies in cerebrovascular disease V. The use of anticoagulant drugs in the treatment of intermittent insufficiency of the internal carotid arterial system. *Mayo Clinic Proceedings*, **30**, 578.

Mitchell, J. R. A. (1968) Platelets and thrombosis. In *Scientific Basis of Medicine Annual Review*. Ch. 16. London: Athlone Press.

Meyer, J. S. & Denny-Brown, D. (1957) The cerebral collateral circulation 1. Factors influencing collateral blood flow. *Neurology* (Minneapolis), **7**, 447.

Meyer, J. S. & Portnoy, H. D. (1958) Localised cerebral hypoglycaemia simulating stroke. *Neurology* (Minneapolis), **8**, 601.

Morax, P. V., Aron-Rosa, D. & Gautier, J. C. (1970) Symptomes et signes ophthalmologiques des stenoses et occlusions carotidiennes. *Bulletin de Societe Ophthalmologique Francais*, Suppl. 1, 169.

Mundall, J., Quintero, P., Kaulla, K. N., Harmon, R. & Austen, J. (1972) Transient monocular blindness and increased platelet aggregability treated with aspirin. *Neurology* (Minneapolis), **22**, 280.

North, R. R., Fields, W. S., De Bakey, M. E. & Crawford, E. S. (1962) Brachial basilar insufficiency syndrome. *Neurology* (Minneapolis), **12**, 810.

Payne, E. E. & Spillane, J. D. (1957) The cervical spine: an anatomico-pathological study of 70 specimens with particular reference to the problems of cervical spondylosis. *Brain*, **80**, 571.

Pearce, J. M. S., Gubbay, S. S. & Walton, J. N. (1965) Long term therapy in transient cerebral ischaemic attacks. *Lancet*, i, 6.

Prineas, J. & Marshall, J. (1966) Hypertension and cerebral infarction. *British Medical Journal*, i, 14.

Rees, J. E., Du Boulay, G. H., Bull, J. W. D., Marshall, J., Ross Russell, R. W. & Symon, L. (1970) Regional cerebral blood-flow in transient ischaemic attacks. *Lancet*, ii, 1210.

Reivich, M., Holling, H. E., Roberts, B. & Toole, J. F. (1961) Reversal of blood flow through the vertebral artery and its effect on cerebral circulation. *New England Journal of Medicine*, **265**, 878.

Russell, R. W. R. (1961) Observations on the retinal blood vessels in monocular blindness. *Lancet*, ii, 1422.

Russell, R. W. R. (1968) The source of retinal emboli. *Lancet*, ii, 789.

Russell, R. W. R. & Green, M. (1971) Mechanisms of transient cerebral ischaemia. *British Medical Journal*, i, 646.

Russell, R. W. R. & Cranston, W. I. (1961) Ophthalmodynamometry in carotid artery disease. *Journal of Neurology, Neurosurgery and Psychiatry*, **24**, 281.

Schwartz, C. J. & Mitchell, J. R. A. (1961) Atheroma of the carotid and vertebral arterial systems. *British Medical Journal*, ii, 1057.

Shanbrom, E. & Levy, L. (1957) The role of systemic blood pressure in cerebral circulation in carotid and basilar artery thromboses. Clinical implications and therapeutic implications of vasopressor agents. *American Journal of Medicine*, **23**, 197.

Siekert, R. G., Whisnant, J. R. & Millikan, C. H. (1963) Surgical and anticoagulant therapy of occlusive cerebrovascular disease. *Annals of Internal Medicine*, **58**, 637.

Sullivan, J. M., Harken, D. E. & Gorlin, R. (1968) Pharmacologic control of thromboembolic complications of cardiac valve replacement. *New England Journal of Medicine*, **279**, 576.

Swash, M. & Earl, J. (1970) Transient visual obscurations in chronic rheumatic heart disease. *Lancet*, ii, 323.

Symon, L. (1969) The concept of intracerebral steal. In *International Anaesthesiology Clinics Cerebral Cirulation*, ed. Mc-Dowall, G. Boston: Little Brown and Co.

Symonds, C. P. (1927) Two cases of thrombosing subclavian artery with contralateral hemiplegia of sudden onset probably embolic. *Brain*, **50**, 259.

Toole, J. F. (1964) Reversed vertebral artery flow: subclavian steal syndrome. *Lancet*, i, 872.

Toole, J. F., Janeway, R., Choi, K., Cordell, R., Davis, C., Johnston, F. & Miller, H. S. (1975) Transient ischaemic attacks due to atherosclerosis. *Archives of Neurology*, **32**, 5.

Toole, J. F. & Tucker, S. H. (1960) Influence of head position upon cerebral circulation. *Archives of Neurology*, **2**, 616.

Torvik, A. & Jorgensen, L. (1964) Thrombotic and embolic occlusions of the carotid arteries in an autopsy material Part 1. Prevalence location and associated diseases. *Journal of the Neurological Sciences*, **1**, 24.

Van der Drift, J. H. A. & Kok, N. K. D. (1973) Clinical pathological correlations in transient cerebral ischaemic attacks. In *Cerebrovascular Disease 6th International Conference, Salzburg 1972*, ed. Meyer, J. S., Lechner, H., Reivich, M. & Eichorn, O. Stuttgart: Thieme.

Vitek, J. V., Halsey, J. H. & McDowell, H. A. (1972) Occlusion of all four extracranial vessels with minimal clinical symptomatology. *Stroke*, **3**, 462.

Whisnant, J. P. (1974) Epidemiology of stroke: emphasis on transient cerebral ischaemic attacks and hypertension. *Stroke*, **5**, 68.

Whisnant, J. P., Metsumoto, N. & Elveback, L. R. (1973) The effect of anticoagulant therapy on the prognosis of patients with transient cerebral ischaemic attacks in a community. *Mayo Clinic Proceedings*, **48**, 844.

Williams, D. & Wilson, T. G. (1962) The diagnosis of the major and minor syndromes of basilar insufficiency. *Brain*, **85**, 741.

Wylie, E. J. & Ehrenfeld, W. K. (1970) *Extracranial occlusive cerebrovascular disease: diagnosis and management*. Philadelphia: W. B. Saunders.

Ziegler, D. K. & Hassanein, R. S. (1973) Prognosis in patients with transient ischaemic attacks. *Stroke*, **4**, 666.

8. Clinical Diagnosis of Completed Stroke

John Marshall

A completed stroke is a common condition; in 1972 45867 people among a population of 49 million in England and Wales were certified as having died from cerebral haemorrhage, thrombosis, or embolism. The mortality from stroke varies greatly according to the pathological cause, but if we take an average figure of 44 per cent (Geltner, 1972), over 100000 people must have experienced a stroke in that year.

DEFINITION

Despite the frequency of stroke, the term itself is a source of confusion. For many people the term stroke is synonymous with hemiplegia and in the absence of the latter a diagnosis of stroke is not made. This usage ignores the fact that vascular lesions may affect any part of the central nervous system so that an isolated hemianopia, dysphasia, or a focal brain stem lesion may also have a vascular cause. Equally, equating stroke and hemiplegia takes no account of the fact that there are many causes of a hemiplegia other than a circulatory disturbance. A stroke is therefore best defined as a focal neurological deficit due to a vascular lesion.

CLASSIFICATION

Within the compass of this definition a classification of practical importance can be constructed. A stroke may first be classified according to its site. Is it in the carotid or is it in the vertebrobasilar territory? Is it massive or localised, is it superficial or deeply situated within the cranial substance? This question affects management because the natural history and the methods of investigation are different. A stroke may also be classified according to the pathological cause—haemorrhage, infarction due to thrombosis or to embolism. Again the type of pathology has a bearing on management.

Finally, a stroke may be classified according to its time course. A deficit which recovers within 24 hours is termed a transient ischaemic attack (TIA); a persistent deficit which takes more than six hours to reach its maximum is called a progressive stroke; a persistent deficit which reaches its peak in less than six hours is labelled a completed stroke. It is with the last of these that this chapter is concerned.

Every endeavour should be made to classify a stroke in each of the three ways described by determining the site of lesion, pathology, and time course, as only in this way can a rational approach to management be achieved.

INITIAL DIAGNOSIS

Whilst it is important in management to attempt to classify a stroke into one of these categories, a completed stroke may constitute a medical emergency; clinical diagnosis must therefore proceed with certain priorities.

The unconscious patient

An appreciable proportion of patients with an acute stroke lose consciousness at the onset of the ictus. In this case an airway must first be established before turning to the cause of coma. It may not be immediately obvious that the patient has had a stroke, and even if he has, there may be some other reason for the loss of consciousness.

There are of course many causes of loss of consciousness, but those in which coma is a late development in the course of an illness need not concern us here. As most strokes develop within minutes or hours, it is with the conditions which cause rapid loss of consciousness that we are mainly concerned. A stroke may, however, develop during sleep, so that the acute nature of the onset may not be apparent.

The commonest cause of acute loss of consciousness which gives rise to diagnostic difficulty is a *head injury*. This situation arises when an elderly person is found lying on the floor unconscious with a bruise or laceration of the face or scalp. In general, all but the most serious head injuries are unlikely to produce a dense focal deficit at the onset. If, therefore, a patient with evidence of head trauma has an obvious hemiplegia, the possibility of an antecedent stroke should be considered.

A condition which may cause temporary difficult is *epilepsy*, particularly if it is associated with a postictal hemiplegia. The loss of consciousness is, however, unlikely to last more than half to one hour. When the patient recovers, he can usually indicate that he suffers from epilepsy so that the recovery of the hemiplegia over the course of a few hours can be awaited. Difficulty also occasionally arises when the onset of a stroke is marked by an epileptic attack. The failure of the patient to recover consciousness within an hour and the absence of a previous history of epilepsy should make the cause of the ictus clear.

A *cerebral tumour* may present as a stroke with or without loss of consciousness. In most general hospital series of emergency admissions of strokes about 5 per cent ultimately prove to have a tumour (Groch, McDevitt, and Wright, 1961). Even in series in which there has been special study and investigation, errors still occur. In a series of 80 acute strokes which were subjected to detailed investigation including angiography, two — initially accepted as strokes — later were shown to have a cerebral tumour (Bull, Marshall, and Shaw, 1960).

Other causes of loss of consciousness need only be considered in those cases in which a stroke may have developed gradually. *Metabolic causes* such as diabetic coma and hypoglycaemia, drug overdose, hepatic or renal failure are in this category; usually there is some preceding history of the underlying disorder and some present evidence as to its nature. These causes of loss of consciousness are not usually missed because of lack of evidence, but because of failure to bear them in mind.

Examination of the unconscious patient

Evidence of neurological deficit and of the site of the lesion may be found even in the unconscious patient. The type and rate of respiration should be carefully noted together with the size and reaction of the pupils. Meiosis and ptosis on the affected side may occur in oculosympathetic palsy. With a contralateral hemiplegia this suggests internal carotid thrombosis; with homolateral bulbar palsy it suggests infarction of the medulla. Pin-point pupils indicate either a lesion in the pons or that the patient has been given morphine. Inequality of the pupils, the larger unreactive to light or reacting sluggishly, is caused by raised intracranial pressure and tentorial herniation. Fixed dilated pupils reflect severe brain stem compression and warn that death is imminent. The oculo-cephalic reflexes (doll's eye movements) should be elicited. Their absence indicates either a primary lesion of the brain stem or secondary compression resulting from a supratentorial lesion. Failure of the eyes to deviate when the ear is irrigated with cold water is also indicative of brain stem damage. In hemisphere lesions involving the frontal lobes or anterior limb of the internal capsule, the head and eyes may be deviated towards the side of the lesion; the corner of the mouth may droop, and the cheek on the weak side blow in and out with respiration. In this case full conjugate lateral deviation of the eyes can be achieved by caloric stimulation.

The affected limbs may lie in an awkward position and a foot-drop may be apparent. When both upper limbs are raised and dropped by the examiner, the paralysed limbs fall in a 'dead-weight' fashion.

It is important to realise that the affected limbs are not spastic at this stage. An initially flaccid paralysis may give way to spasticity after an interval of several days. Similarly the reflexes may be depressed for a time on the affected side. The plantar response will, however, be extensor, but the value of the plantar response as a localising sign may be lost because, when a patient is unconscious, both plantars may become extensor.

If the deficit includes sensory loss, stimulation of the limbs on the affected side may evoke no response or a reflex movement, whereas stimulation of the contralateral side may provoke grimacing and purposive movements. There may be evidence of intracranial bleeding in the presence of neck stiffness.

Ophthalmoscopy may provide important information; although papilloedema may develop when intracranial pressure is raised by a haematoma or by ischaemic oedema, it is very unlikely to appear for some hours. The presence of papilloedema in a patient seen shortly after the onset of a stroke must, therefore, raise the possibility of an alternative pathology such as a neoplasm. Subhyaloid haemorrhage usually shows that there has been subarachnoid bleeding, hence raises the possibility of a cerebral aneurysm. The presence of hypertensive changes in the retinae provides an important clue to the underlying cerebrovascular lesion, particularly as the blood pressure at the onset of a stroke may not be representative of the patient's usual pressure.

Cholesterol emboli in the retinal arteries are an indication of ulcerated atheroma in proximal arteries. Acute retinal ischaemia, occlusion of the central retinal artery, or white moving emboli in the retinal arteries are strong evidence of carotid thrombosis when found in association with a contralateral hemiplegia.

The conscious patient with stroke

When consciousness is retained not only can a more detailed neurological examination be made, but a history is also obtainable. Enquiry should be directed to what the patient was doing at the precise moment of onset of the stroke. Both patients and relatives commonly give misleading accounts. For example, a patient may say he was sitting at the onset, whereas in fact he had just risen from his chair, an action which raises the possibility of a transient orthostatic hypotension. Similarly, a patient

may state that the episode began in bed, whereas the symptoms started immediately on arising out of bed. Alternatively, he may declare the symptoms appeared after he got up when they may have come on overnight. Another source of error is the statement that a stroke developed whilst the patient was in bed, giving the impression he was lying quietly, whereas in fact he was engaged in coitus.

Enquiry as to the precise circumstances in which the stroke developed may be the clue to pathogenesis. A change of posture, as in rising from a chair, may produce hypotension in a patient whose vasomotor reflexes are impaired; diabetes mellitus, tabes dorsalis, sedative or tranquillising drugs, and advancing years may cause this impairment. Cerebral or subarachnoid haemorrhage is more likely to develop during a rise of blood pressure as in sudden exertion, anger, or coitus; it very rarely occurs during sleep except in patients on hypotensive medication.

The symptoms experienced by the patient at the onset of the stroke are also important in determining aetiology. The speed of development of the stroke is of some help; an abrupt onset favours embolism, a rapid onset haemorrhage, and a stepwise and fluctuating onset non-embolic infarction. Loss of consciousness at the onset with recovery after a short interval suggests embolism; persistent and deepening unconsciousness favours haemorrhage, whereas absence of any impairment of consciousness is most common in non-embolic infarction. A seizure at the onset occurs in about 5 per cent of strokes due to emboli or haemorrhage; seizures are very rare in non-embolic infarction. Haemorrhage, either intracerebral or subarachnoid, is almost invariably accompanied by headache at the onset; it tends to be occipital and may be so abrupt as to feel like a blow on the head. The occurrence of headache is not, however, peculiar to haemorrhage; ischaemia due to carotid or basilar occlusion is frequently accompanied by a localised pain in the temporal region which may be of great severity. The cause is probably dilatation of collaterals between the extracranial and intracranial vascular systems.

Vomiting at the onset of a stroke is of great

diagnostic importance as almost invariably it indicates intracranial haemorrhage. For the symptom to carry this connotation it must occur at the onset — say, within 15 minutes. Vomiting at a later stage does not carry the same significance.

Questions should also be directed to elicit any history of cardiac dysrhythmia or anginal pain related to the onset of stroke even if the heart appears normal by the time the patient is seen. The cardiac disturbance may have resulted in a fall in blood flow or may have given rise to emboli.

Questions should also be directed to the weeks or months prior to the stroke. A high percentage of completed strokes due to cerebral thrombosis are preceded by transient ischaemic attacks. A single TIA may have preceded the completed stroke by a matter of hours only, or the patient may have had a number of attacks over the previous weeks or months. The TIAs occur most commonly in the same arterial territory as the subsequent stroke. Preceding TIAs may also be a feature of embolic infarction. The more peripheral in the vascular tree the source of the emboli the more likely they are to lodge at the same site. It is sometimes apparent that whilst the majority of the TIAs have arisen in one site, occasionally another vascular territory has been involved: this is very suggestive of embolism. A history of TIAs does not establish beyond question a vascular aetiology; neoplasms, especially meningiomas, may occasionally be preceded by transient focal symptoms. Nevertheless, a history of preceding TIAs makes a primary vascular cause of a stroke more likely.

Examination of the conscious patient

In addition to the clinical signs which may be elicited in the unconscious patient a more comprehensive examination is now possible.

The field of vision may be examined by confrontation for evidence of a heminaopia. Even when there is no gross field defect evidence of involvement of the visual pathway may be obtained by demonstrating an inattention defect in homonymous half-fields. A patient may detect a moving finger on the affected side but fail to see it if there is simultaneous movement of a finger on the other side. If the eyes are not spontaneously deviated to the side of the lesion, evidence of a defect may still be present in an inability to maintain lateral gaze in one direction. Nystagmus may also be elicited, though interpretation of its significance as a localising sign must be made with caution. Bilateral jerking nystagmus of mild degree is often seen in the presence of a supratentorial lesion, presumably because displacement causes some distortion of the brain stem. Coarse nystagmus, unilateral nystagmus, or nystagmus in the vertical plane point to a brain stem lesion. Voluntary movements of face, tongue, and palate can be tested. The patient's cooperation in assessing power in the limbs and in sensory testing can be obtained and tests of coordination also carried out. During the course of the examination it may become apparent that the patient has a speech disturbance affecting either the content of speech (dysphasia) or articulation (dysarthria); inability to understand the instructions given to him during the examination may point to impairment on the receptive side also. Formal testing may detect minor defects.

General examination is of great importance, particular attention being paid to the heart, for evidence of enlargement, valvular disease, or dysrhythmia. Blood pressure should be measured, but a high reading is not necessarily indicative of hypertensive disease, as the blood pressure may be raised transiently after a stroke The blood pressure should be recorded in both arms as inequality in systolic pressure of more than 15 to 20 mmHg suggests a subclavian stenosis. Absent, delayed, or reduced pulses including superficial temporal carotid and brachial should be noted and the presence of bruits, particularly over the carotid bifurcation and in the supraclavicular fossa, sought. The urine should be examined for glycosuria.

SITE OF LESION

The initial examination of the patient should permit an anatomical diagnosis to be made. Although the many eponymous syndromes described in the past are no longer used, it is important to determine the major vascular territory involved and particularly to distinguish between lesions in the carotid and vertebro-basilar territories. The natural history of vascular events in these two territories differs considerably; this influences the extent of investigation which is appropriate and the need for treatment. Investigation of a stroke may require angiography, hence it is important to know which and how many vascular territories should be studied. Four-vessel angiography is no substitute for precise anatomical diagnosis. Determination by clinical examination of the vascular territory involved enables angiographic study to be planned so as to give the maximum relevant information with least hazard to the patient.

The internal carotid territory

The commonest type of stroke is that loosely referred to as a hemiplegia. This usage is inaccurate because, besides weakness, there is often some degree of sensory loss and hemianopia. If this is the case, the lesion must either be extensive or if localised it must be in the region of the internal capsule, because at no other site are the motor, sensory, and visual pathways so closely related. The motor part of the disability due to a capsular lesion affects upper and lower limbs equally.

Internal carotid occlusion is usually indistinguishable from middle cerebral artery occlusion on clinical grounds since the anterior cerebral territory receives an alternative blood supply via the anterior communicating artery. When on occasions both anterior and middle cerebral territories are involved the infarction is massive and accompanied by brain swelling and coma. Rarely there may be an ipsilateral Horner's syndrome or central retinal artery occlusion.

ANTERIOR CEREBRAL ARTERY

Occlusion of the main trunk of the anterior cerebral artery causes hemiplegia, the leg being weaker than the arm, though the latter may be the more spastic. There is cortical sensory loss in the foot. Urinary incontinence may occur if there is involvement of the paracentral lobule.

Other less constant signs are apraxia of limbs or gait, grasp reflex, paratonic rigidity, and tremor. Some degree of mental impairment is common, and in bilateral infarction profound dementia and akinetic mutism are the rule.

Occlusion of the striate branch of the anterior cerebral artery (Heubner's artery) causes a facio-brachial paralysis, the proximal part of the limb being more affected than the distal; the limb shows rigidity rather than spasticity.

MIDDLE CEREBRAL ARTERY

Occlusion at the origin of the middle cerebral artery causes a paralysis of contralateral face, arm, and leg with cortical sensory loss and, on the dominant side, an expressive dysphasia. The infarct may be large and space-occupying so that coma may be present. Occlusion of the striate branches produces the same picture, but the infarct is smaller and loss of consciousness less common. Extension of infarction posteriorly to the region of the angular gyrus produces a receptive type of dysphasia with in addition dyslexia, dyscalculia, finger agnosia, and right-left disorientation. Involvement of the posterior parietal area of the dominant hemisphere leads to dyspraxia.

On the non-dominant side infarction of the region corresponding to the sensory speech area and posterior parietal lobe produces denial or neglect of the left side of the body or of external space, constructional dyspraxia, and dressing dyspraxia. These features may be overshadowed by a dense hemiplegia but may also be seen without marked weakness in occlusion of the angular or posterior temporal branches of the middle cerebral artery.

The middle cerebral artery territory includes much of the upper part of the optic radiation and a complete or partial homonymous hemianopia involving especially the lower quadrants is a feature of occlusion of the main trunk or of the posterior temporal branch. Central vision is preserved.

Paralysis of conjugate lateral gaze to the side opposite the lesion is a common finding in infarction or haemorrhage involving or undercutting the frontal eye fields. The defect does not persist.

The vertebrobasilar territory

Vascular lesions in the brain stem usually give rise to characteristic signs and symptoms. Unless the lesion is extremely small, one of the cranial nerves is likely to be involved at nuclear level. This will be on the side contralateral to the hemiparesis or hemisensory loss, if either be present. There may be a third or a sixth nerve paralysis or paresis. Sensation—particularly to pin-prick—may be impaired on one side of the face. There may be a facial weakness of lower motor neurone type, the upper and lower parts of the face being equally involved. Dysarthria and dysphagia may be prominent signs.

Vertigo is very common in brain stem lesions, as is nystagmus, but the localising significance of the latter requires care in interpretation. The motor and sensory pathways traversing the brain stem are commonly involved bilaterally, though the deficit may be greater on one side than on the other. Small lesions may, however, cause unilateral motor weakness and sensory loss.

Although cerebellar haemorrhage is not rare, it is unusual for the cerebellum itself to be the site of an infarct; this is because of the abundant anastomoses which are present between the superior, anterior inferior, and posterior inferior cerebellar arteries. Signs of a cerebellar disturbance are, however, common because of involvement of the cerebellar connections in the brain stem. Ataxia of stance and gait are particularly frequent manifestations of a brain stem vascular lesion.

BASILAR ARTERY

Occlusion of the main trunk of the basilar artery produces immediate coma and very small but reactive pupils. There is a flaccid quadriplegia and bulbar palsy. Disturbances of lateral gaze are constantly present. Vital functions—respiration, pulse and temperature control—are disturbed and death usually occurs within a few days. If the lesion is less severe, consciousness may be retained. The patient will then complain of vertigo and will frequently have visual field defects, diplopia, facial paraesthesiae, and dysarthria. Sensation may be preserved even in the presence of complete paralysis. Yet another clevical picture is akinetic mutism; the patient follows a moving object with his eyes but makes no movement voluntarily or no response to stimulation.

Occlusion of the paramedian branches of the basilar artery produces one or other of the classical syndromes: a sixth, seventh, or twelfth cranial nerve palsy with contralateral hemiplegia and sensory loss. Occlusion of the named long circumferential branches causes in the case of the superior cerebellar artery ipsilateral cerebellar ataxia, choreiform movements and Horner's syndrome with loss of pain and temperature sense down the whole of the opposite side, including the face; occlusion of the anterior inferior cerebellar artery causes cerebellar ataxia, Horner's syndrome, loss of pain and temperature sensation over the face, and a lower motor neurone facial palsy all on the side of the lesion with loss of pain and temperature sense over the limbs and trunk on the contralateral side. Occlusion of the posterior inferior cerebellar artery causes cerebellar ataxia, a Horner's syndrome, loss of pain and temperature sensation over the face, and paralysis of the soft palate, pharynx and vocal cord all on the side of the lesion with loss of pain and temperature sensation over the limbs and trunk of the contralateral side.

POSTERIOR CEREBRAL ARTERY

This artery supplies the medial part of the occipital lobe, under surface of the temporal lobe, the splenium of the corpus callosum, and a major part of the thalamus and upper midbrain.

Infarction of the cortical distribution leads to an isolated dense homonymous hemianopia without paralysis or sensory loss. The central part of the visual field is usually spared. Unformed visual hallucinations may be experienced. The occurrence of amnesia indicates infarction of the hippocampus on the dominant hemisphere. Unilateral or bilateral disturbance of visual discrimination, facial recognition, colour, vision, visual orientation, and rarely visual agnosia may all occur, singly or together, in ischaemic lesions of the parastriate cortex.

Isolated dyslexia without dysgraphia is usually found with a right homonymous hemianopia and is due to left posterior cerebral artery occlusion with infarction of the splenium of the corpus callosium.

Infarction of the central territory of the posterior cerebral artery is much less common. The patient experiences a sudden hemianaesthesia involving all sensory modalities accompanied by a mild paraparesis. After an interval spontaneous unilateral pain (thalamic syndrome) and intention tremor may appear. These features indicate infarction of the postero ventral thalamus and subthalamic nuclei. Other branches of the posterior cerebral artery supply the midbrain; the signs indicating infarction of this region are paresis of vertical eye movement, usually bilateral, skew deviation, unreactive pupils, and retraction nystagmus. Third nerve palsy may be seen with either crossed cerebellar ataxia or crossed hemiparesis if infarction involves the cerebral peduncle.

DIAGNOSIS OF PATHOLOGY

Traditionally, strokes have been attributed to haemorrhage, thrombosis, and embolism, and of the three thrombosis was thought to occur most frequently. Because the commonest stroke syndrome is a hemiplegia with sensory loss and and hemianopia the site of thrombosis was presumed to be the middle cerebral artery.

The pathology of the lesion causing the stroke was diagnosed at the bed-side on the basis of simple clinical criteria. A stroke of sudden onset in a hypertensive person rendering him deeply unconscious was attributed to intracerebral haemorrhage. A stroke of sudden onset in a young or middle-aged person with a cardiac lesion such as mitral stenosis or atrial fibrillation was labelled embolic. When these criteria for haemorrhage or embolism were lacking, it was assumed the stroke was thrombotic.

A number of developments have upset this traditional approach. It has been shown at autopsy that a diagnosis based on such clinical criteria was very often wrong. Dalsgaard-Niel-

sen (1956) in Denmark followed 1000 cases to autopsy and showed that the clinical diagnosis of haemorrhage was confirmed in only 65 per cent of cases and that of infarction in only 58 per cent. Similarly, Heasman and Lipworth (1966) in England and Wales found that the diagnosis of cerebral haemorrhage on the death certificate issued for patients dying in hospital was confirmed at autopsy in only 43 per cent of cases. Clearly, using the criteria then available the diagnosis of the pathology of a stroke at the bed-side was subject to considerable error.

Another development undermining the traditional approach has been pathological and angiographic studies which showed that the frequency of the various pathological causes is very different from that expected. Fisher (1954) called attention to the frequency with which lesions at the origin of the internal carotid artery were associated with stroke. In a series of 214 unselected autopsies in patients who died of cerebrovascular disease, stenosis or occlusion of the internal carotid artery was present in 41 (19 per cent). Prior to this Fisher and Adams (1951) in a detailed study of brains with vascular lesions had found thrombosis of the middle cerebral artery to be much less common than anticipated from the clinical diagnosis. Cases diagnosed clinically as middle cerebral thrombosis were found to be either embolic occlusions from the heart or from the internal carotid artery—or were due to occlusions of small striate vessels which required serial sections to find them.

Subsequent workers have confirmed these findings; Blackwood et al. (1969) found that 45 per cent of cerebral infarcts were embolic, the source frequently being clinically unsuspected lesions in the heart. Similarly Jorgensen and Torvik (1966) over a six month period studied at autopsy 320 unselected cases of ischaemic cerebrovascular disease; among these were 82 recent, large infarcts with associated vascular occlusion. Of these 37 (47 per cent) could be identified as embolic and 42 (53 per cent) as thrombotic; (3 were undetermined). The source of the emboli was the extracranial carotid artery in 15 per cent, the majority of the remainder being of cardiac origin. Amongst recent infarcts without associated vascular occlusion, 46 per cent were thought, on the basis of collateral evidence, to have been embolic.

Angiographic evidence has also led to a revision of traditional clinical concepts. Bull *et al.* (1960) examined 80 consecutive cases of acute stroke angiographically and found only eight occlusions of the middle cerebral artery; no abnormality was detected in 45 of the cases, many of these presumably being embolic, the embolus having fragmented by the time the angiogram was obtained.

In the light of these advances the clinical approach to the diagnosis of the pathological nature of the lesion causing a stroke has had to be drastically revised. Haemorrhage must still be differentiated from infarction, but this distinction is made with more circumspection than formerly. Infarction may be thrombotic or embolic in origin, the latter being responsible in a much higher percentage of cases than hitherto thought likely. The diagnosis of embolism is no longer restricted to such obvious cases as a young woman with mitral stenosis and atrial fibrillation and without evidence of generalised vascular disease. The heart is no longer thought of as the sole source of emboli; stenosis or occlusion of the internal carotid artery is recognised as a potential source in about 20 per cent of cases. Finally, an appreciable clinical deficit does not require a sizeable infarct as its cause; a strategically sited lacunar lesion may be responsible.

Most of this new knowledge is important when making a diagnosis at the bed-side. Even with this knowledge clinical diagnosis remains subject to error unless supplemented by some investigations. Examination of the cerebrospinal fluid to exclude the presence of blood is certainly mandatory in more instances especially if any specific therapy is to be employed.

Intracranial haemorrhage (see also Ch. 11)

Massive intracerebral haemorrhage is the diagnosis which can be made with greatest certainty. The patient almost invariably suffers from chronic hypertension and has evidence of hypertensive retinopathy and cardiac enlargement. The onset is sudden with headache and vomiting. Minor episodes preceding the stroke

are rare. The patient becomes progressively obtunded and loses consciousness over minutes or hours. The examination of such a patient has already been described; the points favouring haemorrhage are loss of consciousness, neck stiffness, and conjugate deviation of the eyes to the side of the lesion. Diagnosis should be confirmed by lumbar puncture though the procedure carries a small risk of provoking tentorial herniation.

Echoencephalography is also of value provided it is applied within 24 hours of the onset. Within that period a shift of midline structures indicates a haemorrhage; it is rare for an infarction to produce displacement so rapidly. After the first 24 hours an infarct—because of the development of surrounding oedema—may well produce displacement of midline structures.

Subarachnoid haemorrhage

Differentiation of a subarachnoid bleed from a ruptured intracranial aneurysm or a primary intracerebral haemorrhage is not always easy. The age of the patient is of little help; although the age distribution of patients with primary intracerebral haemorrhage is somewhat higher than of those with primary subarachnoid bleeding, the overlap is so great as to be of no diagnostic help. Most help is obtained from certain features in the clinical picture.

Onset is sudden with headache and vomiting in both. Consciousness, however, is more often preserved with subarachnoid haemorrhage. There is marked neck stiffness in subarachnoid haemorrhage, but in contrast to an intracerebral haemorrhage, signs of a large focal cerebral lesion are usually lacking. Exceptions occur when the aneurysm, instead of bleeding freely into the subarachnoid space, has bled into the brain producing a large intracerebral haematoma. In these circumstances distinguishing between a primary intracerebral haemorrhage which has extended into the cerebrospinal fluid pathway and a primary subarachnoid haemorrhage which has extended into the brain may be impossible on clinical grounds alone.

Another source of difficulty is vasospasm, which commonly occurs when blood surrounds the basal arteries causing an area of focal ischaemia or even infarction. The patient then shows signs of a focal cerebral lesion and the picture may be mistaken for that of an intracerebral haemorrhage. Spasm, however, takes some time to develop so that focal signs are not likely to be present if a patient is seen soon after the onset of a subarachnoid haemorrhage.

The problem can, of course, be best resolved by cerebral angiography, but considerable circumspection is required about when this should be done and to which patients. As primary intracerebral haemorrhage in the region of the internal capsule—which is the commonest site for haemorrhage—is not benefitted by surgery, angiography in this instance serves no useful purpose.

A more superficially placed haematoma may be amenable to surgery and since these two conditions cannot often be differentiated with certainty on clinical grounds alone, angiography is recommended for patients whose condition has stabilised or who show signs of a secondary rise in intracranial pressure after initial stabilisation. Computerised X-ray scanning allows earlier localisation of the haematoma than do other methods. If the clinical picture is strongly indicative of a primary subarachnoid haemorrhage, angiography should be carried out provided the patient's state warrants it. Patients who are alert should have angiography as soon as possible so that if an aneurysm is found, surgery can proceed at once. For patients who are stuporose or comatose, angiography should be delayed, as it may aggravate the patient's condition if carried out at this stage. Delay, of course, carried the risk of recurrent haemorrhage, but this has to be accepted. The patient should be watched closely and angiography performed as soon as his level of consciousness permits.

Cerebral thrombosis

Diagnosis of cerebral infarction and its cause presents more difficulty. Infarction was often attributed to low blood pressure; indeed, when hypotensive drugs became available fear was expressed that their use in patients with cere-brovascular disease would precipitate infarction. In fact, infarction is most often associated with high rather than with low blood pressure. In a series of 134 patients aged 55 years or less diagnosed clinically as having had an infarction, only seven had a blood pressure below that expected for their age and sex; in 22 the blood pressure was within the expected range and 105 had a blood pressure higher than it should have been (Prineas and Marshall, 1966).

Similarly Low-Beer and Phear (1961) found that the blood pressure of patients with cerebral infarction was not in the hypotensive range except when there was an obvious precipitating factor such as myocardial infarction, haemorrhage, postoperative shock, etc. Hypotension as a cause of an infarction should not be diagnosed unless there is clear evidence that there has been a hypotensive episode.

Close study of the patients with raised blood pressure who have experienced a cerebral infarction shows that they can be divided into two groups. There are those in whom the blood pressure, though raised, is not alarmingly high and those in whom the blood pressure is very high. It is difficult to provide a precise cut-off point but a diastolic pressure of 110 mmHg is a useful dividing line. Patients with blood pressure below that level are likely to have predominantly the atherosclerotic type of vascular disease; the prevalence of carotid occlusion in this group is high and the cerebral lesion is likely to be a large infarct. Patients with a diastolic blood pressure over 110 mmHg are likely to have hypertensive vascular disease affecting small vessels. Though carotid stenosis is as common as in the less hypertensive group, carotid occlusion is much less common and the cerebral lesion is likely to be lacunar in type.

Differentiation between these two groups can often be made at the bed-side by paying attention to the level of the diastolic blood pressure. Thus Prineas and Marshall (1966) found that in 81 extracranial arteries visualised angiographically in 47 patients with a diastolic pressure below 110 mmHg who had experienced a cerebral infarction, there were 14 occlusions and 8 stenoses; whereas in 50 extracranial arteries in 30 patients with a diastolic pressure above 110 mmHg, there were no occlusions and three stenoses.

If other features are taken into account besides the blood pressure, differentiation may be even more precise. Extracranial bruits, cholesterol emboli in the retinal vessels, and a focal disturbance in the electrocephalogram point to a large infarction associated with atherosclerotic disease. The clinical deficit is severe and, because of the amount of brain tissue involved, is likely to be persistent. Other indications of cerebral thrombosis are the occurrence of previous transient ischaemic attacks or minor strokes in the same vascular territory, a stepwise or stuttering onset, the preservation of consciousness in the presence of a major deficit, and a clear CSF. On the other hand, the absence of bruits, hypertensive changes in the retinal vessels, clinically or electrocardiographically detectable left ventricular hypertrophy, and a normal or symmetrically disturbed electro-encephalogram indicating a small deep lesion point to a lacunar lesion developing possibly in association with a micro-aneurysm and associated with hypertensive vascular disease.

Cerebral embolism

In many patients the first question to be answered is, 'Is this a primary vascular lesion in the carotid or vertebrobasilar systems or has there been embolisation from outside these systems into a healthy vascular tree?' If the neurological deficits indicate there are scattered cortical lesions involving individual arterial branches, embolisation is highly likely. In many instances the history and examination of the patient gives an indication of the pathological process. Clinical indications of embolism are the very rapid onset of symptoms, the absence of previous minor attacks in most cases, rapid recovery from a severe deficit, evidence of systemic embolism, and a clear CSF. A patient may have an obvious source of emboli such as mitral stenosis with or without atrial fibrillation, a recent myocardial infarct, cardiomyopathy, atrial myxoma, thyrotoxicosis with atrial fibrillation, or following cardiac surgery. Unfortunately, these cases constitute only a minority of cases of stroke due to embolism. This is reflected in the fact that large hospital series of strokes usually report only about 5 per cent as due to embolisation, yet autopsy series report as many as 40 per cent to be embolic (Jorgensen and Torvik, 1966).

Not all of this discrepancy can be accounted for by those emboli which arise in atheromatous lesions at the origin of the internal carotid artery or in one of the great vessels as again autopsy study has shown. The remainder come from the heart in patients in whom this source was not clinically obvious. The patient may be known to have ischaemic heart disease but not of the kind hitherto recognised as producing emboli. Recent work on prolonged cardiac monitoring of active mobile patient has, however, shown that episodes of dysrhythmia are more frequent than hitherto suspected. These may give rise to emboli as may the non-infective type of marantic valvular lesion seen at autopsy in some patients with cerebral infarction.

When there is no clinically obvious source of emboli, although attention should be turned to the possibility of a primary arterial lesion, the possibility of embolisation from an unsuspected cardiac lesion should not be lost sight of. When considering a primary arterial lesion the question must be asked, 'Is the primary vascular lesion in an intracranial or extracranial vessel?' Features favouring a carotid rather than a middle cerebral lesion have already been described, but it may be impossible to make this distinction on clinical grounds alone. If a history of transient ischaemic attacks prior to the stroke can be obtained, differential diagnosis is aided. Episodes of amaurosis fugax point to the internal carotid artery as the site of the primary lesion, a conclusion which is reinforced if a bruit is present. Patients whose preceding TIAs were confined to the cerebral hemisphere, and who do not have a bruit, may have a lesion of the internal carotid but this is less likely than in those with amaurosis fugax.

MANAGEMENT

Precise diagnosis as far as this is possible is important as it influences subsequent management. The first concern, if the patient is unconscious, must be to safeguard the airway. If loss of consciousness persists, survival is unlikely. If consciousness is regained, or was never lost, the concern is with the possible development of raised intracranial pressure. This is most likely to occur as a secondary development in large infarcts. Indication is given by the fact that the patient's condition, after stabilising or even improving for some hours, begins to deteriorate. Focal signs become more prominent and the level of consciousness declines. Immediate measures are required to deal with this situation if it is not to become irreversible.

If the lesion is thought to be embolic, then the question of anticoagulants must arise. There are two schools of thought on this, the one favouring immediate anticoagulation to prevent further embolisation, the other advising delaying the start of treatment for three weeks to avoid the risk of rendering the infarct haemorrhagic. The present author favours the former course provided the cerebrospinal fluid is clear.

When the problems of unconsciousness, cerebral oedema, and the need for anticoagulation have been resolved, decisions about further investigation must await the outcome. Even if there is strong evidence that the lesion is at the origin of the internal carotid artery, there is no immediate call for angiography. If the vessel is already occluded, no good is likely to come from surgery as it is uncommon for it to be possible to re-establish flow at this stage. Even if it is possible, the procedure is dangerous as restoration of flow to an infarcted area usually aggravates the damage. If the vessel is likely to be stenosed and not occluded, it is still advisable to delay angiography. The risks of angiography and endarterectomy are much less if the infarct has had time to heal. Moreover, whether or not these procedures should be undertaken depends upon the degree of recovery the patient makes. Endarterectomy aims to prevent a further stroke, not to treat the present one. If as a result of the present stroke the patient is left severely incapacitated, nothing will be gained by endarterectomy. If, on the other hand, he makes a considerable degree of recovery, the question of angiography must be faced.

Infarction in the brain stem

These considerations apply, with some modification, to infarcts in the vertebrobasilar as in the carotid territory. It is useful to recognise two major anatomical groups. The first is that in which the central part of the brain stem which is supplied by the small paramedian and short circumferential arteries is involved. Consciousness is almost invariably lost or disturbed in the particular manner known as coma vigil or akinetic mutism. Respiration and other vital functions are likely to be involved and the prognosis for life is poor. The second is that group in which the lateral part of the brain stem supplied by branches of the long circumferential arteries is the site of infarction. The classical example of this is the so-called 'posterior infererior cerebellar artery' syndrome. Consciousness is preserved, and prognosis for life and for function are good. In either group massive oedema as a complication is not seen.

There is no indication for angiography in the acute phase. In the patients who recover, the role of angiography is much less than in the investigation of lesions in the carotid territory, being confined largely to those cases in which it is thought that a stenosis of the subclavian artery proximal to the origin of the vertebral was implicated in the causation of the brain stem lesion.

In this connection the word 'complete' to describe a stroke may be misunderstood. The term may be used in two senses. It may describe the time course of a stroke—one that has come on abruptly reached its peak rapidly and left the patient with a persistent deficit. It may also be used to indicate the extent of involvement of an arterial territory. For example, a lesion in the territory of the middle cerebral artery of the dominant hemisphere may produce a hemiplegia without dysphasia or vice versa. The deficit may persist, hence the term complete may be applied in that sense. But the lesion is incomplete in the sense that a further event in that vascular territory could produce more disability. This should be the criterion for angiography in stroke believed to have caused infarction and is one that can only be properly applied about three weeks after the onset. If at this stage it is clear that the patient will make such a degree of recovery that the quality of his life will not be greatly impaired and that a further event involving that arterial territory would greatly increase his degree of handicap, then angiography should be undertaken. If an operable stenosis is found, endarterectomy should be advised.

CONCLUSION

Advance in our understanding of cerebrovascular disease has converted what was a simple problem of clinical diagnosis and management to a complex task. The previous simplicity was more apparent than real, arising from our ignorance of the many types of pathophysiological disturbance included under the heading of stroke. The present complexity can, however, be met by a simple management plan following a critical analytical path. This can be summarised in the following terms:

Is the patient unconscious? If he is, first safe-guard the airway and then consider causes of loss of consciousness other than stroke. Decide which vascular territory is involved, carotid or vertebrobasilar.

Is the lesion a haemorrhage—remembering especially cerebellar and subcortical lesions—or an infarct?

If it is an infarct, is it embolic—from the heart or from the great vessels, particularly the internal carotid artery—or non-embolic?

If it is a non-embolic infarct, is it a large cortical lesion—as is likely in patients with a diastolic blood pressure under 110 mmHg, or a deep lacunar lesion—as is likely in patients with a diastolic blood pressure above 110 mmHg? Finally, has the lesion reached its peak or is it still evolving?

Progress along this path not only leads to rational diagnosis but involves consequences in terms of investigations required and the therapy indicated at a number of points. It is only in this way that our further understanding and improved management of the completed stroke will be achieved.

REFERENCES

Blackwood, W., Hallpike, J. F., Kocen, R. S. & Mair, W. G. P. (1969) Atheromatous disease of the carotid arterial system and embolism from the heart in cerebral infarction: a morbid anatomical study. *Brain*, **92**, 897.
Bull, J. W. D., Marshall, J. & Shaw, D. A. (1960) Cerebral angiography in the diagnosis of the acute stroke. *Lancet*, i, 562.
Cole, F. M. & Yates, P. O. (1967) The occurrence and significance of intracerebral micro-aneurysms. *Journal of Pathology and Bacteriology*, **93**, 393
Dalsgaard-Nielsen, T. (1956) Some clinical experience in the treatment of cerebral apoplexy (1000 cases). *Acta Psychiatrica Scandinavica*, Suppl. 108, 101.
Fisher, C. M. & Adams, R. D. (1951) Observations on brain embolism with special reference to the mechanism of haemorrhagic infarction. *Journal of Neuropathology and Experimental Neurology*, **10**, 92.
Fisher, M. (1954) Occlusion of the carotid arteries—further experiences. *Archives of Neurology and Psychiatry*, **72**, 187.
Geltner, L. (1972) Comprehensive care of cerebrovascular accidents. *Gerontologia Clinica*, **14**, 346.
Groch, S., McDevitt, E. & Wright, I. S. (1961) A long term study of cerebral vascular disease. *Annals of Internal Medicine*, **55**, 358.
Heasman, M. A. & Lipworth, L. (1966) *Accuracy of certification of causes of death.* General Register Office, Studies on Medical and Population Subjects No. 20. London: Her Majesty's Stationery Office.
Low-Beer & Phear, D. (1961) Cerebral infarction and hypertension. *Lancet*, i, 1303.
Jorgensen, L. & Torvik, A. (1966) Ischaemic cerebrovascular diseases in an autopsy series Part 1. Prevalence, location and predisposing factors in verified thrombo-embolic occlusions, and their significance in the pathogenesis of cerebral infarction. *Journal of Neurological Sciences*, **3**, 490.
Prineas, J. & Marshall, J. (1966) Hypertension and cerebral infarction. *British Medical Journal*, i, 14.

9. Management of Acute Cerebral Infarction

E. C. Hutchinson

Information on the immediate mortality of cerebral infarction cannot be precise. The two main sources of information are from epidemiological studies of unselected populations and reports derived from general hospital records. The accuracy of data from the first source is frequently questioned, and the patients studied in the second are often highly selected.

It is now traditional for clinicians to question the accuracy of the diagnosis of the cause of death in epidemiological studies. The epidemiologists' reply that there is clear evidence that the gains and losses in terms of accuracy of diagnosis of cause of death will balance out if the standard of medical care and reporting is high (Acheson, 1966; Kurtzke, 1969). One important point established by epidemiological studies and not sufficiently emphasised in the reported studies on hospital patients is that cerebral infarction and cerebral haemorrhage are predominantly diseases of old age. In their studies in Oxford, Acheson and Fairbairn (1970) examined the age incidence of cerebral vascular disease in hospital and in the general population and demonstrated clearly that the incidence of cerebral infarction rises rapidly with increasing age. In males of the 55 to 65 age group the rate per 1000 of cerebral infarction was 1.35 whereas in the over 75 age group the rate per 1000 was 11.43.

In attributing death directly to cerebral infarction it is usual to take a period of four weeks from the acute episode. This is certainly realistic, but it obscures one important fact. Death in hemisphere infarction in the first week is usually due to massive cerebral oedema; in the next three weeks death is commonly due to systemic complications. This will be amplified later.

The mortality figures in the first four weeks given by Whisnant *et al.* (1971) appear to be as reliable as any, firstly, because they relate to the population of Rochester, Minnesota, where the standards of medical care available from the Mayo Clinic are excellent; secondly, the autopsy rate in the general population is high.

Using traditional clinical grounds for differentiating between cerebral haemorrhage, embolism, and thrombosis, there were 412 patients between the years 1945 and 1955 who presented with a 'cerebral thrombosis'. The death rate at the end of one month in these patients was 27 per cent. In giving these figures the authors stress the overdiagnosis of cerebral haemorrhage shown by the death certificate. The vital statistics for the United States during the period of study gave a ratio of 2.5 :1 of cerebral haemorrhage to 'cerebral thrombosis'; in the population of Rochester over this period the same ratio was 0.15 :1. No doubt this degree of over-reporting of cerebral haemorrhage holds good for the Western world as a whole.

The figure of 27 per cent mortality in the first month probably approximates to the true figures, and this is supported by a general hospital population study where little or no selection of admissions to hospital is practised. Carter (1964), in a personally observed series of 612 patients with stroke, found that 26 per cent died within four weeks of the onset.

MANAGEMENT

Management of acute cerebral infarction in the first four weeks may be considered under the two major headings of clinical observation and treatment. The subdivision, though useful, is somewhat artificial as certain observations, such as dehydration hypernatraemia, may lead to immediate treatment.

As a background to both observation and treatment it is necessary to consider the clinical implications of the pathological changes which occur in hemisphere infarction. This in its turn leads on to a consideration of the problem of brain herniation occurring as a consequence of a rapidly developing space occupying lesion which, in this instance, is a cerebral infarct.

Cerebral oedema

The cause of cerebral oedema in cerebral infarction is the subject of a recent contribution by O'Brien, Waltz, and Jordan (1974). They examined the distribution of water in the brain in experimental animals after occlusion of a major cerebral artery. They found that oedema occurred following experimental infarction in both the ischaemic and the non-ischaemic hemisphere, but in every specimen the water content was greatest in the infarcted brain. The increased water content was apparent four hours following occlusion and was maximal within two days. This time sequence has clinical importance.

The sequence of events following an expanding lesion of one hemisphere is now well recognised. Immediately, the ipsilateral lateral ventricle is compressed, the third ventricle is then distorted, and there is a shift of the mid-line structures away from the lesion. Following these changes internal herniae of the brain occur at several well-recognised sites.

Herniation of the cingulate gyrus under the inferior margin of the superior falx may occur but is of little importance to the clinician. More important is the herniation of the medial portion of the temporal lobe, predominantly the uncus and the hippocampal gyrus, which is displaced over the free edge of the tentorium where it may compress the mid-brain in its transverse axis. Subsequently the aqueduct is distorted and the contralateral cerebral peduncle is pushed against the free edge of the tentorium on the opposite side, thus producing early signs of a contralateral third nerve palsy. These findings are illustrated in Figure 9.1.

Further increase in the size of the space occupying lesion results in a downward displacement of the diencephalon, midbrain, pons, and medulla—a process referred to as central transtentorial herniation. Ultimately, the combination of a downward displacement together with the fixed position of the basilar artery and its branches results in stretching and tearing of small vessels which, if unrelieved, culminates in haemorrhage in the midbrain and pons. The unchecked downward shift of the mid-line structures finally results in tonsillar herniation of the cerebellum through the foramen magnum.

In infratentorial lesions a rapidly expanding lesion, such as a cerebellar haemorrhage or infarct, will cause death within a few hours due to compression of the essential mid-line structures from below, the so-called reversed tentorial herniation.

The above changes in the intracranial structures in response to a space occupying lesion have been clearly recognised in cerebral tumours and other space occupying lesions. It is now appreciated, however, that the same sequence of events occurs in cerebral infarction.

Cerebral oedema secondary to cerebral infarction has been recognised by pathologists for many years, but the credit for drawing attention to its clinical importance belongs to Shaw, Alvord, and Berry (1959). They reported an investigation in which the purpose was to establish the prevalence of brain herniation and the temporal pattern of its development in cerebral infarction.

They studied 15 patients who came to postmortem and the criteria for inclusion in the study were precise. They required that each patient should present with a sudden hemiplegia and that, at autopsy, infarction should involve the classical distribution of the whole middle cerebral artery territory, thus indicating that infarction was due to occlusion of both the cortical and subcortical branches. They also required that actual occlusion of the middle cerebral should be demonstrated and that the infarct should be almost entirely ischaemic in type with little or no secondary haemorrhage which would complicate the assessment of the oedema.

Fifteen patients whose autopsy findings satis-

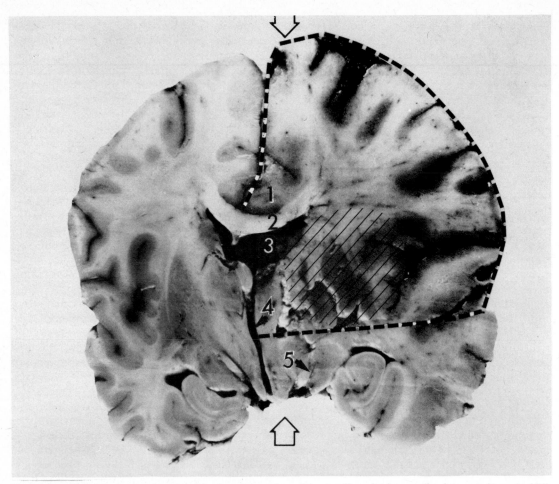

Fig. 9.1 Acute infarction and oedema resulting from internal carotid artery thrombosis spreading into anterior and middle cerebral arteries. *Arrows* indicate approximate position of original mid-line. *Cross-hatch* indicates area of encephalomalacia. *Broken line* indicates extent of oedema which causes:
1. Herniation of cingulate gyrus.
2. Downward displacement and rotation of corpus callosum.
3. Distortion of body of lateral ventricle.
4. Narrowing and displacement of third ventricle.
5. Herniation of uncus of temporal lobe.

fied these criteria died within periods ranging from 18 hours to three months after the onset of infarction. They subdivided the patients into two groups. The first group comprised patients who died after a relatively short duration of the illness in periods ranging from 18 hours to $4\frac{1}{2}$ days. The second group were patients where life was sustained for two weeks or more after the initial infarct. This sub-grouping was shown to be of importance to the clinician.

In patients dying within the first few days there was clear evidence that death was due to hemisphere oedema with brain stem compression. In all but one there was encephalomalacia with oedema of the grey matter, together with a loss of demarcation between grey and white matter. The ipsilateral ventricle was distorted and there was considerable displacement of the mid-line structures. Uncal herniation was consistently noted and found to be of the order of

10 to 12 mm of brain tissue. Tonsillar herniation was observed in three cases; they noted only one example of cingulate gyrus herniation.

The clinical findings were not recorded with the same precision as the pathological changes. All patients rapidly became unconscious or were extremely drowsy soon after the onset of the infarct, and thereafter conscious levels deteriorated as time progressed. Pupillary abnormalities were noted in some and comprised either ipsilateral, bilateral, or (in one patient) contralateral pupillary dilatation. Variations in pulse rate and blood pressure were not striking and no consistent pattern emerged. The cerebrospinal fluid (CSF) pressure in two patients was recorded as 200 mm H_2O in one and 510 mm H_2O in another.

The patients in the second group—that is, patients who died in more than two weeks— proved an interesting and important clinical contrast. The same basic pathology was found in terms of arterial disease in that the same major arteries were occluded, but the evidence of cerebral oedema and its effects could no longer be demonstrated. The cause of death was not directly related to involvement of the brain but was due to complications such as nephritis, uraemia, and bronchopneumonia. The clinical records of these patients did suggest that there had been signs of developing cerebral oedema initially, but they found them difficult to interpret in satisfactory detail.

To establish the temporal pattern they used reported cases from the literature, together with their own material, and thus had 25 cases who satisfied the strict criteria. They then plotted the shift of the mid-line in millimetres against the duration of the infarct, which was known in every case. They found a consistent pattern showing a rapid development of oedema within the first 24 hours, then a shift of the mid-line, which reached its maximum at the fifth day. The oedema then subsided, and by 20 days there was no evidence of any deviation of the mid-line.

A study by Ng and Nimmannitya (1970) substantially confirmed the findings of Shaw et al. (1959). The also confined their observations to cerebral oedema, brain herniation, and cerebral infarction. They confirmed the important point that in every case either occlusion of the main trunk of the middle cerebral artery or extensions of thrombus from internal carotid artery occlusion in the neck had occurred. In contrast, occlusions of the subdivisions of the middle cerebral and anterior cerebral arteries did not lead to significant oedema. They also found that brain stem oedema secondary to the compressive effects of the expanded, infarcted hemisphere was noted in no less than 26 of the 45 patients and in some were associated with frank ischaemic changes and haemorrhage.

Clinical observations

The clinical observations which are necessary for the adequate care of patients with an acute cerebral infarction may be considered under two headings. The first is concerned with monitoring the central nervous system. The second deals with the complications arising in the general care of the patient.

MONITORING THE CENTRAL NERVOUS SYSTEM

The sequence of events described as a result of the developing cerebral oedema can be recognised by careful monitoring of the developing signs of brain stem involvement which are superimposed on the initial focal signs of brain infarction.

For practical purposes the two types of brain displacement and herniation which are important to the physician are the development of downward transtentorial descent of the brain stem and uncal herniation. In cerebral infarction the former, because of its frequency, is the more important. In 67 cases of documented examples of supratentorial lesions causing one or other type of brain stem compression described by Plum and Posner (1972), there were 11 cases of massive cerebral infarction, and all caused downward displacement of the brain stem. They did not encounter any isolated examples of uncal herniation. However, since localised intracerebral haemorrhage may be impossible to differentiate from infarct the clinical picture of uncal herniation will also be considered briefly.

Three sets of observations need to be made on a patient with progressive brain stem involvement in order to appreciate the significance in pathological terms. These are the level of consciousness, the oculovestibular reflex, and the oculocephalic reflex.

Levels of consciousness

Any experienced physician can detect an alteration in the level of consciousness without necessarily being unduly troubled by philosophical or neurophysiological definitions. It is well recognised that an appreciation of any change in the level of consciousness is an essential part of the assessment of the patient.

Oculovestibular reflex

The reflex is induced by caloric stimulation. Its importance is that in an unconscious patient with developing brain stem compression due to a hemisphere lesion, there occurs firstly an impairment of the reflex and secondly its abolition. Abolition indicates pontine involvement which may not be reversible. In other causes of coma, such as barbiturate poisoning, the oculovestibular reflex is abolished early, and in the absence of focal signs such abolition should suggest a metabolic cause. Fisher (1967) observed that in 100 personal cases the presence of full reflex eye movements to caloric stimulation in association with signs of hemiparesis indicated with certainty that the cause of the coma lay in the hemisphere and not in the brain stem.

In the semiconscious or unconscious patient the reflex is elicited with ice-cold water. The ears are first examined to exclude a local lesion; a small rubber catheter is placed in the external auditory meatus, and 200 ml of cold water are introduced.

The normal response is the development of nystagmus with the slow component towards the irrigated ear and the fast component away from it. The response lasts about three minutes. When brain stem function is disturbed by progressive compression the fast component becomes impaired. When it finally disappears the slow component carries the eye towards the irrigated ear where it usually remains for three to four minutes. With progressive compression of the brain stem the reflex is abolished.

Oculocephalic reflex

This reflex has been variously referred to as the 'proprioceptive head turning reflex' or 'doll's-head eye phenomenon.' It is elicited by holding the eyelids open and briskly rotating the head from side to side. The normal response is conjugate deviation of the eyes to the side opposite that to which the head is turned. The second part of the examination is to flex the head briskly and then extend it. The normal response is for the eyes to elevate when the head is flexed and to deviate downwards when the head is extended. The eyes will return rapidly to the resting position after the head is moved even though the position of flexion and extension is maintained. The examiner assesses the presence or absence of vertical deviation of the eyes. Another method used to assess the preservation of upward gaze is the elicitation of the corneal reflex while holding the eyelids open; it is of course essential that reflex blinking has not already been abolished. If upward movement is preserved eliciting the corneal reflex will cause the eyes to deviate upwards.

SIGNS OF BRAIN STEM COMPRESSION

Once one is familiar with the technique of carrying out the simple clinical tests described, it is possible to use them in the management and study of coma.

Plum and Posner (1972) in their excellent monograph on stupor and coma divide the stages of brain stem involvement into four categories, namely, the diencephalic stage, the midbrain-upper pons stage, the lower pons-upper medullary stage, and finally the terminal medullary stage. What follows is a brief resumé of their observations.

CENTRAL TRANSTENTORIAL HERNIATION

Diencephalic stage

With compression of the diencephalon the overall level of consciousness will deteriorate and Cheyne-Stokes respirations may appear. The pupils are small (1 to 3 mm) but will respond to a bright light. The eyes may be deviated from the onset of the ictus conjugately towards the site of the infarcted hemisphere, but if they are not, the usual roving eye movements of light coma are present and will be only weakly interrupted by the doll's head manoeuvre. Even though there is some disturbance of gaze the eyes still respond briskly and in a normal fashion with passive side-to-side rotation.

Eliciting the oculovestibular reflex will evoke a full conjugate, slow tonic movement to the side irrigated but possibly with some impairment of the fast component at this stage. Some impairment of upward gaze may also be observed by the methods already noted. At this stage of coma it is still possible for full neurological function to return providing the underlying lesion either regresses or responds to treatment.

Midbrain-upper pontine stage

If further descent of the brain stem occurs early ischaemic changes in the pontine structures will take place, and with this progression disturbance of vegetative function now becomes apparent. Cheyne-Stokes respiration or other abnormalities of respiration may on occasion be replaced by genuine central neurogenic hyperventilation (P_aCO_2 low, Po_2 normal). The oculovestibular reflexes are now difficult to elicit but may be present in a modified fashion.

At this stage attacks of decerebrate rigidity may occur spontaneously in response to the unavoidable stimuli of nursing and medical procedures. The pupils, which were previously small, are now dilated to about 3 to 5 mm and are fixed to light.

Lower pons-upper medullary stage

The progressive ischaemia resulting from descent of the brain stem may now go on to necrosis and haemorrhage and at this stage any return of function is most unusual. Respiration is quiet with periods of apnoea. The pupils are usually pin points and fixed to light in the mid-position. The oculovestibular reflexes have now disappeared. Flaccid quadriparesis is usually superimposed upon the original hemiplegia caused by the cerebral infarction.

Medullary stage

This stage is familiar to all and represents the stage immediately prior to death. There is irregular respiration with frequent apnoea, the pulse

becomes slow, and respiration finally ceases. At this stage the pupils are widely dilated and fixed. Although a semblance of life may be retained by sustaining the blood pressure, death is inevitable after this stage.

UNCAL HERNIATION

Pathologists commonly observe lateral displacement of the mid-line, downward displacement of the brain stem, and displacement of the uncal and hippocampal gyrus over the free edge of the tentorium all in the same specimen. To the clinical observer, however, it is important to differentiate between early uncal herniation and downward displacement of the brain stem. There is one very good reason for this, namely, that in early uncal herniation the diencephalon may not be affected. At this stage the only abnormalities are ipsilateral pupillary dilatation associated with signs of a hemisphere lesion but unaccompanied by disturbance of consciousness, which is a feature of a diencephalic lesion. There is no significant disturbance of extraocular movements or alteration of the oculovestibular responses.

Recognition of early uncal herniation, whatever the cause may be, is important, for although there may be no initial drowsiness a sudden precipitate descent into the midbrain stage may occur with little or no warning. Thereafter the process is that observed in association with the later stages of downward herniation. It is certainly true that uncal herniation is much more commonly seen with neoplasm than with vascular lesions of the hemisphere.

OTHER DISTURBANCES OF GAZE IN VASCULAR LESIONS

The importance of observations on reflex eye movements in coma due to hemisphere lesions has been stressed. There are other disturbances of gaze which are useful from time to time in the anatomical localisation of vascular lesions. Fisher (1967) observed that in haemorrhage into the putamen there is a hemiparesis with the eyes deviated conjugately to the opposite side. In thalamic haemorrhages there may be a hemiparesis but the eyes are deviated downwards 'as if they were peering at the nose.' There is impairment of vertical eye movements and the pupils are 2 mm in size and unreactive. In cerebellar haemorrhage there can be forced conjugate lateral deviation of the eyes away from the side of the lesion and a paralysis of conjugate lateral gaze to the side of the lesion or sometimes a VI nerve palsy. There is no pyramidal paresis of the limbs. The pupils are of average size and react normally to light.

Ocular bobbing

Ocular bobbing is a term first used by Fisher (1961) to describe a distinctive spontaneous movement of the eyes which may occur in the unconscious patient. To fulfill the criteria it is essential to demonstrate, by eliciting the oculo-vestibular reflex, that there is paralysis of horizontal conjugate gaze. The bobbing consists of a brisk conjugate downward jerking of the eyes followed by a slow return to the mid-position. The rate of movement is between two and four per minute. It is a striking sign but its slow rate may make it difficult to recognise; it is by no means so rare as the literature would suggest. The importance of recognising ocular bobbing is that it is most commonly associated with intrinsic vascular lesions of the brain stem and is, therefore, a valuable localising sign.

There are a variety of other spontaneous eye movements which have been reported in the literature in disturbances of the brain stem, cerebellum, and their connections. One of these is opsoclonus, which is defined as a constant conjugate chaotic movement of the eyes. Boddie (1972) reported a patient where he observed 'ocular bobbing' change, after some weeks, to opsoclonus. The underlying lesion in the patient was probably a restricted pontine haemorrhage diagnosed on clinical grounds. He felt that ocular bobbing and opsoclonus ultimately may be shown to have a common patho-physiological basis.

CLINICAL COURSE

The clinical course of patients with cerebral infarction is too well known to be described in any considerable detail. It is, however, important to distinguish between hemisphere infarction and infarctions of the brain stem and cerebellum because of their implications in terms of management.

Hemisphere infarction

The clinical course in established infarction of the hemispheres may be summarised. Firstly some 70 per cent of patients will survive the acute stage with varying degrees of disability. In fatal cases death in the first few days may be equated with cerebral infarction and cerebral oedema as a result of occlusion of major intracranial vessels such as the middle cerebral, and both the subcortical and cortical branches will be involved. The mode of dying will usually be that of brain stem compression.

Survivors of the first week after the acute infarct may die of associated vascular disease affecting the coronary circulation, from pulmonary infarction, from renal failure, or from other co-existing chronic disease (Shaw et al., 1959, Ng et al., 1970).

Hind brain

The most devastating form of infarction of the hind brain is basilar artery occlusion with extensive infarction of the mid-pontine area. This frequently causes death, and if the infarcted area extends into reticular substance then coma may be present from the onset. If the infarct is situated lower in the pontine area, then the patient may present the distressing clinical syndrome which has been described by Plum and Posner (1972) as the 'locked-in syndrome'. The clinical state is one of quadriplegia with inability to move even the bulbar muscles but the patient is entirely appreciative of his surroundings. This latter point is important on a humane basis for it is important to distinguish this state from akinetic mutism where the patient has little or no awareness of the surrounding world.

One particular type of infarction in the hind brain circulation, although rare, requires special attention. It is eminently responsive to surgical treatment with survival of the patient and, in some cases, with very little in the way of residual disability. This condition is massive cerebellar infarction.

Massive cerebellar infarction

Lehrich, Winkler, and Ojemann (1970) reviewed the literature up to that time and added four personal cases to the 12 already described. The clinical syndrome of massive cerebral infarction is one of an acute onset suggesting a vascular lesion, but this is rapidly followed by the signs of a developing infratentorial lesion with progressive deterioration of consciousness. Ocular gaze palsies may be present with ipsilateral cerebellar ataxia. If the lesion is allowed to progress contrast studies will show an acute obstructive hydrocephalus and the clinical signs will indicate brain stem compression.

Decerebrate posturing of the limbs may appear at this stage, and the signs of brain stem compression already described are obvious. Untreated, death is the rule.

Examples of this syndrome may closely simulate cerebellar haemorrhage or any acute brain stem infarction such as may follow basilar artery occlusion. This is shown by the following personal case.

Case report

Male, aged 24. Admitted 29.7.71. Discharged 20.8.71

On the morning of admission the patient complained of sudden acute vertigo and vomiting. He was unable to stand without assistance because of unsteadiness of his trunk. There was no headache immediately but on admission to hospital three hours later he complained of a right temporal headache.

On admission the blood pressure was 130/80. There were no abnormal signs on general examination. The patient was alert and speech and memory were normal. There was no neck stiffness. The only abnormality in the cranial nerves was a marked nystagmus to the right and on upward and downward gaze. The nystagmus had a rotatory component. In the limbs there was minimal bilateral ataxia but no paresis and no sensory loss. The reflexes were brisk throughout and the plantar responses were indefinite.

Investigations. CSF resting pressure 120 mm of water, clear colourless fluid, acellular, protein 45 (mg/100 ml) W.R. negative. Serum electrolytes, blood sugar, blood cholesterol, were all within normal limits.

The diagnosis of an intrinsic brain lesion was made, and in view of his relative youth the possibility of acute demyelination was considered.

After remaining unaltered for two days he suddenly complained of occipital headache. He was sweating profusely and his general condition deteriorated. He was drowsy but his speech was normal. The nystagmus was as noted on admission, but there was now some restriction of upward gaze. The plantar responses now showed an extensor plantar on the right but the left was still indefinite. For the first time some neck stiffness was noted. Within two hours upward gaze was further restricted and there was a divergent squint with diplopia.

In view of the signs at the onset and the clinical deterioration without obvious pyramidal weakness the diagnosis of an intrinsic brain stem lesion was abandoned and a vertebral angiogram was carried out.

This showed a large space occupying lesion in the right cerebellar hemisphere with displacement of the right superior cerebellar artery (Fig. 9.2).

Following angiography there was a further deterioration of consciousness and the pulse rate fell to 50 per minute. The pupils were still reacting to light. The following morning there was a further decrease in the level of consciousness but the patient still responded to commands. There was bilateral ptosis and a divergent squint. Upward movement of the eyes was now absent.

Urgent exploration of the posterior fossa was carried out by Mr J. W. McIntosh on 2.8.71. A preliminary Myodil ventriculogram was done; this showed that the Myodil was held up in the fourth ventricle, which in its turn was displaced forward and to the left. At operation, when the dura was opened, marked swelling and herniation of the right cerebellar tonsil was noted. Soft material in the right cerebellar hemisphere was removed by suction and the tonsillar herniation through the foramen magnum was reduced. Histology showed that the softened tissue was a cerebellar infarct.

Subsequent detailed search for a possible cause of infarction failed to reveal a source of emboli or primary arterial disease.

He was discharged home 22 days after admission and had returned to work within two months. When finally reviewed on 17.4.72 he was well and working full time. No abnormal signs were detected in the central nervous system.

General care

So far attention has been focused on the neurological problems of detecting the changes occurring in established cerebral infarction. Other factors are of equal importance, notably the the monitoring and possible manipulation of the blood pressure, the prevention of fluid and electrolyte disturbance, and the maintenance of an adequate oxygen supply. Subsidiary considerations include the management of convulsions, the necessity for angiography, and the need for surgical treatment.

BLOOD PRESSURE

A fall in blood pressure is not a feature of uncomplicated acute cerebral infarction, and the presence of hypotension should immediately prompt a search for the underlying cause. This will commonly be found to be due to myocardial infarction, pulmonary embolus, or internal bleeding. On occasions septicaemia has been

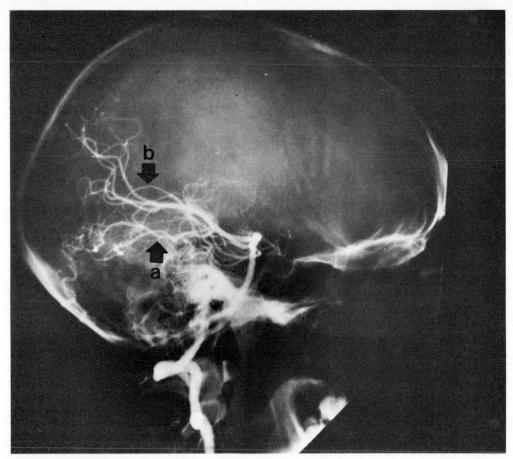

Fig. 9.2 Vertebral angiogram in massive infarct of right cerebellar hemisphere.
a = Left superior cerebellar artery in normal position.
b = Elevation of right superior cerebellar artery.

recorded as the underlying cause of the hypotension (Shaw *et al.*, 1959, Ng *et al.*, 1970). Any
of these conditions can cause hypotension which
may precipitate cerebral infarction. It is rarely
difficult to demonstrate the cause of the hypotension by routine clinical methods.

It is now believed that frequent recording of
the systemic blood pressure does not make any
major contribution to the assessment of brain
stem ischaemia secondary to a hemisphere space
occupying lesion. The classical signs of falling
pulse rate and rising blood pressure are no
longer regarded as reliable signs of increased
intracranial pressure (Plum and Posner, 1972).

In the more general context of raised intracranial pressure Miller and Adams (1972) observed
that bradycardia and increased arterial tension
are frequently absent even with an intracranial
pressure in excess of 75 mmHg (1000 mm H_2O).

However, combined clinical and pathological
studies have thrown some interesting light on
variations of the blood pressure in association
with vascular lesions. Ito, Omae, and Katsuki
(1973) reported on the results of autopsies on
108 patients of whom 51 were found to have
cerebral haemorrhage and 57 cerebral infarction. The vascular lesions affected the hemispheres or the brain stem but not the cerebellum.

The blood pressure readings were available in all patients.

Their conclusions were quite precise. In lesions which were situated either rostral to the midbrain or were in the medulla oblongata there was no associated elevation of the blood pressure. An elevation of the blood pressure did occur with primary pontine lesions whether they were due to haemorrhage or infarction or where cerebral haemorrhage extended into the fourth ventricle or the pons. Blood pressure elevations were more marked in tegmental pontine lesions than in lesions affecting the basilar pons. They concluded that caudal brain stem lesions, especially in the pons, had a causal role to play in blood pressure elevation following cerebral vascular accidents.

Induced hypertension

The belief that elevating the systemic arterial blood pressure—and thus altering the perfusion pressure of the brain—may be beneficial in cerebral ischaemia is not new. Shanbrom and Levy (1957), Farhat and Schneider (1967), and Wise (1970) have all published observations on its effects. Wise, Sutter, and Burkholder (1972) published an interesting study on the treatment of brain ischaemia with vasopressive drugs.

They studied 13 consecutive normotensive patients with signs of focal brain ischaemia who were seen within four hours of the onset of the ictus. The blood pressure in these patients was elevated by drugs from a mean of 158/85 to 170/100, and in five of these neurological function improved. Although this is a small series the case histories given are remarkable.

The first patient, a man of 54, recovered neurological function on elevation of the blood pressure from 125/80 mmHg to 170 mmHg within minutes. The neurological defect recurred no less than five times when the blood pressure was allowed to subside to its original level. Although not quite so dramatic as this, the observations in four other cases showed similar changes which would be difficult to explain by chance alone. These findings are not unexpected, for Ross Russell (1970) has demonstrated in the experimental animal that after regional occlusion the pial vessels in the ischaemic area and surrounding zones behaved passively in response to changes in blood pressure.

Management of established hypertension

A commoner clinical problem is the patient presenting with hypertension and focal neurological signs. The level of the blood pressure is of no value in differentiating between cerebral haemorrhage and cerebral infarction as the classical studies of Aring and Merritt (1935) have shown.

The clinico-pathological study of Hudson and Hylan (1958) complements this study. In 100 autopsies a well documented clinical history of hypertension was available. They recognised a group of patients who survived cerebral haemorrhage but in only half of these was the CSF bloodstained at the time of the acute episode. They rightly emphasised the considerable difficulty in differentiating between non-fatal cerebral haemorrhage and cerebral infarction.

There is developing evidence from pathological and clinical studies (Cole and Yates, 1967; Acheson, 1971) that a significant proportion of patients presenting with focal cerebral lesions and a diastolic blood pressure over 110 mm will have sustained a localised cerebral haemorrhage. On clinical grounds, however, it may be impossible to differentiate for certain between an infarct and a localised haemorrhage and, therefore, an empirical approach is necessary. The dangers of treating hypertension in the acute phase of ischaemic cerebral infarct have undoubtedly been overemphasised. If there is evidence of focal vascular hemisphere lesion without signs of secondary brain stem involvement and if there is a history of significant, pre-existing hypertension which can be established either from previous blood pressure readings, from ECG, or from radiological studies of the heart, then the blood pressure can be controlled immediately. If careful clinical supervision is maintained significant side effects are rare and can be easily corrected. It is true that blood pressure elevation secondary to brain stem infarction may lead to difficulties. But if care is taken to exclude patients where there is the possibility of a space-occupying lesion in the posterior fossa, and if similar care is used in reducing the blood pressure, then again the majority of harmful side-effects can be avoided.

FLUIDS AND ELECTROLYTES

Disturbances of fluid and electrolyte balance must always be considered as a serious potential hazard to patients with disturbance of their conscious level (Sambrook, Hutchinson, and Aber 1973). Attention to the basic principles covering the daily requirements of water (2000 to 3000 ml), sodium (80 to 120 m.Eq), potassium (60 to 90 m.Eq) and calories (2500 to 3000) will maintain a satisfactory metabolic nutritional state in the majority of patients.

It should be emphasised that the above values are basal daily metabolic requirements and do not take into account other losses of biological fluids which may occur at the time of the acute episode through vomiting or during a period of prolonged treatment. Any such losses will require to be taken into account, and careful charting of the daily intake and output (with biochemical analysis of the latter) from all sources should be established for the semi-comatose or unconscious patient as soon as possible. Daily records of weight will often prove valuable in helping to assess fluid requirements.

Attention to serum and urine osmolality will aid the recognition of inappropriate ADH secretion and its differentiation from other states of hyponatraemia. On the other hand hypernatraemia and hyponatraemia are alleged to represent genuine disturbances of sodium and water homeostasis resulting from 'cerebral injury' which cannot be accounted for by inadequate attention to the intake and output balance (Welt, Seldin, German, and Peters, 1952; Cort, 1954; Taylor, 1961; El-Zayat and El-Danasoury, 1972).

The clinical importance of recognising disturbances of electrolyte metabolism is emphasised when one examines the case reports of neurological abnormalities in hyponatraemia. Convulsions and drowsiness are well-recognised clinical expressions of a low serum sodium, but their occurrence without appreciation of the possible role of disturbed electrolyte levels could easily confuse the management of these patients.

Epstein, Levitin, Glaser, and Lavietes (1961) described a 16-year-old girl who on one occasion was deeply unconscious with pin point pupils and divergent squint, neck rigidity, flaccid limbs, and bilateral extensor plantar responses. The cause was hyponatraemia and there is little doubt that such a clinical picture presenting without knowledge of the disturbance of serum electrolytes could cause considerable diagnostic confusion.

MAINTAINING OXYGEN SUPPLY

The maintenance of adequate blood oxygenation is essential in all patients in coma regardless of the cause.

In the majority of patients with a restricted neurological lesion due to cerebral infarction the maintenance of an adequate airway presents no problems. If infection or pulmonary infarction develops or is superimposed on pre-existing chronic lung disease, then appropriate antibiotic therapy may be necessary.

In patients where consciousness is impaired the problems are very different. If clinical signs of hypoxia are present then the immediate administration of 100 per cent oxygen is advisable, thereafter maintaining the blood oxygen level by monitoring the arterial gases where this is appropriate. The precipitating cause for the hypoxia will usually be due to one of two causes. The first is an obstructed airway, the second incipient respiratory failure due to brain stem involvement.

The obstructed airway can usually be dealt with by adequate care of the upper respiratory airway maintained by simple suction. If the obstruction is in the bronchial tree then bronchoscopy may be necessary to achieve an adequate airway. Clearly it is a matter of clinical judgement whether this should be undertaken if the chances of survival are negligible.

A similar caution applies to heroic methods such as tracheostomy. It is general experience that modern methods of resuscitation have led to a far more widespread use of intubation and tracheostomy than in the days when these procedures were reserved for upper airway obstruction.

The decision to advocate tracheostomy in a

patient with an extensive cerebral infarction requires justification, and the limited amount of information available on the subject would offer slender support for such action.

Lancaster (1973) published the results of tracheostomy in patients with 'stroke'. Twenty-five patients were reviewed, but there were only 12 survivors from the acute stage. Of the 12 survivors eight died within 10 weeks of discharge and one within six months. All the other patients surviving required continuous nursing care. Two patients made a good recovery and indicate one of the two exceptions where assisted respiration may be justified.

These two patients presented with pontine lesions. In infarcts of the lateral medullary area some patients may appear—and are in fact—desperately ill for a period of time. Total dysphagia may render it difficult if not impossible to maintain adequate respiration and nutrition because of retained pharyngeal secretion; here assisted respiration by means of endotracheal intubation or tracheostomy may be justified and necessary for a time because of the remarkable capacity for recovery some of these patients show.

The other exception to the use of controlled respiration is where a trial of hyperventilation is being carried out in an attempt to influence the blood supply to the ischaemic area. This will be considered later.

EPILEPSY

The incidence of convulsions in occlusive cerebral vascular disease has been variously estimated at 7.7 per cent per 1000 patients by Louis and McDowell (1967) and 5 per cent by Moskowitz, Lightbody, and Freitag (1972) in the first two years of the natural history.

Dodge, Richardson, and Victor (1954) as a result of a pathological study of six cases of cerebral infarction confirmed previous views that involvement of the cortex was important in the pathogenesis of epilepsy in this condition.

The figures of Aring and Merritt (1935) still appear to be as reliable as any relating to the incidence of epilepsy in the acute phase of cerebral infarction. They observed a 6.6 per

cent prevalence in pathologically proven cases of 'cerebral thrombosis'. Convulsions at the onset of cerebral haemorrhage were more than twice as frequent (14.8 per cent).

The development of major convulsions in the acute stage of cerebral infarction demands treatment directed to the control of the convulsions and the maintenance of an adequate airway to avoid hypoxia. The latter has already been discussed.

Anticonvulsant treatment is neither more or less difficult than in other forms of epilepsy. The intravenous use of diazepam (Valium 5 mg) is usually sufficient to achieve control. In the event of further intravenous diazepam being necessary then the modern intravenous cannulae, which permit the administration of continuous intravenous fluids and intermittent intravenous injections, are valuable.

Jacksonian epilepsy, and rarely 'epilepsia partialis continuans', may occur at the onset of an infarct. Both should be treated with routine anticonvulsants such as primidone or phenytoin as much for the comfort of the patient as anything else. The former will commonly respond briskly to treatment, the latter slowly if at all but will usually regress within a few days. If it does not then revision of the diagnosis will almost certainly be necessary.

VASCULAR SURGERY AND ANGIOGRAPHY

In the early days of extracranial vascular surgery carotid surgery in the acute stage of cerebral infarction was frequently practised. Enthusiasm has now waned. Fields (1973) with considerable experience in this field indicated that extracranial vascular surgery carried out in the acute phase is attended by a mortality of 50 per cent. Since this is considerably more than the anticipated mortality with conservative treatment there does not appear to be any real justification for its practice.

In established cerebral infarction arteriography should no longer be necessary in the majority of patients for the purpose of diagnosis. It then follows that there is no place for cerebral angiography in the management of established cerebral infarction in the acute phase since angiography should only be practised prior to surgery.

There are two groups of patients, both presenting with hemisphere lesions, where angiography may become essential. In the first group the history may be so obscure, either due to aphasia or because of an inadequate history from relatives, that it may be impossible to obtain a picture of the evolution of the ictus and therefore be confident on clinical grounds of the diagnosis of cerebral infarction. In the second group of patients there may be a rapid progression of the physical signs associated with a deteriorating level of consciousness, sometimes associated with papilloedema, where a decision to carry out angiography cannot be deferred. Only then can one be reasonably certain that an eminently treatable neurosurgical lesion, such as an intracranial cyst or a subdural haematoma, is not overlooked.

In this small group of patients the commonest vascular lesion demonstrated is an occlusion of the internal carotid artery at its origin, usually without evidence of collateral flow.

NEUROSURGERY

In hemisphere infarction it is probably true that neurosurgical treatment is rarely if ever attempted. Decompression by means of a fairly large bone flap and the removal by suction of all necrotic material has been advocated in certain cases by Greenwood (1968). However, his initial experiences would hardly encourage enthusiastic support. Ten patients were submitted to operation. Four died, three were left with severe disability, and three had 'moderate and acceptable neurological deficit'.

The one urgent condition of an established stroke which will require neurosurgical assistance is that of massive cerebellar infarction. The syndrome has already been described. Having established the diagnosis, then the urgency for neurosurgical treatment can only be compared with the necessity for early operation for extradural haematoma at any site.

DIABETES MELLITUS

The routine screening for diabetes mellitus should be obligatory in all forms of ischaemic vascular disease. The reported incidence of diabetes mellitus in the general population is often an index of the degree to which the diagnosis has been pursued. The Royal College of General Practitioners' survey in 1962 reported an incidence of 3.3 per cent in 18 532 patients. In contrast Sharp, Butterfield, and Keen (1964), in a population of 25 701 using where appropriate a battery of investigations, observed an incidence in the population of 12 per cent.

The true frequency of diabetes mellitus in established cerebral infarction is not clearly defined. That selection of cases tends to exaggerate the prevalence of diabetes mellitus is suggested by the experience of Silverstein and Doniger (1963); in patients with arteriographic evidence of arterial occlusion a prevalence of 32 per cent was observed. In contrast Goldenberg, Alex, and Blumenthal (1958) in 3470 autopsies found an overall prevalence of diabetes mellitus of 7.6 per cent. There was no evidence of a higher prevalence of diabetes mellitus in patients with established cerebral vascular disease.

The age of onset of the stroke may well be important, however, for in a review by Louis and McDowell (1967) of 'young strokes' they observed a prevalence of diabetes mellitus of 42 per cent, the diabetes developing either before, during, or in the immediate follow-up period after the acute episode.

The importance of routine screening for diabetes mellitus in the acute management of the established stroke is emphasised by the report of Anderson (1974). He described three patients with acute focal signs in the central nervous system presenting as emergencies. In each patient diabetes mellitus was demonstrated, and following treatment full and rapid resolution of signs occurred in two.

McCurdy (1970), discussing the relatively recently recognised entity of hyperosmolar hyperglycaemic non-ketotic diabetic coma, felt that the high mortality was related not only to the absence of the classical signs of diabetic ketosis in this condition but also to the tendency to diagnose a cerebral vascular accident because of focal neurological signs and the patient's age.

TREATMENT

Attempts to minimise the disastrous effects of acute cerebral infarction may be considered under five headings:

1. Attempts to control cerebral oedema.
2. The use of vasodilators.
3. The use of hyperventilation.
4. The use of anticoagulants.
5. The use of low molecular weight dextran.

Cerebral oedema

Attempts to control cerebral oedema date back to the original observations of Weed and McKibben (1919). One of the nicest examples of serendipity is the result of their decision to observe changes in the concentration of sodium and chloride in the cerebrospinal fluid following the injection of hypertonic saline. Shortly after the intravenous injection of hypertonic sodium chloride they found that CSF could not be obtained from the subarachnoid space. They immediately appreciated the significance of this observation and the results are now well known. A sustained rise in CSF pressure occurred with hypotonic solutions whereas with hypertonic solutions there was an initial rise of CSF pressure followed shortly by a marked fall. These observations initiated numerous attempts to control cerebral oedema over the next few decades.

Many substances attained temporary popularity but most have had the disadvantage that following the control of raised intracranial pressure there has been a 'rebound phenomenon' within a matter of hours and the CSF pressure has returned to its original level or even higher. Intravenous urea remained popular for a considerable time but later it was realised that it also showed a delayed rebound phenomenon. There was also clinical evidence of toxicity of urea, particularly in high concentration, and so it lost popularity in clinical practice.

Hypertonic mannitol solution was introduced and is still useful in certain circumstances. Wise and Chater (1962) described its use in 70 patients with various intracranial lesions, and with a 20 per cent solution they found it to be an effective method for achieving temporary control of raised intracranial pressure.

For obvious reasons the majority of attempts to control cerebral oedema were carried out in patients where the oedema is secondary to tumours in the hemisphere or the posterior fossa. However there have been studies which have attempted to influence the course of established hemisphere infarction in the acute stages with measures designed to reduce cerebral oedema. Two substances worth examining are glycerol and corticosteroids.

GLYCEROL

Meyer, Charney, Rivera, and Mathew (1971) reported on 36 patients with acute cerebral infarction who were treated with glycerol in a dose of 1.2 g per kg of body weight every 24 hours in a 10 per cent solution of saline or in dextrose and water. Treatment was started within 72 hours of the onset. The mortality was 11 per cent and the deaths were confined to those patients who were in coma when treatment was begun. In all other patients neurological improvement was observed at the end of four days of treatment. There were no toxic side effects and it was noted that glycerol administration was associated with a fall in the CSF pressure without evidence of a rebound phenomenon.

In a further report Meyer, Fukuuchi, Shimazu, Ohuchi, and Ericsson (1972) described the intravenous use of glycerol and its effect on hemisphere blood flow and brain metabolism in patients with an acute cerebral infarction. Seventeen patients were studied and the estimations were carried out within two weeks of the infarct in all but three patients. Arterial oxygen uptake, CO_2 tension, and pH were recorded throughout the observations and hemisphere blood flow was calculated by the hydrogen electrode technique.

During the infusion the hemisphere blood flow increased in all but one patient and a mean increase in blood flow of 8 per cent was considered to be significant. The effect on blood flow, however, was transient. The central venous pressure and the intracranial venous pressure both increased significantly during the infusion, but on completion the intracranial venous pressure fell below the pre-infusion levels.

The mean CSF pressure did not change during the infusion but decreased significantly afterwards. They noted striking changes in the EEG during the infusion and in the majority of patients neurological function also improved. They concluded that the expansion of the perivascular space by removal of the oedema fluid within the glial cells seemed to be the primary factor in causing an increase in hemisphere blood flow.

Their conclusion was that their clinical and experimental observations gave some credence to the view that the intravenous use of glycerol was a useful form of therapy in patients with acute cerebral infarction.

CORTICOSTEROIDS

The effectiveness of steroids in the control of cerebral oedema was soon appreciated. Galicich, French, and Melby (1961) reviewed the literature up to that time and described the use of dexamethazone in 14 patients with raised intracranial pressure due to tumour. They observed a dramatic improvement with relief of signs and symptoms of raised intracranial pressure. In two cases they obtained angiographic proof of decrease in the size of the intracranial mass as a result of steroids which they felt was due to a decrease in the oedema surrounding the tumour.

Russek, Zohman, and Russek (1954) were the first to report the use of cortisone in the acute treatment of 'apoplectic stroke' in 12 patients. Three patients with cerebral haemorrhage died without benefit. In the remaining nine patients they were enthusiastic about the results. The rapid resolution of symptoms in response to steroids caused them to state that 'cortisone accompanied in one day what ordinarily might take several weeks of conservative treatment'. The dose used was 300 mg orally over 48 hours reducing to 50 mg daily at the end of the first week. Roberts (1958) considered that steroid therapy in acute and subacute vascular accidents, particularly when there was clinical evidence of brain stem involvement, made a positive contribution to treatment.

Dyken and White (1956) did not share this enthusiasm. They reported on 36 patients whom they divided into two groups according to the severity of the stroke, the age at onset, and the blood pressure. Seventeen patients were treated with 300 mg of cortisone daily and 19 patients received a placebo. Thirteen deaths occurred in the treated group and 10 in the placebo group. After studying the clinical results of the survivors they detected a trend indicating that cortisone 'may be a dangerous drug to use in cerebral vascular disease'.

The experiments of Plum, Alvord, and Posner (1963) also demonstrated that steroids had little value in controlling the effects of experimental ischaemia. They gave dexamethasone to rats both before and after a controlled ischaemic insult. They found that mortality during anoxia was significantly elevated among animals treated with corticoids, and in the surviving animals treatment with steroids did not appear to have any significant effect on the clinical outcome, the extent and degree of cerebral oedema, on the cerebral electrolyte content, or on the extent of cerebral vascular damage.

The use of steroids in cerebral infarction has been re-examined in the past five years but conclusions as to their benefit are still diametrically opposed.

Patten et al. (1972) carried out a double blind study on a group of patients with a sudden focal neurological deficit of less than 24 hours' duration. The patients were assigned randomly to treated and control groups. Neurological examination was carried out by skilled observers at intervals over three weeks after admission, and assessment was based on a scoring system. The dose of steroids was 16 mg daily of dexamethasone for 10 days followed by a gradual reduction to zero over the next week; at the conclusion of the study 17 patients had acted as controls and 14 patients were treated.

The scoring system indicated that the patients treated with steroids had improved their functional status by an average of 12 per cent whereas the placebo group had deteriorated to a similar degree. When they considered 15 patients who were severely affected by the initial infarct the benefit of steroids was, they felt, even more clearly demonstrated since the treated group improved 23 per cent whereas the placebo group deteriorated 14 per cent. These results were statistically significant. They concluded, not unnaturally, that dexamethasone was a useful adjunct to the treatment of patients with stroke and its effect was due to controlling the amount of cerebral oedema secondary to massive cerebral infarction.

Bauer and Tellez (1973) also reported a double blind trial using dexamethasone in 50 cases with cerebral infarction. They were quite unable to detect any difference between the treated and the untreated patient. They fully appreciated the discrepancy between their findings and those of Patten *et al.* (1972) and indicated that if there was any difference in case material between the two groups of patients then their own patients were probably more severely ill than in the trial of Patten *et al.* (1972).

If this were true then their results might have been expected to parallel those of Patten *et al.* (1972), who observed the best results in the most severely affected cases. No obvious reason other than unwitting case selection can be put forward to explain these widely discrepant results.

Vasodilators

The lack of agreement on the effectiveness of agents designed to reduce cerebral oedema is mirrored in the opinions expressed on the use of vasodilators. Waltz (1971) writes 'present evidence provides no support for the use of vasodilators in the treatment of acute cerebral ischaemia'. McHenry (1972), discussing the merits of cerebral vasodilatation in cerebral infarction, wrote 'one cannot accept the pessimism that there is no hope from more thorough evaluation and more aggressive management of the acute stroke'.

The heart of the disagreement lies in the recent advances in knowledge which have been achieved by the methods of studying regional blood flow following cerebral infarction. A detailed treatment of this topic is given in Chapter 5. It only needs to be restated briefly that following ischaemia there may be adjacent areas of vasomotor paralysis with abolition both of the normal response to CO_2 and to

variations in systemic blood pressure. It has been argued that, because of impaired vasomotor control, increasing the cerebral blood flow by any means may deviate blood from the ischaemic areas achieving a result which is the reverse of that intended (intracerebral steal'). The question of how serious or how frequent is this phenomenon is still debated.

Cerebral vasodilatation can be induced in two ways. The first is the utilisation of the well-known response of the cerebral circulation to hypercarbia. The second is the administration by the arterial, venous, or oral route of drugs capable of inducing vasodilatation.

THE EFFECT OF CO_2 INHALATION

The introduction by Kety and Schmidt (1945) of an ethically acceptable method of measuring the total cerebral blood flow in man was the start of the unravelling of the dynamic events which may follow cerebral infarction. The remarkable rapidity with which total cerebral blood flow can be restored following carotid artery occlusion was shown by the acute experiments of Shenkin *et al.* (1951) in carotid artery occlusion carried out for intracranial aneurysms, and their observations have been expanded experimentally by Symon *et al.* (1963) and Eklof and Schwartz (1969).

The demonstration by Kety and Schmidt (1948) that 7 per cent CO_2 in inspired air could double the cerebral blood flow inevitably led to the examination of the possibility that CO_2 may contribute to the treatment of cerebral vascular disease. It was soon shown that the response to CO_2 of the cerebral circulation affected by occlusive vascular disease is not a simple one. Fazekas and Alman (1964) in patients with angiographically proven occlusive vascular disease of the major vessels of the neck observed that there were two recognisable groups of patients. There were those who responded in a normal, or near normal, fashion to inspired CO_2 by increasing the cerebral blood flow; in other patients, apparently affected in an identical manner, there was no useful response. This observation indicated, they believed, an exhaustion of the homeostatic reserves and concluded there was a potential danger in the use of CO_2 in cerebral vascular disease whether the disease be in the acute or chronic phase.

A clinical evaluation of the effects of 5 per cent CO_2 inhalation was carried out by Millikan (1955). Two hundred and seventy-five patients formed the basis of his observations of whom 50 were given CO_2 and 225 were untreated. Although the design of the trial was not ideal by modern standards he could find no evidence of any benefit from the administration of CO_2.

McHenry *et al.* (1972) carried out regional blood flow studies on normal subjects, on patients with diffuse cerebral arterial disease, and on patients with known focal vascular disease which had been demonstrated by angiography. Five per cent CO_2 was administered and the effects on the regional blood flow were studied. In the normals there was the anticipated increase in the cerebral blood flow. The response in diffuse cerebral vascular disease was much less, showing a mean increase of 28 per cent as compared with 60 per cent in the normal. In patients with focal vascular lesions hypercarbia increased the mean cerebral blood flow but there was a less marked response in the focal areas of ischaemia. They felt that 'intracerebral steal' was a rare occurrence. For this reason they believed that the dangers of increasing cerebral blood flow by vasodilatation had been overstressed.

They did, however, conclude that on the evidence of clinical and experimental studies which had been carried out there could be no support for the view that CO_2 makes a contribution to the treatment of acute cerebral infarction. The fact that both the mean arterial pressure and cardiac output was significantly increased was, they felt, another good reason for not advocating the use of CO_2 in treatment. Few would disagree with this conclusion.

VASODILATATION BY DRUGS

Many substances have been examined for the ability to produce cerebral vasodilatation. Papaverine is a well-established cerebral vasodilator and has been examined in some detail. Its use has been alternatively recommended and condemned and the observations on this drug illustrate well the areas of contention which apply to all vasodilator drugs acting directly on the cerebral blood vessels.

Papaverine

Jayne, Scheinberg, Rich, and Belle (1952) demonstrated that intravenous papaverine hydrochloride could significantly increase cerebral blood flow. Using the nitrous oxide method they found a significant mean increase in cerebral blood flow. Since they detected no concomitant change in the mean arterial pressure or the pH of the blood they deduced that this was a direct cerebral vasodilatory effect by the drug.

Experimental evidence cited by Meyer, Teraura, Sakamoto, and Hashi (1971) indicated that oral papaverine may also be capable of increasing cerebral blood flow. In baboons, within 20 to 60 minutes after the oral administration of the drug, cerebral blood flow increased and the A-V oxygen difference decreased to a significant degree. They found no significant change in the systemic blood pressure.

The clinical use of papaverine hydrochloride in the treatment of stroke had already been reported by Meyer, Gotoh, Gilroy, and Nara (1965). They studied a series of 70 cases, 30 of whom received intravenous papaverine and 36 acted as controls. They used a scoring system based on physical signs which they said were objective and reproducible within one point by different observers.

They monitored the cerebral arterio-venous oxygen difference and combined this with a clinical assessment of the two groups. Following papaverine they found a significant increase in the oxygen uptake of the brain and in the treated group they found a significantly greater clinical improvement than in the control group.

McHenry, Jaffe, and Kawamura (1970) examined the effects of papaverine on regional blood flow in focal vascular disease. They examined six patients with focal cerebral vascular disease demonstrated by angiography. After basal cerebral blood flow measurements they gave 100 mg of papaverine intravenously over a 30 minute period and, 50 minutes after this, again assessed the hemisphere and regional blood flow.

Before papaverine, in all six cases, the individual regional blood flow values in the area which was shown to be abnormal by angiography were all below the limits of normal as was the total hemisphere blood flow in each patient. After papaverine the mean cerebral blood flow for the whole group was increased by 18 per cent per 100 g of brain per minute, an increase which was significant. In addition to this, eight of the individual regional values for cerebral blood flow over an angiographically abnormal area also increased significantly.

They emphasised that whilst they found no evidence of a decrease in flow in ischaemic areas in their patients they could not coincidentally find evidence that papaverine improved neurological function.

Olesen and Paulson (1971) studied the effects of intracarotid injection of 10 mg of papaverine on regional blood flow in 27 patients. In patients without focal flow abnormalities the regional blood flow showed a uniform increase which averaged 93 per cent. In patients with focal flow abnormalities the flow values were subnormal in the whole hemisphere and where an ischaemic focus occurred the response to papaverine was decreased, or demolished. In one instance they obtained a clear-cut example of 'intracerebral steal' occurring where the reduction of flow in focal areas simultaneously occurring with flow increase in non-focal areas.

Examining all the experimental evidence they concluded that the existence of an 'intracerebral steal' had been frequently demonstrated and 'that it probably occurs frequently in apoplexy after papaverine injection'. Therefore, they believed the rationale of such treatment was open to serious doubt.

Again there is the dilemma, as with agents for reducing cerebral oedema, of reconciling diametrically opposed views on the value of vasodilators in cerebral infarction. Conclusions from studies of variations in the response of the cerebral circulation in areas of focal ischaemia can only complement well designed clinical studies. They cannot replace them. At the moment the information from trials is too limited to allow useful conclusions to be drawn.

HYPERVENTILATION AND INDUCED HYPOCARBIA

The belief that increasing the CO_2 content in the inspired air and thus producing hypercarbia may in fact be harmful in cerebral infarction resulted in the examination of the possibility that hypocarbia induced by hyperventilation may be beneficial.

Soloway, Nadel, Albin, and White (1968) demonstrated that reducing the P_{CO_2} to 25 mm restricted the area of infarction following experimental occlusion. Battistini, Casacchia, and Bartolini (1969), also in experimental animals, showed that, after ischaemia, hyperventilation either restored the circulation in a large part of the ischaemic area or prevented a progressive decrease in blood flow. Soloway, Moriarty, Fraser, and White (1970) on the basis of experimental data suggested that time may be all-important. In experiments where there was a delay in inducing hypocarbia for more than one hour after the occlusion a subsequent period of three to four hours of hypocarbia produced no beneficial effect on the extent of the infarct. If this observation is ultimately shown to be applicable to patients with cerebral infarction then the results may well be disappointing.

A clinical trial of hyperventilation in the acute stroke has been reported by Christensen (1970) where 42 patients with an acute stroke were treated with prolonged hyperventilation. The interval between the onset and the commencement of treatment was, with few exceptions, less than 24 hours.

The procedure was that the patients were ventilated through an endotracheal tube for 72 hours. The patients were randomised and in those assigned to the hypocarbic group they aimed to obtain an arterial P_{CO_2} of about 25 mmHg. In the 'untreated' group the respirator was adjusted to give an arterial P_{CO_2} of 40 mmHg.

When they compared patients with an occluded internal carotid artery they could find no difference between the treated and untreated group; in patients with occlusion of the middle cerebral artery they found the mortality was decreased in patients treated with hypocarbia. Among patients without evidence of arteriographic occlusion there was a reduction of the mortality but no effect on the result in terms of improved neurological function.

Overall, although they emphasised that the numbers were too small for valid statistical analysis, they felt that their results suggested that hypocarbia had beneficial effects on acute brain lesions by reducing the mortality. They admitted that the results were not impressive and did not, in their view, justify prolonged hypocarbia as a routine treatment in all patients with acute stroke. The treatment is difficult to perform and there are complications. Nevertheless, they felt that it was possible to select cases of stroke for treatment by induced hypocarbia and these would be the relatively young patients without cardiac or pulmonary disease and with evidence of a very recent stroke.

Anticoagulants

There is sufficient information available now on the use of anticoagulants in the management of the completed stroke due to occlusive vascular disease to refer to them only briefly. It is generally agreed that anticoagulants are contraindicated.

Millikan (1971) discussed the use of anticoagulants in various types of occlusive cerebral vascular disease. He reviewed five contributions where the clinical condition of completed stroke was observed and where controls were compared with the treated patients.

It is clear from the results obtained that there was little or no evidence that the treated group fared better than the controls in terms of recurrence of cerebral infarction; there is also the potential hazard of cerebral haemorrhage. With the growing awareness of the importance of localised intracerebral haematoma as a cause of focal cerebral vascular disease there can be little justification for treatment with anticoagulants in the acute phase of the completed stroke.

Anticoagulants may, however, have a part to play in the management of progressive cerebral infarction (stroke in evolution), that small minority of patients in whom neurological deficit becomes worse during a period of observation of some hours. The mechanism of progressive ischaemia is thought to be extension or propaga-

tion of thrombus, e.g. up the internal carotid artery to involve the terminal branches. The diagnosis of progressive cerebral infarction should be made with great caution since it may resemble closely a subdural or intracerebral haematoma or even a cerebral tumour. Patients with stroke may also deteriorate from extracerebral causes such as cardiac failure or hypoxia.

In cerebral ischaemia progression is usually stepwise or fluctuating with periods of improvement but this is not always the case. Either the carotid or vertebrobasilar territory may be involved. CSF examination and EMI scanning is advisable in case of doubt.

This is a difficult group in which to assess the effects of anticoagulants. The degree of ultimate disability in treated and control groups have been compared (Baker et al., 1962) and the proportion of patients showing progression was somewhat less in the treated group. More significantly, the death rate from cerebral infarction was also reduced by treatment (Carter, 1961).

Because of the urgency of the situation the anticoagulant used is intravenous heparin for the first 48 hours (10000 units over six hours by continuous infusion). Treatment is continued with warfarin or subcutaneous heparin (5000 units six hourly) for two weeks.

In the management of patients with recent cerebral infarction secondary to embolism from the heart the role of anticoagulants is to lessen the risk of repeated embolism rather than to effect the outcome of the existing stroke (see Chap. 14). Heparin is administered as soon as the diagnosis is made, is replaced after 48 hours by warfarin and the latter drug is continued indefinitely, under laboratory control.

Low molecular weight dextran

The importance of changes in the microvasculature in determining the extent of ischaemia has been reviewed by Wells (1964). Aggregation and thrombosis of the blood components in the microcirculation and an increased viscosity due to haemoconcentration are all features which may occur. Evidence has accumulated that the use of intravenous low molecular weight dextran may be useful in combating these changes by its action in expanding plasma volume rather than by a specific effect on viscosity.

Gilroy, Barnhart, and Meyer (1969) reported on a clinical trial of 100 patients with acute cerebral ischaemia and infarction due to atherosclerotic thrombo-embolism. All patients had sustained a severe neurological deficit without improvement 24 to 72 hours before entering into the study. The patients were divided into treated and control groups on a randomised basis. Initially the treated group were given 500 ml of dextran 40 over an interval of an hour. This was followed by a slow intravenous infusion of dextran 40 at the rate of 500 ml every 12 hours. They used a scoring system already referred to (Meyer *et al.*, 1965) and found that in the treated group there was a significant improvement in mental state and total neurological function. This improvement in the treated group was significantly better than in the untreated group. They also studied variations in platelet behaviour and demonstrated that in patients with an acute stroke platelet aggregation was increased in the venous blood. Low molecular weight dextran caused the platelet abnormality to return to normal.

The future

The undoubted advances in knowledge of the haemodynamic changes following cerebral ischaemia which have been made over the past 25 years have not been paralled by advances in treatment. There appear to be several possible reasons for this.

One is that acute cerebral infarction, lacking the emotive appeal of cardiac infarction, has not attracted the attention it deserves as a cause of disability in the community. This may be due, in part, to lack of knowledge of the facts. If the incidence for subarachnoid haemorrhage, cerebral haemorrhage, and cerebral thrombosis are considered together, then 20 per cent of attacks occur in the ages covering the working life. It is true that 40 to 50 per cent of the patients remain in hospital for more than one month but this is independent of age (Acheson and Fairbairn, 1970). There can be little justification, therefore, for regarding cerebral infarction as the province of the geriatric service alone.

A further reason which may not encourage active therapy is the understandable feeling that the majority of patients presenting with cerebral infarction are suffering from the end result of a long process of vascular degeneration. This cannot be denied. What needs to be debated is the view that there is little hope that treatment can make anything more than a marginal contribution to limiting the effects of acute cerebral infarction. It is certain that in a restricted number of infarcts in the vertebro-basilar circulation of the type already referred to it may be necessary to call on the full resources of intensive care units to achieve the best results and that these may approximate to full recovery.

Admittedly, these opportunities are rare and a much commoner problem are patients who sustain a cerebral infarct for the first time, but in whom the occlusion does not involve a whole arterial territory and thus results in the rapid development of cerebral oedema with a fatal outcome within a few days. The wide discrepancy between the views of various observers on the value of treating cerebral oedema or using vasodilators can only be accounted for by an insufficient volume of clinical evidence.

A case can be made for setting up in selected hospitals responsible for acute admissions 'stroke units' where the medical and nursing staff can develop the appropriate skills necessary to the assessment and management of a clinical problem which is frequently complex. Only then will it be possible to evaluate, in unequivocal terms, the potential lines of treatment. It may be that when a definitive assessment is available the final decision will be that the only hope lies in preventative measures such as the adequate control of hypertension and the prevention of atheroma. The evidence presently available, however, does not warrant pre-empting this conclusion by advocating a policy of therapeutic nihilism.

REFERENCES

Acheson, J. (1971) Factors affecting the natural history of focal cerebral vascular disease. *Quarterly Journal of Medicine*, **40**, 25.

Acheson, R. M. (1966) *Mortality from cerebrovascular disease in the United States*. Public Health Monograph, **76**, 23.

Acheson, R. M. & Fairbairn, A. H. (1970) Burden of cerebrovascular disease in the Oxford area in 1963 and 1964. *British Medical Journal*, ii, 621.

Anderson, J. M. (1974) Diabetic ketoacidosis presenting as neurosurgical emergencies. *British Medical Journal*, iii, 22.

Aring, C. D. & Merritt, H. H. (1935) Differential diagnosis between cerebral haemorrhage and cerebral thrombosis. A clinical and pathological study of 245 cases. *Archives of Internal Medicine*, **56**, 435.

Baker, R. N., Broward, J. H., Fang, H. C. *et al.* (1962) Anticoagulant therapy in cerebral infarction: report of a cooperative study. *Neurology* (Minneapolis), **12**, 823.

Battistini, I. N., Casacchia, M. & Bartolini, G. (1969) Effects of hyperventilation on focal brain damage following middle cerebral artery occlusion. In *Cerebral Blood Flow*. New York: Springer Verlag.

Bauer, R. B. & Tellez, H. (1973) Dexamethasone as treatment in cerebrovascular disease. 2. A controlled study in acute cerebral infarction. *Stroke*, **4**, 547.

Boddie, H. G. (1972) Ocular bobbing and opsoclonus. *Journal of Neurology, Neurosurgery and Psychiatry*, **35**, 739.

Carter, A. B. (1961) Anticoagulant treatment in progressing stroke. *British Medical Journal*, ii,70.

Carter, A. B. (1964) *Cerebral infarction*. New York: MacMillan.

Christensen, M. S. (1970) Stroke treated with prolonged hyperventilation. In *Brain and Blood Flow*. Proceedings of the Fourth International Symposium on the Regulation of Cerebral Blood Flow, ed. Ross Russell, R. W. London: Pitman.

Cole, F. M. & Yates, P. O. (1967) The occurrence and significance of intracerebral micro-aneurysms. *Journal of Pathology and Bacteriology*, **93**, 393.

Cort, J. H. (1954) Cerebral salt wasting. *Lancet*, i, 752.

Diabetes Survey Working Party (1962) Report of a working party appointed by the Royal College of General Practitioners. *British Medical Journal*, i, 1497.

Dodge, P. R., Richardson, E. P. & Victor, M. (1954) Recurrent convulsive seizures as a sequel to cerebral infarction. A clinical and pathological study. *Brain*, **77**, 610.

Dyken, M. & White, P. T. (1956) Evaluation of cortisone in treatment of cerebral infarction. *Journal American Medical Association*, **162**, 1531.

Eklof, B. & Schwartz, S. I. (1969) Effects of critical stenosis of the carotid artery and compromised cephalic blood flow. *Archives Surgery*, **99**, 695.

El-Zayat, A. & El-Danasoury, M. (1972) Dysnatremia and cerebrovascular accidents. *Journal of Egyptian Medical Association*, **54**, 68.

Epstein, F. H., Levitin, H., Glaser, G. & Lavietes, P. (1961) Cerebral hyponatremia. *New England Journal of Medicine*, **265**, 513.

Farhat, S. M. & Schneider, R. C. (1967) Observations on the effect of systemic blood pressure on intracranial circulation in patients with cerebrovascular insufficiency. *Journal of Neurosurgery*, **27**, 441.

Fazekas, J. F. & Alman, W. R. (1964) Maximal dilatation of cerebral vessels. *Archives of Neurology*, **11**, 303.

Fields, W. S. (1973) Selection of stroke patients for arterial reconstructive surgery. *The American Journal of Surgery*, **125**, 527.

Fisher, C. M. (1961) *Pathogenesis and Treatment of Cerebrovascular Disease*, ed. Fields, W. S. Springfield, Illinois: Thomas.

Fisher, C. M. (1967) Some neuro-ophthalmological observations. *Journal of Neurology, Neurosurgery and Psychiatry*, **30**, 383.

Galicich, J. H., French, L. A. & Melby, J. C. (1961) Use of dexamethasone in treatment of cerebral oedema associated with brain tumours. *Lancet*, i, 46.

Gilroy, J., Barnhart, M. I. & Meyer, J. S. (1969) Treatment of acute stroke with dextran 40. *The Journal of the American Medical Association*, **210**, 293.

Goldenberg, S., Alex, N. & Blumenthal, H. T. (1958) Sequelae of arteriosclerosis of the aorta and coronary arteries. A statistical study of diabetes mellitus. *Diabetes*, **7**, 98.

Greenwood, J. (1968) Acute brain infarction with high intracranial pressure: surgical indications. *Johns Hopkins Medical Journal*, **122**, 254.

Hudson, A. J. & Hyland, H. H. (1958) Hypertensive cerebrovascular disease: a clinical and pathologic review of 100 cases. *Annals of Internal Medicine*, **49**, 1049.

Ito, A., Omae, T. & Katsuki, S. (1973) Acute changes in blood pressure following vascular diseases in the brain stem. *Stroke*, **4**, 80.

Jayne, H. W., Scheinberg, P., Rich, M. & Belle, M. S. (1952) The effect of intravenous papaverine hydrochloride on cerebral circulation. *Journal of Clinical Investigation*, **31**, 111.

Kety, S. S. & Schmidt, C. F. (1945) The determination of cerebral blood flow in man by use of nitrous oxide in low concentrations. *American Journal of Physiology*, **143**, 53.

Kety, S. S. & Schmidt, C. F. (1948) Nitrous oxide method for the quantitative determination of cerebral blood flow in man. Theory procedure and normal valves. *Journal of Clinical Investigation*, **27**, 476.

Kurtzke, J. F. (1969) *Epidemiology of Cerebrovascular Disease*. New York, Berlin, Heidelberg: Springer Verlag.

Lancaster, M. G. (1973) Tracheostomies and stroke. *Stroke*, **4**, 459.

Lehrich, J. R., Winkler, G. F. & Ojemann, R. G. (1970) Cerebellar infarction with brain stem compression. Diagnosis and surgical treatment. *Archives of Neurology*, **22**, 490.

Louis, S. & McDowell, F. (1967) Epileptic seizures in non-embolic cerebral infarction. *Archives of Neurology*, **17**, 414.

McCurdy, D. K. (1970) Hyperosmolar hyperglycemic nonketotic diabetic coma. *Medical Clinics of North America*, **54**, 683.

McHenry, L. C. (1972) Cerebral vasodilator therapy in stroke. *Stroke*, **3**, 686.

McHenry, L. C., Jaffe, M. E. & Kawamura, J. (1970) Effect of papaverine on regional blood flow in focal vascular disease of the brain. *New England Journal of Medicine*, **282**, 1167.

McHenry, L. C., Goldberg, H. I., Jaffe, M. E., Kenton, E. J., West, J. W. & Cooper, E. S. (1972) Regional cerebral flow. Response to carbon dioxide inhalation in cerebrovascular disease. *Archives of Neurology*, **27**, 403.

Meyer, J. S., Charney, J. Z., Rivera, V. M. & Mathew, N. T. (1971) Treatment with glycerol of cerebral oedema due to acute cerebral infarction. *Lancet*, ii, 993.

Meyer, J. S., Gotoh, F., Gilroy, J. & Nara, N. (1965) Improvement in brain oxygenation and clinical improvement in patients with strokes treated with papaverine hydrochloride. *Journal of American Medical Association*, **194**, 109.

Meyer, J. S., Teraura, T., Sakamoto, K. & Hashi, K. (1971) The effect of pavabid (oral papaverine) on cerebral blood flow and metabolism in the monkey. *Cardiovascular Research Center Bulletin*, **9**, 105.

Meyer, J. S., Fukuuchi, Y., Shimazu, J., Ohuchi, T. & Ericsson, A. D. (1972) Effect of intravenous infusion of glycerol on hemispheric blood flow and metabolism in patients with acute cerebral infarction. *Stroke*, **3**, 168.

Miller, D. & Adams, H. (1972) *Scientific Foundations of Neurology*, ed. Critchley, M., O'Leary, J. L. & Jennett, B. London: Heinemann.

Millikan, C. H. (1955) Evaluation of carbon dioxide inhalation for acute focal cerebral infarction. *Archives of Neurology and Psychiatry*, **73**, 324.

Millikan, C. H. (1971) Reassessment of anticoagulant therapy in various types of occlusive cerebrovascular disease. *Stroke*, **2**, 201.

Moskowitz, E., Lightbody, F. E. H. & Freitag, N. S. (1972) Long term follow up of the post-stroke patient. *Archives of Physical Medicine and Rehabilitation*, **53**, 167.

Ng, L. K. Y. & Nimmannitya, J. (1970) Massive cerebral infarction with severe brain swelling. A clinico-pathological study. *Stroke*, **1**, 158.

O'Brien, M. D., Waltz, A. G., Jordan, M. A. (1974) Ischaemic cerebral edema. *Archives of Neurology*, **30**, 456.

Olesen, J. & Paulson, O. B. (1971) The effect of intra-arterial papaverine on the regional cerebral blood flow in patients with stroke or intracranial tumour. *Stroke*, **2**, 148.

Patten, B. M., Mendell, J., Bruun, B., Curtin, W., Carter, S. (1972) Double-blind study of the effects of dexamethasone on acute stroke. *Neurology*, **22**, 377.

Plum, F., Alvord, E. C., Posner, J. B. (1963) Effect of steroids on experimental cerebral infarction. *Archives of Neurology*, **9**, 571.

Plum, F. & Posner, J. B. (1972) *Diagnosis of Stupor and Coma*, 2nd edn. Philadelphia: Davis.

Roberts, H. J. (1958) Supportive adrenocortical steroid therapy in acute and subacute cerebrovascular accidents with particular reference to brain-stem involvement. *Journal of American Geriatrics*, **6**, 686.

Ross Russell, R. W. (1970) A microangiographic study of experimental cerebral ischaemia and of the effects of blood pressure changes. In *Brain and Blood Flow*. Proceedings of the Fourth International Symposium on Regulation of Cerebral Blood Flow, ed. Ross Russell, R. W. London: Pitman.

Russek, H. I., Zohman, B. L. & Russek, A. S. (1954) Cortisone in the immediate therapy of apoplectic stroke. *Journal American Geriatric Society*, **2**, 216.

Sambrook, M. A., Hutchinson, E. C. & Aber, G. M. (1973) Metabolic studies in subarachnoid haemorrhage and strokes — 11. Serial changes in cerebrospinal fluid and plasma urea electrolytes and osmolality. *Brain*, **96**, 191.

Shanbrom, E. & Levy, L. (1957) The role of systemic blood pressure in cerebral circulation in carotid and basilar artery thromboses. Clinical implications and therapeutic implications of vasopressor agents. *American Journal of Medicine*, **23**, 197.

Sharp, C. L., Butterfield, W. J. H. & Keen, H. (1964) Diabetes Survey in Bedford. *Proceedings of the Royal Society of Medicine*, **57**, 193.

Shaw, C. M., Alvord, E. C. & Berry, R. G. (1959) Swelling of the brain following ischaemic infarction with arterial occlusion. *Archives of Neurology*, **1**, 161.

Shenkin, H. A., Cabieses, F., Van-Den Noordt, G., Sayers, P., Copperman, R. (1951) The hemodynamic effect of unilateral carotid ligation of the cerebral circulation of man. *Journal of Neurosurgery*, **8**, 38.

Silverstein, A. & Doniger, D. E. (1963) Systemic and local conditions predisposing to ischaemic and occlusive cerebrovascular disease. *Journal of the Mount Sinai Hospital, New York*, **30**, 435.

Soloway, M., Nadel, W., Albin, M. S. & White, R. J. (1968) The effect of hyperventilation on subsequent cerebral infarction. *Anesthesiology*, **29**, 975.

Soloway, M., Moriarty, G., Fraser, J. G. & White, R. J. (1970) The effect of delayed hyperventilation on experimental middle cerebral artery occlusion. In *Brain and Blood Flow*. Proceedings of the Fourth International Symposium on the Regulation of Cerebral Blood Flow, ed. Ross Russell, R. W. London: Pitman.

Symon, L., Ishikawa, S., Lavy, S. & Meyer, J. S. (1963) Quantitative measurement of cephalic blood flow in the monkey. *Journal of Neurosurgery*, **20**, 199.

Taylor, W. H. (1961) Hypernatraemia in cerebral disorders. *Journal of Clinical Pathology*, **15**, 211.

Waltz, A. G. (1971) Studies of the cerebral circulation. What they have taught us about stroke? *Mayo Clinic Proceedings*, **46**, 268.

Weed, L. H. & McKibben, P. S. (1919) Pressure changes in the cerebro-spinal fluid following intravenous injection of solutions of various concentrations. *American Journal of Physiology*, **48**, 512.

Wells, R. E. (1964) Rheology of blood in microvasculature. *New England Journal of Medicine*, **270**, 832.

Welt, L. G., Seldin, D. W., Nelson, W. P., German, W. J. & Peters, J. P. (1952) Role of the central nervous system in metabolism of electrolytes and water. *American Medical Association Archives of Internal Medicine*, **29**, 355.

Whisnant, J. P., Fitzgibbons, J. P., Kurland, L. T., Sayre, G. P. (1971) Natural history of stroke in Rochester, Minnesota, 1945 through 1954. *Stroke*, **2**, 11.

Wise, G. (1970) Vasopressor drug therapy for complications of cerebral arteriography. *New England Journal of Medicine*, **282**, 610.

Wise, B. L. & Chater, N. (1962) The value of hypertonic mannitol solution in decreasing brain mass and lowering cerebro-spinal fluid pressure. *Journal of Neurosurgery*, **19**, 1038.

Wise, G., Sutter, R. & Burkholder, J. (1972) The treatment of brain ischemia with vasopressor drugs. *Stroke*, **3**, 135.

10. Cerebral Ischaemia in Hypertension

J. C. Gautier

The adverse effects of high blood pressure on life expectancy are well established (Leishman, 1959; Hodge, McQueen, and Smirk, 1961) and cerebral arterial accidents rank in second place among the causes of death in hypertensives (Breckenridge, Dollery, and Parry, 1970). Furthermore beneficial results of treating hypertension have been repeatedly reported (Hamilton, Thomson, and Wisniewski, 1964; Veterans Administration Cooperative Study Group on Antihypertensive Agents, 1967; Breckenridge et al., 1970). The improved prognosis resulting from antihypertensive treatment also holds true after a cerebral arterial accident (Marshall and Kaeser, 1961; Marshall, 1964; Cambier and Gautier, 1965).

Large and small cerebral haemorrhages are almost entirely confined to hypertensives (Cole and Yates, 1968) and it is likely that the merits of reducing hypertension result largely from a decrease in haemorrhagic accidents (Breckenridge et al., 1970; Beevers et al., 1973). However there is also a strong case for hypertension as a significant aetiological factor in cerebral infarction. A prospective study has proved that hypertension is the most common and potent precursor of atherothrombotic brain infarction (Kannel, Wolf, Verter, and McNamara, 1970; Kannel, 1971). The fact that hypertension is a major risk factor in brain infarction has been confirmed in other surveys (Whisnant, 1974; Shekelle, Ostfeld, and Klawans, 1974). In a postmortem controlled series Low-Beer and Phear (1961) showed that patients who die from cerebral infarction have on average a higher blood pressure than the normal population.

This is hardly surprising when it is known that arterial hypertension aggravates atherosclerosis (see below). In addition, hypertension appears to be linked to the development of microinfarcts or lacunes which outnumber all other cerebrovascular lesions combined (Fisher, 1969).

Macro- and microinfarction are the main topics of the present chapter. However a brief account will be given of the much rarer diseases Binswanger's encephalopathy and arteriopathic Parkinsonism. Although hypertensive encephalopathy is not strictly an ischaemic disorder and might more correctly be called a hyperaemic disorder (see below), it is convenient to deal with it here.

A short account of the cerebral blood flow disorders and pathological lesions in hypertension is relevant at this stage. An attempt is made to review cerebral arterial lesions in hypertension on the premise that although lesions of large and small arteries are morphologically quite different, there are basic physiopathological and pathological similarities between them.

HYPERTENSION AND THE CEREBRAL CIRCULATION

In acute and chronic hypertension the arteries are subjected to a physical stress which is responsible for a variety of lesions in vessels from the size of the aorta to the smallest intracerebral arteries. However, since the bulk of cerebrovascular resistance depends upon the small (pial and intracerebral) arteries (Figs. 10.1 and

Author's note: I wish to thank Professors P. Castaigne and F. Lhermitte for essential support in cerebrovascular studies, and Professor R. Escourolle for the use of every facility in the Charles Foix Neuropathological Laboratory.

Figures 10.3, 10.4, 10.5, 10.9, 10.13, and 10.14 have been reproduced through the courtesy of Drs F. B. Byrom and C. Miller Fisher and with the kind permission of Heinemann Medical Books Ltd., London and Springer Verlag, Berlin.

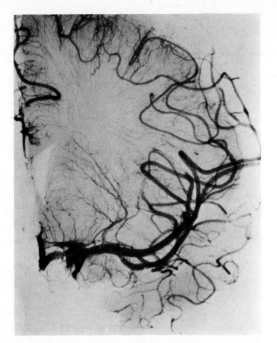

Fig. 10.1 Intracerebral arteries in human brain coronal section. Arteries injected with lead carbonate. Author's specimen.

10.2) lesions most specific to arterial hypertension are to be expected and are indeed mainly present on these vessels. For anatomical features of these vessels, see Vander Eecken (1959), Baker and Iannone (1959a, b), and Russell (1963). Due to their size and distribution to nervous tissue there are fundamental similarities in behaviour between retinal and the small intracerebral arteries. Therefore much has been gained and is to be gained from the study of the

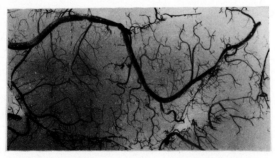

Fig. 10.2 Pial arteries of human brain. Arteries injected with lead carbonate. Author's specimen.

retinal circulation in hypertension. Since there is no anatomic way to distinguish between arteries and arterioles (Kernohan, Anderson, and Keith, 1929; Cook and Yates, 1972) the word arterioles will not be used here.

Intra-arterial pressure is one of the main stimuli responsible for the tone of arteries by stretching the muscular coat or media of the vessel wall. A rise in intra-arterial pressure causes arterial constriction while a decrease in pressure causes dilatation (Bayliss, 1902). It is not within the scope of this paper to discuss whether arterial vasoconstriction is a primary or secondary event in essential hypertension. Suffice it to say that the basic concomitant arterial reaction in hypertension is arterial constriction. This can be witnessed in retinal arteries in man (Harnish and Pearce, 1973) and in rat mesenteric and retinal arteries (Byrom, 1954) and in cerebral arteries of various species (Byrom, 1954, 1969; Meyer, Waltz, and Gotoh, 1960a). In man, angiograms in hypertensives may be highly suggestive of arterial constriction.

For the sake of clarity the circulatory and structural consequences of hypertension will be considered under three categories keeping in mind that there may be some overlapping and oversimplification.

Mild and moderate hypertension

In mild and moderately severe hypertension of some duration diffuse narrowing of the arteries is present. Besides degenerative changes involving hyperplasia of connective tissue and damage to the elastica, the characteristic structural feature is hypertrophy of the muscle cells of the media (Russell, 1963; Cook and Yates, 1972) with an increase in the size of their nuclei. Such muscular hypertrophy may be likened to left ventricular hypertrophy. Histological criteria which are proposed for this 'hypertonus' are distortion of smooth muscle cells and their nuclei, progressive deformation of the internal elastic lamina, crowding of endothelial cells (Van Citters, Wagner, and Rushmer, 1962), crowding and spiral twisting of the nuclei of the muscular cells (Rodda and Denny-Brown, 1966a).

In patients with mild or moderately severe chronic hypertension without cerebral complications the cerebral blood flow remains normal. Chronic arterial constriction is the basis of autoregulation of the cerebral blood flow. A similar autoregulation, i.e. myogenic, is likely to be present in the human retinal arterial circulation (Russell, 1973). There is, however, a lower level of cerebral arterial pressure below which the cerebral autoregulation becomes inadequate and blood flow decreases. In normotensives this lower limit of autoregulation is 60 to 70 mmHg (Lassen, 1959). An increase in oxygen extraction compensates for this decrease in blood flow but only down to a second limit, corresponding to a pressure of 35 to 40 mmHg, below which symptoms of cerebral hypoxia appear. It is of interest for the clinician to keep in mind that in patients with untreated hypertension the lower limit of the autoregulatory range is higher than in normotensives (Finnerty, Witkins, and Fazekas, 1954; Lassen, 1959). In one study the average value for this lower limit of autoregulation in severe hypertensives was 120 mmHg and the limit for brain hypoxia was on average 68 mmHg (Strandgaard, Olesen, Skinhøj, and Lassen, 1973). Such a shift to a higher level of autoregulation in hypertensives may be explained by the hypertrophy of the small arteries walls (Folkow, 1971). It suggests that therapeutic lowering of arterial hypertension should be gradual and cautious (Strandgaard et al., 1973), a fact in keeping with clinical experience.

Acute hypertension

In acute severe hypertension extreme arterial constriction is to be expected. This indeed occurs but it is important to realise that, at least after some time, it appears as a *segmental* constriction (Figs. 10.3 and 10.4). This has been the source of terms such as vasospasm and probably of much confusion in understanding the disorders of the cerebral circulation in such circumstances. Since the first observations in retinal and pial arteries in man and animals the segmental arterial constriction has been held responsible by many authorities for ischaemia

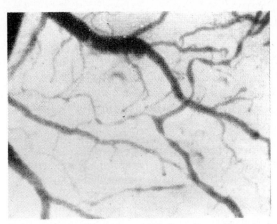

Fig. 10.3 Reversible change of calibre in small cerebral arteries of rat in severe uncomplicated hypertension (× 26). Light ether anesthesia (B.P. 240 mm). Gross irregularity in calibre of small arteries, veins normal.

resulting in damage to the vessel wall and consequently to the tissues supplied by the damaged arteries (Fog, 1939; Byrom, 1954; Meyer *et al.*, 1960b; Rodda and Denny-Brown, 1966b; Dinsdale, Robertson, and Haas, 1974). However, in the first reports of these carefully designed experiments it had also been mentioned that there existed *dilated* arterial segments as well as constricted ones (Byrom, 1954). By injecting intravitam trypan blue Byrom (1954) found

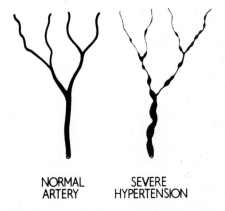

NORMAL   SEVERE
ARTERY   HYPERTENSION

Fig. 10.4 The typical picture of dilatation, tortuosity, irregularity of largest vessels, tight uniform constriction of smallest vessels, and alternating constriction and dilatation of intermediate vessels. (Figures 10.3 and 10.4 are from F.B. Byrom (1969) *The Hypertensive Vascular Crisis*, London: Heinemann. Reproduced by courtesy of the author.)

conspicuous rounded blue areas on the surface of the brain (Fig. 10.5), a finding which implied a break in the blood brain barrier (BBB). The blue areas of cerebral tissue were found to contain a considerably higher content of water than control tissue, i.e. they were oedematous. This seemed to account for the cerebral oedema in human hypertensive encephalopathy (see below). However it now appears that the leakage of fluid through the arterial wall may not take place in the constricted but in the *dilated* arterial segment. This was elegantly demonstrated by Giese (1966) in a series of experiments with serum labelled with a fluorescent dye and carbon-labelled plasma. This crucial evidence was subsequently confirmed by using Evans blue albumin as an index of breakdown of the BBB and ^{125}I-antipyrine and ^{3}H-ethanol as indicators of blood flow (Johansson, 1974). In short during acute very high hypertension there is a forced arterial dilatation resulting in a 'breakthrough' of autoregulation (Lassen and Agnoli, 1972) and in a pronounced increase in blood flow. This pressure-forced arterial dilatation leads to BBB damage with focal leakage of fluid through the walls of the overstretched arteries (Johansson, Li, Olsonn, and Klatzo, 1970) and formation of cerebral oedema (Johansson, 1974; Johansson, Strandgaard, and Lassen, 1974). The characteristic arterial lesion (Figs. 10.6 and 10.7) is necrosis of medial muscle fibres with the presence of erythrocytes and of a substance staining pink with eosin, bright red with PAS, and purple with PTAH. This has been termed hyaline or fibrinoid necrosis (Byrom, 1969; Wilson, 1969). Both hyaline and fibrinoid changes are due to the presence within the vessel wall of material which has the histochemical immunological and ultramicroscopic features of fibrin (Adams, 1967).

In hypertensive monkeys ultrastructural studies of retinal arteries showed seeping of plasma and fibrin deposits into the vessel wall ('insudation or plasmatic vasculosis'). Eventually the muscle cell cavities in the basement membrane contained only plasma, fibrin, muscle cells debris, and lipid, and in some cases large numbers of platelets and occasional red cells. The pathway of the plasma leakage through the

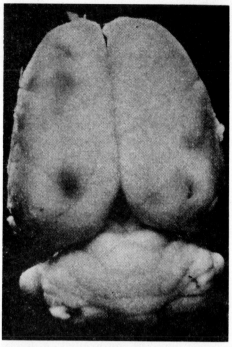

Fig. 10.5 Brain of a rat with encephalopathy, killed soon after an intravenous injection of trypan blue, showing rounded areas of staining on the surface of the cerebral cortex. (From F. B. Byrom (1969) *The Hypertensive Vascular Crisis*. London: Heinemann. Reproduced by courtesy of the author.)

endothelium could, however, not be demonstrated (Garner and Ashton, 1970).

With regard to moderately severe hypertension in which hypertrophy of the media is the characteristic lesion (see above) it is of interest to note that the arterial disorders of acute severe hypertension, namely focal leakage of plasma, occurs in experimental animals (i.e. in previously normotensive animals) and are almost restricted to clinical conditions in which there is an abrupt onset of severe hypertension in a previously normotensive patient (e.g. in acute glomerular nephritis or toxaemia of pregnancy). Hypertensive encephalopathy is rarely encountered in other hypertensive conditions; for instance, there was only one case of hypertensive encephalopathy in 190 cases of established malignant hypertension (Clarke and Murphy, 1956), and experimentally hypertensive encephalopathy is rare when blood pressure is

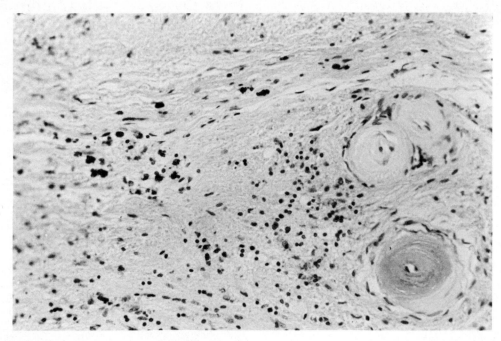

Fig. 10.6 Arterial hyalinosis, at bottom. Two hyalinised occluded arteries, above. On the left, haemosiderin-laden macrophages. H. E. × 120. Female, aged 60 (B.P. 250/150).

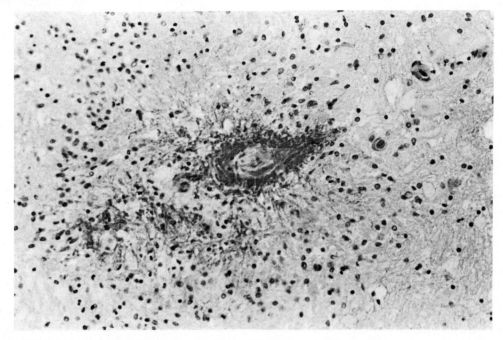

Fig. 10.7 Fibrinoid necrosis of intracerebral artery. H.E. × 120. Same case as Figure 6.

increased in a step-wise fashion (Häggendahl and Johansson, 1972). This may be due to the hypertrophy of the muscular coat with an increased resistance to overstretching.

Chronic hypertension

In chronic severe hypertension there exists two distinct though related cerebral arterial changes, namely, aggravation of atherosclerosis and the development of specific lesions on the small intracerebral arteries.

AGGRAVATION OF ATHEROSCLEROSIS BY HYPERTENSION

Experimental, clinical, and pathological studies indicate that hypertension accelerates the onset and accentuates the progress of atherosclerosis (*see* Baker, Resch, and Loewenson, 1969). Fisher *et al.* (1965a) found that stenosis of the cervical and cerebral (i.e. Circle of Willis and stems of the main intracranial arteries) arteries was more frequent and more severe in hypertensives than in normotensives. Increased calcification of the carotid syphon was clearly associated with hypertension (Fisher *et al.*, 1965b). Russell (1963) and Baker *et al.* (1969) found that the severity of atherosclerosis of the Circle of Willis was more pronounced where hypertension had been present. Multiple stenoses of arterial branches on angiography and yellow specks on the leptomeningeal arteries at autopsy are almost a hallmark of severe long-standing hypertension. Fisher (1961a) reported that in his material it had been extremely easy to find hypertensive atherosclerotic cases while it had taken several months to find an adequate sample of normotensive cases with severe cerebral atherosclerosis or hypertensive cases without atherosclerosis. In some hypertensive patients, a particular type of atherosclerosis of cerebral arteries is present characterised by scaleriform, i.e. ladder-like yellow or orange bars (Arab, 1957)(Fig. 10.8).

However, besides aggravating atherosclerosis hypertension exerts a second and most important effect, the production of lesions on smaller arteries. In normotensives atherosclerosis implicates arteries 0.2 or more millimetres in diameter, namely, from vessels of the size of those

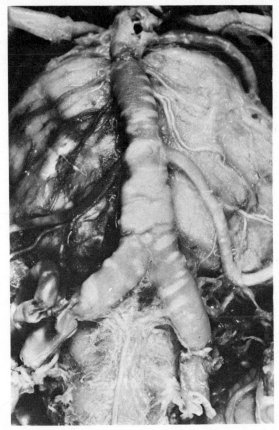

Fig. 10.8 Scaleriform atherosclerosis of vertebral and basilar arteries. Arteries injected with lead carbonate. Author's specimen.

which penetrate the basal ganglia and pons to the common carotid arteries in the neck (Adams, 1955). Hypertension extends the atheromatous process, seeming to force the fatty deposits upon vessels of lesser size. For instance the penetrating arteries of the internal capsules, basal ganglia, and pons tend to be involved only in patients subject to hypertension, the diabetic being a possible exception (Adams and Fisher, 1961b). Examples of this may be found in intracerebral and retinal arteries. In a study of the arterial lesions underlying 50 lacunes Fisher (1969) reported three cases in which a focal plaque consisting of fatty macrophages had encroached upon or occluded the lumen of the feeding artery. The lesion was typical of microscopic atherosclerosis in small cerebral arteries. It is of interest to note that the involved arteries were larger than in any of the other lacunes, namely 500, 400, and 300 μm, respectively. Atherosclerosis is lacking on retinal arteries since, except for the central retinal artery, all are less than 100 μm in diameter (Adams, 1955). However in hypertensives atherosclerotic lesions of the retinal arteries have been demonstrated (Harnish and Pearce, 1973; patients E and G). Moreover it should be noted that in Harnish and Pearce's patient E an atherosclerotic lesion was present post-mortem where a soft exudate had been observed during life. If it is accepted that soft exudates are likely to represent focal leakage of plasma, it appears that there may be relations between the most acute and the most chronic arterial lesions.

SPECIFIC HYPERTENSIVE LESIONS ON INTRA-CEREBRAL ARTERIES

In chronic severe hypertension, arterial lesions specific to hypertension are present which to some extent are restricted to cerebral arteries. Unlike arteries of other organs which divide regularly into smaller branches, penetrating or nutrient cerebral arteries enter the brain from main stems or large pericerebral branches (Duret, 1874) (Fig. 10.2). Most of the hypertensive lesions lay in the territories of the basal perforating arteries, and it has been suggested that this could be due to the proximity to large arteries where a high pressure or marked fluctuations in pressure would be more likely to be transmitted to smaller vessels (Russell, 1963). It may be that at the base of the brain the small nutrient arteries are subjected to especially high pressure by virtue of their origin at right angles from the major arterial trunks and that a gradual reduction of pressure is lacking (Fisher, 1961b). Whatever the truth in these considerations, it must be recognised that with regard to atherosclerotic thrombosis the behaviour of penetrating arteries at the base of the brain is different from that of pial arteries on the convexity (Fisher, 1961b), a fact which suggests significant differences in the regime of blood flow.

Intracerebral arterial lesions found chiefly in hypertensives are of two main kinds: (1) lipo-hyalinosis and (2) miliary aneurysms. Both have in common, it should be noted at once, to be present on small arteries in the range of 40 to 300 μm diameter.

Lipohyalinosis is a word coined by Fisher (1972) to refer to cerebral arterial lesions correlating chiefly with hypertension and which had been described under various names: fibrinoid necrosis, hyaline arterionecrosis, atherosclerosis of small arteries, hyaline fatty changes, plasmatic vascular destruction, hyalinosis, angionecrosis, fibrinoid arteritis (see Fisher, 1972), segmental arterial disorganisation (Fisher, 1969). The essential pathological process may be summarised as follows (Fig. 10.9): mural destruction, focal expansion of the vessel, fatty macrophages or foam cells frequently present in the disorganised wall, thrombotic occlusion haemorrhagic extravasation and fibrinoid deposit (Fisher, 1969, 1972). The term lipohyalinosis stresses the fact that such lesions stain readily for fat, and it should be reminded that Charcot and Bouchard (1868) had commented on the presence of fatty granulations in some of the lesions. By some features, e.g. fibrinoid deposit, focal enlargements (Fisher [1972] went as far as to use the term 'miliary aneurysms in lipohyalinosis'), lipohyalinosis, is reminiscent on one hand of lesions resulting from arterial overstretching under high blood pressure. On the other hand the presence of a lipid-staining material as a prominent constituent of arterial segmental disorganisation strongly suggested to Fisher (1969) that there exists a relation with the fatty plaque of atherosclerosis, a view with which the author entirely agrees. Fisher's (1969, 1972) evidence for this is worth to be quoted here: (1) severe atherosclerosis of the cerebral arteries accompanies lacunar infarcts (of which lipohyalinosis is the commonest cause); (2) in hypertension the smaller surface cerebral and cerebral arteries are affected by atherosclerosis, hence atherosclerosis of the very small intracerebral twigs might also be expected; (3) it may be significant that vessels larger than 200 μm display atherosclerosis rather than lipohyalinosis and the reverse is also true; (4) the presence of fat combined with macrophages hints that the lesion may be related to atherosclerosis; (5) in hyper-

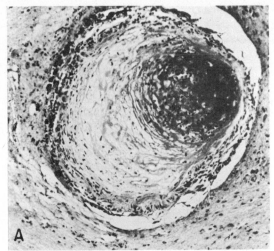

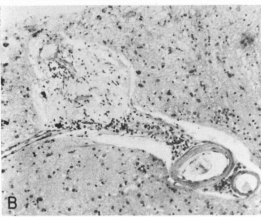

Fig. 10.9A. Segmental disorganisation (angionecrosis) with local enlargement of the artery to three times the normal diameter of 130 μm. The dark material is fibrinoid staining (H.E.).

B. Old segmental enlargement of an 80 μm artery consisting of a nodule of collagenous connective tissue. The edge of the lacune is seen above. (Courtesy of Dr. C. Miller Fisher, 1969.)

tension atherosclerotic nodules may be found with concomitant evidence of leakage of red blood cells; (6) in cases showing disorganisation of the smaller twigs plaques filled with typical fatty macrophages were often found in the immediate larger parent branches.

Miliary aneurysms were described by Charcot and Bouchard (1868) (Fig. 10.10) then more or less discarded or misinterpreted during almost

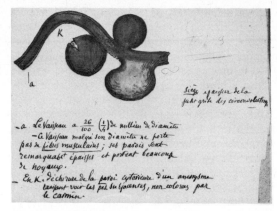

Fig. 10.10 Original drawing and notes by Charcot of miliary aneurysms (Musée de la Salpêtrière).

a century. By micropaque injections and pathological observations Russell (1963) put them back into the limelight of neurology. Cole and Yates (1967a) showed that they are hypertension and age-dependent. Fisher (1972) gave a detailed study based on serial sections. Apart from their significance in hypertensive arterial lesions, miliary aneurysms must be considered here for they are likely to be a cause, admittedly an infrequent one, of small infarcts in hypertensives patients (Charcot and Bouchard, 1968; Russell, 1963; Fisher, 1972). The significance of miliary aneurysms with regard to lipohyalinosis must now be considered. Fisher (1972) described saccular and fusiform asymmetric miliary aneurysms but thought that both kinds are closely related and have much in common. He apparently considered lipohyalinosis as a variety of aneurysm and commented that all three types of aneurysms are tied to hypertension, involve arteries of the same size and location and small extravasations of red blood cells occur around each, clearly suggesting a relationship. Although he did not find intermediary forms, he obviously felt that there exists a strong possibility that they all have a common origin and that the three types of aneurysms might really be variations of the same process. If this were true it could be assumed that in hypertensive cerebral arterial disease there is a change in the morphology of lesions where arteries become less than about 300 μm in diameter, i.e. frank atherosclerosis disappear while lipohyalinosis and miliary aneurysms appear. However, this change is probably more apparent than real for atherosclerosis is likely to be closely related to lipohyalinosis while miliary aneurysms may well be closely related to lipohyalinosis. Moreover cerebral arterial lesions in moderately severe or very severe hypertension display mixed features of both aggravated atherosclerosis and overstretching of the vessel wall with resultant enlargement and leakage of plasma. For the student of hypertensive arterial cerebral lesions it is likely that there is a continuum of lesions from the large to the smallest arteries with variations presumably due to differences in pressure and structure of the vessel wall.

HYPERTENSIVE ENCEPHALOPATHY

Acute cerebral disorders in Bright's disease, mainly convulsions and blindness, were at first ascribed to uraemia ('convulsive uraemia'). However, at the turn of the century it became apparent that they could result from vascular disturbances due to a rise in systolic pressure (Pal, 1905). Oppenheimer and Fishberg (1928) coined the term hypertensive encephalopathy to account for the recurrent fits in a case of acute nephritis with raised blood pressure. They discarded the current views on pathogenesis, namely renal insufficiency or chloride retention, to conclude that hypertension was responsible for the nervous disorders, most likely through 'a widespread and perhaps universal peripheral vasoconstriction'. In the late 1930s and 1940s the nervous lesions were emphasised in French literature under the term of acute meningo-cerebral oedema (oedème aigu cérébro-méningé) (Alajouanine and Hornet, 1939; Milliez, 1943) Eventually hypertensive encephalopathy superseded other appellations but came to be used in a restricted sense, i.e. to refer to largely reversible cerebral disorders associated with raised blood pressure in the absence of evidence of cerebral thrombosis or haemorrhage (Jellinek et al., 1964).

Cases of hypertensive encephalopathy have been most frequently associated with acute nephritis and toxaemia of pregnancy. In a series of 225 patients with nephritis admitted to the London Hospital in the years before the Second World War hypertensive encephalopathy occurred in 11, an incidence of 6.4 per cent (Wilson, 1963). A few cases have been reported in association with phaeochromocytoma (Milliez, 1943; Graham, 1951) and lead poisoning. As already mentioned the condition appears to be infrequent in the course of malignant hypertension (see above). A case of Jellinek et al. (1964) was due to renal arterial occlusion. Meyer (1961) mentioned porphyria as a rare cause. There seems to be few doubts that the condition was formerly overdiagnosed (Ziegler, Zosa, and Zideli, 1965). Nowadays although Finnerty recently claimed to have treated 'over 400 patients with various types of hypertensive encephalopathy with diazoxide' (Finnerty, 1972) the condition appears to be very uncommon since conditions which lead to it are either naturally rare or have become rare with the advent of efficient treatments of hypertension. However, a few cases continue to be reported (Strandgaard, Olesen, Skinhøj, and Lassen, 1973; Jewett, 1973) and it may well be that in some parts of the world hypertensive encephalopathy is still frequent.

Disorders of cerebral blood flow with a breakthrough in autoregulation, overstretching of arteries and focal damage to BBB have been mentioned earlier. Cerebral lesions of oedema have been reported by Blackfan (1926) who demonstrated the presence of a medullary pressure cone and consequently concluded that lumbar puncture, which was formerly advocated by some authors as a therapeutic procedure, 'should be used guardedly'. Alajouanine and Hornet (1939) stressed that there was at postmortem a great quantity of CSF around the brain and that the latter was swollen with flattened gyri and a conspicuous superficial vasodilatation. Arteries, capillaries, and veins appeared to be distended and Virchow-Robin spaces were greatly distended with the presence of an amorphous material which had the features of an albumin-fibrin coagulum. There was in addition a characteristic shredded appearance (état effiloché) of the nervous tissue with acute swelling of the oligodendroglia, sometimes clasmatodendrosis, and ischaemic changes of neurones. The lesions were most marked in cortex and basal ganglia.

The full crisis of hypertensive encephalopathy is often heralded by weakness, apathy, headache, drowsiness, and vomiting concomitant with a severe rise in blood pressure. Convulsions are common, either generalised or focal. In the absence of treatment they are usually recurrent. Loss of vision is a second main feature. Hypertensive changes in the fundi are frequently lacking (Milliez, 1943; Jellinek et al., 1964), a fact that again sets hypertensive encephalopathy apart from malignant hypertension and obviously suggests occipital blindness. This is supported by cases in which homonymous hemianopia has been recorded. Drowsiness may lead to coma. Various focal cerebral disturbances may occur, e.g. transient paralysis and aphasia. Stiffness of the neck is frequent (Milliez, 1943). The cerebrospinal fluid pressure is usually raised, although this is inconstant. A rise in the CSF protein content is also usual but may also be absent. The cell count is normal.

The electroencephalogram in Jellinek et al.'s (1964) cases showed in the acute stage bilaterally synchronous often rhythmic occipital sharp and slow activity. The alpha rhythm was lost or impaired during the period of blindness. Some records showed in addition focal abnormalities elsewhere.

Hypertensive encephalopathy is, as already mentioned, generally concomitant with a severe rise in blood pressure but it must be stressed that this is not always true. The condition may occur with rather moderate hypertension.

The clinical disorder may lead to deep coma and death or rapidly regress. Sequelae have been recorded, e.g. intellectual impairment and epilepsy (Jellinek et al., 1964). More often emergency therapy (see below) brings dramatic relief by lowering blood pressure. The cerebral disorders may disappear very quickly in a matter of hours or even minutes.

Hypertensive encephalopathy must be differentiated from: (1) infarction due to occlusive arterial disease and haemorrhage; (2) subarachnoid haemorrhage; (3) cerebral abcess or tumour which by raising intracranial pressure could determine hypertension. Finnerty (1972) stated that acute anxiety states with labile hypertension and acute pulmonary oedema due to hypertensive heart disease may require differentiation from hypertensive encephalopathy.

The treatment is essentially based on a prompt lowering of hypertension. It has been recently reviewed by Finnerty (1972). From this and present knowledge it would appear that three main drugs are available: diazoxide, trimetaphan camphor sulfonate, and furosemide. (For detailed pharmacological properties see Finnerty, 1972.) If such drug facilities are not available in emergency situations it should be remembered that venesection was formerly used with success. For reasons stated above, vasodilator drugs such as papaverine and hypercapnia should be avoided.

LACUNES. ETAT LACUNAIRE

The term 'lacunes' (Latin, lacuna, -ae: a hole or small cavity) was first used by Durand-Fardel (1843, case 78) in the macroscopic description of the striate bodies of a 77-year-old man whose brain showed a wide variety of ischaemic and haemorrhagic lesions. The term 'état lacunaire' was introduced by Pierre Marie (1901) to refer to the chronic condition of patients affected by lacunes. Marie reported clinical and pathological observations from 50 patients and Ferrand added 38 cases in his monograph which appeared the following year (Ferrand, 1902). For review of what could be called the 'first historical period' of lacunes see Ferrand (1902) and Fisher (1965a). Between the First and Second World Wars a number of clinico-pathological cases were reported, although according to the fashion of the time, nervous lesions and their clinical counterparts and not arterial lesions were the chief interest of the authors. After Foix and Hillemand's (1925) description or the patterns of arterial anatomy in the brain stem, studies took into account the localisation of the lesions in the newly defined territories, but again, arterial lesions were too often missed or mentioned without precise qualifications. During the 1940s and 1950s the advent of angiography into clinical use strongly focused interest upon extracranial arteries and for a time lacunes were the poor relative of cerebral arterial disease. This is no longer the case and for this a special tribute must be paid to Fisher's pathological (1961a, 1965a, 1969, 1972) and clinico-pathological studies.

Lacunes (Figs. 10.11 and 10.12) are small infarcts, mostly found in the chronic or healed stage when they appear as irregular trabeculated usually pale cavities. When of recent origin they show liquefaction necrosis. In the acute stage the area of temporary ischaemia is considerably larger than the scar, possibly two or three times (Fisher, 1961a) a fact that may account for the partial recovery of clinical episodes resulting from lacunes. The dimensions of lacunes range on average from 0.5 to 15 mm in diameter but it would be unwarranted to draw a firm line between lacunes and infarcts. To emphasise the unusual size of the larger lacunes Fisher (1965a) suggested to qualify those 10 mm or more in diameter as 'giant' and suggested that preferably the nature and site of the lesion rather than its size should be the chief criterion. However, such qualifications leave the student of cerebral lesions undecided on many of the cases reported in the literature. The author of the present paper believes that the term 'lacune' should be restricted to lesions which can be ascribed to permanent or transient occlusion of *intracerebral* arteries. Admittedly, however, a small number of lacunes may be due to transient occlusion of the mouth or extracerebral part of the penetrating arteries by transient occlusion of their large parent vessel, e.g. in cardiac embolism.

In a series of 1042 consecutive post-mortems in a general hospital, 114 brains (11 per cent) had one or more lacunes. Seventy-one were male, 43 female (Fisher, 1965a).

The primary or immediate causes of lacunes are likely to be reflected in Fisher's (1969) series of the arterial lesions underlying lacunes: 40 were due to occlusive segmental arterial disorganisation or lipohyalinosis (see above) (Figs. 10.13 and 10.14), two resulted from thrombosis in an assymmetric fusiform micro-aneurysm,

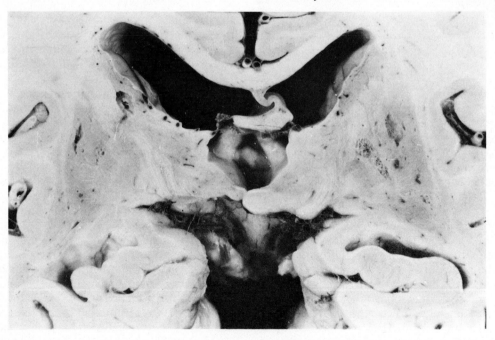

Fig. 10.11 Lacunes in basal ganglia and internal capsule. Moderate ventricular enlargement. The left mamillary body is atrophied.

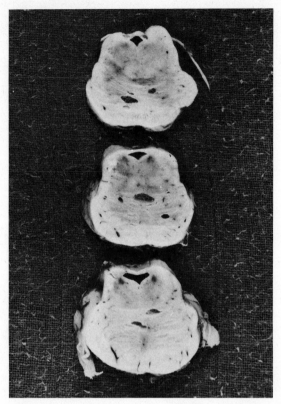

Fig. 10.12 Lacunes in basis pontis. Same case as Figure 10.11. Male, aged 53 (B.P.: 230/125).

three from typical microscopic atherosclerosis in small cerebral arteries, in four the nature of the lesion was questionable, albeit in three there was some disorganisation of the wall. Finally, in the fiftieth lacune the nutrient artery was patent and possible embolism with transient occlusion had to be considered.

In the series of 114 patients with lacunes (Fisher, 1965a) correlations were sought for various pathological conditions. It was concluded that lacunes were not related to carotid disease or cerebral embolism (although there may be exceptions to this) or diabetes. On the other hand a strong correlation was found with cerebral, i.e. intracranial atherosclerosis, and in approximately 50 per cent of patients with lacunes atherosclerotic lesions extended up to the small pial cerebral and cerebellar arteries. This, as already mentioned, closely parallels

hypertension and indeed the strongest correlation for lacunes was found to be hypertension which was documented in 111 out of 114 patients (in two BP was unknown, one was normotensive and had been treated for neurosyphilis, possibly meningovascular syphilis).

In all studies the first preferential site for lacunes has been found to be the lenticular nucleus, particularly the putamen (Fig. 10.11) followed by pons (Fig. 10.12), thalamus, and caudate nucleus. However it must be stressed that lacunes are by no means rare in the white matter of the brain. Among 100 lacunes in Ferrand's (1902) series, 13 were in the white matter of the brain, and among 376 lacunes of Fisher's (1965a) series 89 (23 per cent) were either in the internal capsule or corona radiata or corpus callosum or white matter of cerebral lobes. Regarding the lacunes of the internal capsule Ferrand (1902) aptly remarked that lacunes usually do not occur in the internal capsule but rather in adjacent lenticular nucleus, thalamus, or caudate nucleus whence they encroach upon the internal capsule (Fig. 10.11), and moreover that it is unfrequent that all capsular fibers are interrupted, a fact that may obviously have some clinical implications. Conversely lacunes appear to be absent from cortex, rare in cerebellum, and absent from medulla oblongata and spinal cord.

It is a common belief that lacunes are very numerous in any one patient but this is far from being always the case. In Ferrand's (1902) 88 patients a single lacune was present 14 times (15.9 per cent) and in Fisher's (1965a) 114 patients 29 (25.4 per cent) had also a single lesion. Among the 114 patients 54 had one or two lacunes, i.e. nearly half the total number of patients. Sixty patients had more than two lacunes; among these 2 had 14 and 2 had 15 lesions. Thus more often than is commonly believed lacunes allow a precise clinico-anatomical correlation, a point which will be commented on further. Unfortunately lacunes are often associated with haemorrhages as well as infarcts. In Marie's (1901) series of 50 brains there were haemorrhages in 16 and infarctions in seven. In Fisher's (1965a) series of 114 brains, haemorrhages were associated with lacunes in 35 per cent and infarction in 26 per cent. Also Marie (1901) mentioned that in four brains there existed in the cortex of the frontal or temporal poles, on one or both sides, '*état vermoulu*', i.e. worm-eaten condition, consisting of a circumscribed destruction of the cortex with presence of small pits. Although Marie's description does not suggest the usual site of granular atrophy it would seem that this is a likely diagnosis for '*état vermoulu*'.

The clinical picture of lacunes and *état lacunaire* according to Marie (1901) and Ferrand

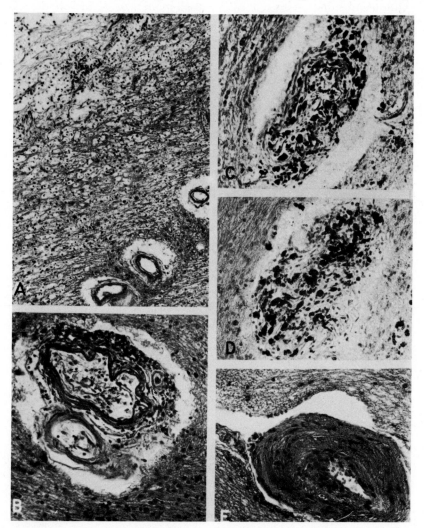

Fig. 10.13 Diseased artery running to 5 × 5 mm lacune in pontine base. Five different levels.
A. Section No. 38 showing three small arteries adjacent to lacunes.
B. Section No. 300. Arteries joining are occluded by fine connective tissues.
C. Section No. 357. Artery disorganised and enlarged, lumen obliterated. Many hemosiderin-filled macrophages. Artery is normally 160 μm.
D. Section No. 381. Chief segment of disorganisation.
E. Section No. 677. Artery entering subarachnoid space acquires lumen. Sections are approximately 10 μm thick. The vascular arrangement is pictured diagrammatically in Figure 10.14.

(1902) was mainly that of an hemiplegia of sudden onset, most often without loss of consciousness. After a few hours or days paralysis improved to a great extent but recovery remained usually incomplete. Useful clinical tests for minimal motor skill deficit were to ask the patient to button and unbutton his coat with either hand and for minimal facial paresis to ask the patient to wink either eye. It was frequently noted that one eye could easily be closed alone while this was impossible on the side of the facial paresis. In addition, it was noted that hemianesthesia was rare, and hemianopia was not observed. Dysarthria was common but aphasia was not encountered. No contracture of the limbs occurred. Walking was very characteristic, consisting of *marche à petits pas de Dejerine*. Psychic functions were impaired, pseudobulbar palsy was common.

It is usual in medicine that the earliest descriptions give an account of a disease in its fully developed form. Since Marie's and Ferrand's descriptions of *état lacunaire*, numerous attempts have been made to isolate clinical disorders that could be related to specifically located lesions. Many of the infrequent classical eponymic syndromes of the brain stem listed in the textbooks of neurology were the result of small infarcts or lacunes. In the present chapter a short account will be given only of the most frequent of them.

Fisher and Curry (1965) reported 50 clinical cases of pure motor hemiplegia, meaning that there were no clinical signs other than a complete or incomplete paralysis of face, arm, and leg at any time in the illness. All patients except four were hypertensive, hypertension being defined as blood pressure above 150/90 mmHg. One patient (case 10) had atrial fibrillation. In nine cases a post-mortem examination of the brain was performed. In five cases there was an infarct of the internal capsule (as well as of the adjacent basal ganglia), in three there was a lacunar infarct on one side of the basis pontis, not crossing the

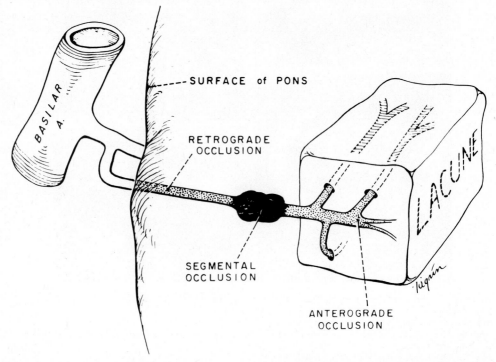

Fig. 10.14 Diagram of pons showing relation of lacune to vascular lesion described in Figure 10.13. (From C. M. Fisher (1969) The arterial lesions underlying lacunes. *Acta Neuropathologica*. (Berlin), **12**, 1. Reproduced by courtesy of the author.)

mid-line nor reaching into the middle cerebellar peduncles. Capsular cases appear to be similar to those reported by Foix and Lévy (1927) under the term 'ramollissements sylviens profonds partiels', i.e. incomplete deep basal infarcts (in the basal territory of the middle cerebral artery, see Fig. 10.1). Pontine cases resemble those previously reported by Lhermitte and Trelles (1934) under the term of 'hemiplégie protubérantielle', i.e. pontine hemiplegia. The same authors reported cases of 'paraplégie protubérantielle', i.e. pontine paraplegia resulting from bilateral small infarcts in basis pontis.

In the capsular as well as in the pontine cases of Fisher and Curry there was hemiparesis or hemiplegia. The extraocular movements may help to distinguish capsular from pontine lesions. In capsular cases, even in the presence of a severe hemiplegia, there usually was no paralysis of gaze; conjugate lateral gaze away from the hemiplegic side was sometimes easier than in the opposite direction. By contrast in one case of pontine lesions conjugate eye movements were easier towards the hemiplegic side. This sign, however, had disappeared within 24 hours.

The prognosis for recovery of the neurological deficit and surviving the illness appeared to be good. Usually recovery began within two weeks and advanced more quickly in the leg than in the arm. There was, however, a tendency to bilateral occurrence. Fisher and Curry concluded that in such cases angiography is not indicated and anticoagulant therapy probably not efficacious. It should be added—and this will hold true for other lacunar syndromes— that since nearly all patients are chronic hypertensives anticoagulant therapy should be considered dangerous for the reason that miliary aneurysms are very likely to be present.

Fisher (1965b) reported 26 patients with a symptomatology limited to a persistent or transient numbness and mild sensory loss over one entire side of the body, including the face arm and leg. There was no motor deficit and other symptoms and signs were absent. All patients except one had hypertension defined as blood pressure above '150/90 mmHg. A post mortem study of the brain was obtained in one

patient showing a single lacune 7 mm in diameter situated in the postero-ventral (sensory) nucleus of the thalamus and it was postulated that in most of the other cases of pure sensory stroke the responsible lesion also lay in the thalamus. Pure hemisensory strokes were nearly always benign and in none of the typical cases were they a harbinger of hemiplegia or other severe accident. It was inferred that the thalamic lesion resulted from thrombotic occlusion of a penetrating artery on the basis of hypertension and atherosclerosis. Therefore it was advised that anticoagulants be withheld and angiography not undertaken.

Pure sensory stroke is reminiscent of the thalamic syndrome, although in the three cases reported by Dejerine and Roussy (1906) there was mild hemiplegia and choreic-athetosic movements in addition to sensory disorders, and the infarcts were a little more extensive involving the adjacent internal capsule and lenticular nucleus. On the other hand Garcin and Lapresle (1954, 1960) reported two patients in whom the sensory deficit affected only the lips and hand or part of the hand. In both cases the causal lesion was a lacunar infarct partially involving the ventral posterior lateral nucleus of the thalamus.

Fisher and Cole (1965) reported 14 patients in whom arm and leg on one side showed a combination of severe cerebellar-like ataxia and pyramidal signs. The leg was weak more distally than proximally and in some cases only the toes and ankle were involved. The arm showed little or no weakness. The face was spared and usually there was no dysarthria. A Babinski sign was always present and the deep reflexes were exaggerated. Walking was impossible or almost so without support. Sensation was intact in all but one case. Two patients had nystagmus. Twelve of the 14 patients were hypertensive. The only available post-mortem brain examination was undecisive for there were at least 11 old lesions in the brain, most of them taking the form of lacunes. A clinical case closely resembling this had been reported by Nicolesco, Cretu, and Demetresco (1932). Fisher and Cole (1965) were inclined to believe that a supratentorial lesion of the crural pyramidal fibres was responsible for the clinical picture and that it possibly lay in the posterior-superior part of the internal capsule or in the adjacent corona radiata. In 12 of the 14 patients recovery was almost complete, and it was concluded that angiography and any therapy carrying a significant risk (anticoagulants had been used) are to be avoided.

Fisher (1967) reported some 20 patients with mild stroke consisting chiefly of dysarthria and clumsiness of one hand. The cardinal features of the syndrome included, in addition, central weakness of one side of the face, deviation of the tongue on protrusion, a trace of dysphagia, a wavering ataxia on the finger-nose test not clearly cerebellar in type, mild imbalance on walking, possibly enhanced tendon reflexes on the affected side, a Babinski sign, and reduced arm swing. Hypertension was almost always present. One patient with right-hand clumsiness came to post-mortem examination due to a pancreatic carcinoma. The lesion held responsible for the nervous disorders was a lacune on the left side of the base of the pons in its top-most 5 mm. It was situated deeply, almost reaching the medial lemniscus. The cavity lay close to the mid-line and its broadest part may have crossed slightly to the other side. The cause of the lacune was likely to be thrombosis but the possibility of an embolus could not be excluded. The prognosis of this syndrome for virtually complete recovery appeared to be good. Angiography it was deemed is unnecessary and anticoagulants were not warranted.

Pseudobulbar palsy refers to a clinical condition in which there is paralysis or paresis of those muscles that control movements of the lips, tongue, pharynx, larynx, i.e. muscles that subserve mainly talking and swallowing. According to Broadbent's hypothesis (later demonstrated), 'the more muscles are bilateral in their action the more equally are the muscles of both sides represented in each side' (quoted by Jackson 1874–1876). Therefore muscles innervated from the medulla receive impulses from both hemispheres. This implies that pseudobulbar palsy results from lesions on both corticobulbar tracts, and the word pseudobulbar implies that the lesions are situated above the medulla. For reviews of early cases and of the concept of pseudobulbar paralysis see Comte (1900) and Thurel (1929).

Pseudobulbar palsy of arterial origin is usually due to successive lacunar infarcts resulting in *état lacunaire*. Although the levels of blood pressure are not mentioned in many of the early cases it may be reasonably assumed that patients did not differ from others with lacunes, i.e. they were hypertensives. Present experience supports this view. It is generally admitted that multiple lacunar infarcts involve both internal capsules and/or basis pontis, two elective sites for lacunes (see above).

The clinical picture (Fig. 10.15) includes poor mimicry at rest, often facial assymmetry due to uneven facial paresis (since the nuclei of the facial nerve are also often deprived of their normal innervation), drooling of saliva. Most characteristic is a dysarthria with paralytic and dystonic components. Speech is slurred, consonants especially labials and dentals being affected; palilalia may occur (Thurel, 1929, Brain, 1961). Loss of emotional control is common with outbursts of so-called spasmodic laughing or more often weeping. Disorders of swallowing may appear less severe although death may be due to choking as mentioned by Hughes, Dodgson, and MacLennan (1954) and supported by the author's experience. Impairment of memory and dementia may be present but not necessarily even in severe cases (Hughes *et al.*, 1954).

The limbs are generally clumsy and mildly paretic with bilateral extensor plantar response, but contracture is usually slight with *marche à petits pas*. Double severe hemiplegia is exceptionally rare; urgency of micturition is common.

There is no doubt that pseudobulbar palsy deserves further studies of the kind that Fisher performed for other lacunar states. In the present state of knowledge the term refers to a galaxy of symptoms and signs which could most probably be broken down into more specific syndromes. Two well-identified syndromes must be mentioned: (1) pseudobulbar palsy resulting from lesions of both rolandic opercula and adjacent part of the third frontal gyrus (Foix, Chavany, and Marie, 1926; from the short extraneurological notes of this paper it is likely that both

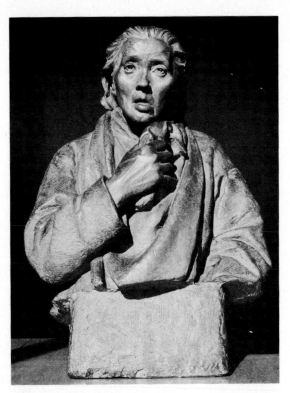

Fig. 10.15 Pseudobulbar palsy (Musée de la Salpêtrière).

infarcts were of cardiac embolic nature) and (2) pseudobulbar palsy due to pontine infarcts with additional cerebellar disorders (Lhermitte and Trelles, 1934; Thurel, 1928).

Another quite different cerebral disorder has been recently tentatively ascribed to lacunes; Earnest *et al.* (1974) reported two hypertensive patients with symptoms and signs suggesting normal pressure hydrocephalus. Pneumoencephalograms showed enlarged lateral and third ventricles in both cases. A right ventriculoperitoneal shunt in the first patient and a right ventriculojugular shunt in the second one were performed. The first patient improved and did not die until three years later, after the onset of cerebral symptoms from myocardial infarction with cardiac failure plus evidence of new cerebral lesions. The second patient did not improve and died four weeks after the neurosurgical procedure. Post-mortem studies showed numerous lacunes in both cases. Earnest *et al.* suggested that many infarcts in the periventricular matter and basal ganglia could reduce tissue bulk and tensile strength allowing the ventricles to enlarge under the stress of increased intraventricular cerebrospinal fluid pulse pressure of hypertensive vascular disease. The enlarged ventricles could then be subject to an increased total intraventricular force setting up a progressive ventricular enlargement. With enlargement of the ventricles ballooning of the hemispheres could compromise the convexity subarachnoid space by compression against the calvarium, so reducing cerebrospinal fluid drainage and causing a communicating hydrocephalus with convexity or incisural block and abnormal isotope cisternogram (Earnest *et al.*, 1974). Enlargement of the ventricles (Fig. 10.11) is no new fact in *état lacunaire*. Marie (1901) reported that 'a common feature of lacunar brains was a dilatation of the cerebral ventricles . . . which may be fairly pronounced. It has been mentioned by authors in the first half of the nineteenth century under the name of senile hydrocephalus'. Ferrand (1902) stated that ventricular dilatation may reach such proportions as 'to reduce to almost nothing' the white matter of centrum ovale. Granted that ventricular dilatation is likely to be common in *état lacunaire* it must be recognised that its mechanisms and consequences are poorly understood and that it deserves further study.

Undoubtedly the last word has not been said about lacunes. Studies of recent years have shown that there certainly is much more to be discovered about these disorders by painstaking clinical and pathological correlations. To be sure the results may be disappointing when lacunes are too numerous to allow any correlation. On the other hand asymptomatic lacunes or at least lacunes which go by without recognised clinical disorders do exist. Fisher (1968) reported the case of a fit man, aged 71, who attended the Neurological Clinic because of a brief dizzy spell. A detailed neurologic examination showed no defect. Five days later the patient died unexpectedly as the result of a myocardial infarction and neuropathological examination showed the presence of 44 lacunes in the cerebral hemispheres and brain stem. It is reasonable to hope that detailed study of such cases may one day yield further information.

ARTERIOPATHIC DEMENTIA

Dementia in late adult life and in the elderly is one of the most challenging problems of modern neurology. Among people over the age of 65, 10 per cent may be estimated to show signs of organic dementia (Kay, Beamish, and Roth, 1964). Approximately 63 per cent of the elderly who are institutionalised in the United States have dementia (Wang, 1969). Dementia, that is, a permanent and irreversible mental deterioration, is a syndrome with many varied causes, and the part played by vascular disease as an aetiological factor is fairly reflected in the following three series of patients of differing origins.

(1) In a pathological study of 50 brains of demented old patients confined to a mental hospital or geriatric unit, (Tomlinson, Blessed, and Roth, 1970) 50 per cent were considered to be cases of senile dementia showing the histological features of Alzheimer's disease, the majority with no or small ischaemic lesions. Only 12 per cent appeared to be definitely and solely produced by cerebral softenings (arteriosclerotic dementia) although a further 5 per cent were possibly of similar origin. Mixed cases with the pathological features of both senile and arteriosclerotic disease accounted for 8 per cent with certainty and probably for a further 10 per cent. One case of Wernicke's encephalopathy was seen and one was possibly of traumatic origin. Five cases were not classified. Sex differences were rather striking since 15 of the 16 females were cases of senile dementia while in the males arteriosclerosis probably caused or contributed to the dementia in 50 per cent.

(2) In a retrospective clinical study of 106 patients referred to the National Hospital, Queen Square, with a presumptive diagnosis of dementia (Marsden and Harrison, 1972) 84 were considered demented. In 48 of these 84 (57 per cent) no firm aetiological diagnosis could be achieved although many of these patients were presumed to have Alzheimer's disease or Pick's disease. An aetiological diag-

nosis was deemed to have been reached in 36 patients (43 per cent) among whom eight, i.e. about one-fifth, were classified as arteriosclerotic dementia. Seven of these eight were hypertensives.

(3) In Kay et al.'s studies of institutionalised and non-institutionalised people over the age of 65 living in Newcastle-upon-Tyne 5 per cent of cases of dementia (out of a total of 10 per cent) were alleged to be cases of cerebral arteriosclerosis.

Thus the commonest type of dementia of late age is the progressive mental deterioration characterised by failure of memory, disorientation, and confusion ending in a profound dementia with an average duration of two to five years. At post-mortem examination this condition correlates with the presence of numerous senile plaques, neurofibrillary changes, and granulovacuolar degeneration in cortex and basal ganglia. Such pathological features are found both in Alzheimer's disease, which typically appears between the age of 50 and 60 (presenile dementia), as well as in senile dementia. Whether both conditions are a continuum or separate entities is a matter for debate in pathology (McMenemey, 1963). All available evidence indicates that pre-senile and senile dementia are correlated neither with atherosclerosis nor with hypertension (Arab, 1954; Fisher, 1968) although Alzheimer changes may of course co-exist with infarcts in some patients.

It should also be mentioned that arterial lesions different from atherosclerosis, miliary aneurysms and lipohyalinosis have been described in senile brain, mostly from demented patients. They have been referred to as amyloid meningopathy (Divry, 1941–1942), congophile angiopathy (Pantelakis, 1954), or dyshoric angiopathy (Surbek, 1961). It may well be that not all of these lesions are of the same nature. It seems that the pial and cortical arteries are mainly affected, their walls being infiltrated by a substance with variable tinctorial affinities. The amyloid nature of this substance has been questioned. Whatever the case, both Pantelakis (1954) and Surbek (1961) concluded that hypertension played no aetiological role.

The arterial lesions responsible for arteriopathic dementia are of atherosclerotic or lipo-hyalinotic nature, but contrary to general opinion cerebral atherosclerosis *per se* is not responsible for dementia by a gradual restriction of the blood supply to the brain. CBF and cerebral metabolic rate of oxygen decreases little if at all with age. Cerebral arteries react normally to changes in P_aCO_2 and arterial blood pressure in arteriosclerotic dementia. When the reactivity of cerebral vessels is impaired this may be ascribed to a recent infarct or to small vessel disease. Areas of decreased CBF may be found in arteriosclerotic dementia, but again this is in accordance with previous findings in cerebral infarction. In brief, CBF and arterial reactivity are not significantly disturbed in arteriosclerotic dementia unless there is evidence of infarction or small vessels lesions (Simard *et al.*, 1971; Olesen, 1974; Hachinski, Lassen, and Marshall, 1974). This is supported by the clinical observation that whatever the state of atherosclerotic cerebral arteries hypotension is an exceptional cause of focal disorders (Gautier, 1970).

Thus the loose term 'cerebral atherosclerosis' used to describe mental deterioration in old people is probably almost always a misdiagnosis, and apart from precluding correct therapeutic measures it may have disastrous consequences when it results in the failure to recognise treatable conditions such depression, subdural haematomas, benign tumours, or communicating hydrocephalus.

Arteriopathic dementia, indeed, results from focal lesions and it has been concisely defined by Fisher (1968) 'as a matter of strokes large and small'. Recently Hachinski *et al.* (1974) have defined as multi-infarct dementia a condition in which dementia may be the dominant symptom but besides which there are focal neurological signs and symptoms, a step-wise deterioration and often hypertension. This group of patients is of special interest at present since many of the large cerebral infarcts due to atherosclerosis result from extracranial lesions (Lhermitte and Gautier, 1975), some of which could probably be prevented by surgery or antithrombotic drugs; in addition hypertension which aggravates atherosclerosis and is responsible for the

lesions underlying lacunes, may be controlled if detected in time.

Small or large infarcts concomitant with mental deterioration may result from various pathological conditions: *état lacunaire*, watershed infarction, multiple infarcts. In such conditions with numerous or extensive infarcted areas it is often difficult or impossible to ascertain the significance of single lesions. On the other hand aphasic, apraxic, agnosic, amnestic disorders and disorders of attention have been correlated with discrete cerebral infarcts. Although none of these latter disorders should be diagnosed as dementia, all of them may be part of the clinical picture of mental deterioration. Therefore knowledge of their pathological basis may assist clinico-pathological correlation in multi-infarct dementia.

Mental deterioration occurs in most cases of *état lacunaire*. Comte (1900) observed that in pseudobulbar patients memory is generally severely impaired and intelligence weakened. Ferrand (1902) was also impressed by the memory disorders and stressed the point that a severe mental deterioration may co-exist with a slight hemiplegia. It should not be forgotten, however, that the reverse may be true. As previously mentioned, Hughes *et al.* (1954) reported that emotional lability was usually associated with intellectual deterioration but that the two processes did not run parallel in every case. Furthermore intellectual deterioration did not necessarily run parallel with the severity of the pseudobulbar palsy. Thus two patients who could no longer express themselves in speech maintained prolific correspondence with their relatives and could answer questions rationally and communicate their requests by writing. Fisher (1968) defined the mental changes in the lacunar state in its basic form as impaired memory, slowness, decreased spontaneous activity and difficulty in handling complex tasks. He reported the interesting observation that spasmodic laughing and crying is very frequent in vascular disease and almost always absent in senile dementia.

No comprehensive clinicopathological correlations of dementia in *état lacunaire* is yet available. The problem is a formidable one for apart from lacunes, haemorrhagic lesions and/or large infarcts are often present and both lacunes and Alzheimer's changes may be present. However, Ferrand's (1902) and Hughes et al.'s (1954) 'dissociated' cases allow reasonable hope that a few cases of état lacunaire could allow useful clinicopathological correlations for the understanding of dementia.

The clinical diagnosis generally offers no difficulty since the typical symptoms and signs of pseudobulbar palsy are present. It is very rare indeed that the characteristic stepwise evolution with successive small strokes is not found in the history. This together with the presence of arterial hypertension clinches the diagnosis. However it would be obviously better to recognise earlier symptoms. Relatives not infrequently mention changes of mood, decrease in working capacities, lack of interest for usual hobbies in the months or weeks preceding the first definite stroke. This warrants further research since earlier treatment of hypertension might improve the prognosis.

Watershed infarction may occur in unilateral but chiefly in bilateral internal carotid artery occlusion. Cerebral lesions extend along the borders of the territories of the anterior, middle, and posterior cerebral arteries in a sickle-shaped fashion. They result apparently from falls in perfusion pressure in the distal parts of the arterial tree. The pial arteries, in the damaged areas, appear either as white threads (Lhermitte et al., 1970) or are patent (see below). Fisher (1968) mentioned that occasionally mental symptoms predominate in the clinical picture with slowing up, decreased spontaneous activity, grasp reflexes, dyspraxia, slow stepped gait, and incontinence, all pointing to a frontal deficit. There may be visual disturbances, elements of dysphasia and forgetfulness indicating a more posterior localisation. Fisher reported an example of this type of dementia in a man aged 68 who for four months had shown personality changes such as selfishness, overeating, impoliteness, clumsiness, falling down without being able to arise by himself, spilling food unnoticed, slowness, episodic difficulty in speaking, and urinary incontinence. On examination the patient stared vacantly into space, spoke in a quiet

voice, forgot quickly, and was clumsy in all movements. There was a left internal carotid artery occlusion and a watershed infarct in the left cerebral hemisphere. Castaigne et al. (1963) reported the case of a 51-year-old man with bilateral internal carotid artery occlusion, the distal end of the occlusion being below the ophthalmic artery on both sides. The patient survived for two years and died from cancer of the colon. Neuropathological examination showed bilateral watershed lesions, more marked on the left cerebral hemisphere. On the left side the posterior cerebral artery as well as anterior and middle cerebral arteries arose from the internal carotid artery. The pial arteries were patent, thin-walled, and stained pale pink with eosin. Clinically deep reflexes were brisk on both sides; there was a bilateral Babinski sign and marche à petits pas. The appearance and demeanour of the patient were quite remarkable. He had a mask-like face with an impressive absence of mimicry. Day after day he lay for hours on his bed, motionless, head and eyes turned towards the left. At long intervals he winked or sighed or made a few clumsy movements with both hands. However, when encouraged he appeared well orientated in time and space. He could name objects and colours and recognised faces. He clumsily and slowly but correctly carried out spoken commands. There was no severe ideomotor apraxia. In Pierre Marie's test of the three papers two out of the three orders were correct. However as soon as the examination ended the patient reverted to his motionless attitude.

Patients who have survived cardiac arrest during surgery or in the course of heart disease are now frequently observed in intensive therapy wards. Coma after cardiac arrest carries a poor prognosis and a significant proportion of those who survive have a persisting neurological deficit including mental deterioration, which may, however, eventually improve (Bell and Hodgson, 1974). Global severe reduction or arrest of cerebral perfusion may of course produce extensive lesions of cerebral hemispheres, but successive brief failures of perfusion pressure may result in watershed lesions particularly in the border zones between middle and posterior cerebral arteries (Romanul and Abramowicz, 1964). A few patients, generally after a period of occipital blindness and decerebration, are hallucinated, restless, and delirious.

Torvik *et al.* (1971) reported three cases of slowly progressive dementia in elderly patients with generalised thrombosis of arteries and veins, rarely exceeding 0.5 mm in diameter. Such thrombosis was present throughout the body, but the main ischaemic lesions were present in the brain, particularly along the watershed zones. In addition there was ischaemic disease of the peripheral nerves and vascular disease of the legs. There was no sign of primary vascular disease and the mechanisms of thrombus formation remained obscure. Blood pressure was mentioned in patient 3 only (190/125). In patients 1 and 2 the heart weighed 270 and 400 g, respectively.

Multiple infarcts were the pathological condition underlying arteriopathic dementia in Tomlinson *et al.*'s (1970) series of 50 brains of old demented people. As previously mentioned there were six definite and three further probable cases of arteriopathic dementia (eight men, one woman), while in four definite and five further probable cases, both lesions of arteriopathic dementia and Alzheimer's changes could have been held responsible for the clinical disorders. Pathological findings in the nine (six definite and three probable) cases of 'pure' arteriosclerotic dementia are outlined in the paper. The salient features appear to be that there were bilateral extensive cortico-subcortical infarcts involving in most cases the parieto-temporal regions. It should be noted that in six of the nine cases the corpus callosum was involved. In most of the cases there were in addition scattered small foci of infarction of the white matter which may well have been lacunes although this term was not used. Curiously enough, since *état lacunaire* is common in old demented people, no case of this condition was reported in this series.

Tomlinson *et al.* (1970) compared their findings with those from a previously studied series of brains of 28 non-demented old people who were referred to as controls (Tomlinson, Blessed, and Roth, 1968). It is of obvious interest that they found that 16 of the 50 dements had considerable areas of ischaemic destruction readily detectable on gross examination prior to cutting the brain as against 2 of the 28 controls (significant at the 5 per cent level). Further, in the dements total destruction of the territory supplied by a major cerebral artery occurred six times and was not present in the control group. Involvement of the frontal lobes in ischaemic lesions of more than minute amount was not encountered in the controls but was seen seven times in the dements. Considerable ischaemic destruction of the hippocampus and adjacent limbic structures was found seven times in the dements and in none of the controls. Considerable destruction of the corpus callosum was only seen in the dements. In addition, Tomlinson *et al.* (1968, 1970) made an attempt to quantify the amount of brain tissue which had been destroyed by infarction. The mean volumes of 48.9 ml in the demented and 13.2 ml in the control group are not statistically different. However, infarction of more than 20 ml was significantly more common in the demented group and only 2 of the 28 controls showed more than 50 ml infarction whereas 16 of 50 dements exceeded this figure (statistically significant), and softening greater than 100 ml was confined to the demented cases. It is difficult at present to assess the significance of such quantifications of infarcted tissue. It is to be expected that larger infarcts will produce more disturbances than smaller ones. However, in the dementia of *état lacunaire* the amount of destroyed tissue is relatively small. Further research is certainly warranted; it may be that careful study of the lesions in a few cases as was performed, for instance, in the disconnexion syndromes, may prove the most rewarding approach to the understanding of the *mechanisms* of arteriopathic dementia. Nevertheless, Tomlinson *et al.*'s series (1968, 1970) demonstrates that multiple large and small infarcts are a cause of dementia and a cause which could well be amenable to preventive therapy.

Multi-infarct cases are most often of cardiac or atherosclerotic *embolic origin*, the embolic material being thrombus, i.e. a conglomerate of platelets, fibrin and red cells. Cholesterol embolism from atherosclerotic plaques has been reported both in the retinal and cerebral circulation (Russell, 1969; Gautier, 1970). McDonald (1967) reported two hypertensive patients whose cerebral small arteries, mainly in the white matter, were stuffed with cholesterol emboli. One of the patients had a fluctuating condition with disorientation and confusion. The source of embolism was ulcerative atherosclerosis of the aortic arch. In the second patient, the source was an atherosclerotic lesion at the origin of the left internal carotid artery.

Fat embolism may be responsible for mental confusion and retrograde amnesia (Sevitt, 1960). It is of interest that systemic embolism is nearly always associated with a heavy degree of pulmonary embolism at necropsy. Bourgeois and Blanc (1966) reported two cases and collected 30 cases in the literature on neurological and psychiatrical sequelae of fat embolism. In cases of mild severity the only symptom may be agitation, confusion, and clouding of consciousness, raising obvious diagnostic difficulties when there has been concomitant cranial trauma. In cases surviving coma severe dementia is possible although far from constant.

A short review with references will now be given of clinico-pathological correlations of disorders of cognitive functions with discrete cerebral infarcts, intending to help in further analysis of cases of arteriopathic dementia.

Dementia with *thalamic lesions*, i.e. 'thalamic dementia', has been reported in cases of tumour, degenerative diseases, Creutzfeld-Jakob disease and lesions of arterial origin. Schuster (1936–1937) is credited with reporting the first 'vascular' case in a woman aged 49 who developed mood changes, indifference, and dullness with conservation of some intellectual function. Neuropathological examination showed infarction in the territory of the thalamo-tuberal arteries. Castaigne *et al.* (1966) reported two further cases with bilateral infarction in the territory of the retro-mamillary arteries. In both cases the salient features of the dementia were impairment of memory and attention.

Lesions which determine aphasias, apraxias, and agnosias have been the subject of extensive literature. They were reviewed in Foix (1928) classical paper, and in recent years comprehensive studies are those of Geshwind (1965) and Meyer (1974). The point of interest here is whether there is an intellectual impairment in aphasic patients. Weisenburg, McBride and Roe, later Teuber and Weinstein, Newcombe (see Meyer, 1974) adduced psychometric evidence that in aphasia, especially of the receptive type, performances are impaired in nonverbal as well as in verbal tests. All stressed that performances in nonverbal tests were more affected in temporo-parietal than in more rostral lesions. On the other hand Tissot, Lhermitte, and Ducarne (1963) in a study of 218 cases of aphasia with the Wechsler-Bellevue test found no correlation between the performance IQ and the severity of aphasia. They concluded that the performance IQ in the Wechsler-Bellevue test was more a measurement of apraxia than of intelligence. In addition, in non-apraxic aphasic patients the scatter was quite different from that of demented patients (Tissot, 1966).

Studies in *Korsakoff's psychosis* led to recognition of the significance of lesions of the mamillary bodies, of certain thalamic nuclei, and of the terminal part of each fornix in retrograde and anterograde amnesia. Studies of the memory disorders following bilateral temporal surgical removal led to recognition of 'the significance of the hippocampal formation in amnesia for recent events. In summary there is now evidence suggesting the presence of a circuit starting from the hippocampal gyrus to the hippocampus then via the fornix to the mamillary bodies. From the latter the mamillo-thalamic tract reaches the anterior nuclear complex of the thalamus, which in turn projects to the cingulate gyrus. Connections between the cingulate and hippocampal gyri 'loop the loop'. Brierley (1966) reviewed the various lesions determining memory disorders. Escourolle and Gray (1975) analysed their material and reviewed the literature with respect to vascular lesions of the circuit. It appears that reported cases of bilateral cingular infarction are poorly documented on lesions of the fornix. In four cases with normal fornix and mamillary bodies the clinical picture was that of akinetic mutism while in one case with lesions of the fornix there were in addition impairment of attention, disorders of behaviour and amnesia predominantly retrograde with confabulation. In bilateral thalamic lesions involving both mamillothalamic tracts anterograde amnesia may be a prominent clinical feature (Castaigne *et al.*, 1966, case 1; Escourolle and Gray, 1975, case 1). Occlusion of both posterior cerebral arteries resulting in bilateral infarction of the inferomedial portions of the temporal lobes and hippocampal formation, fornix and mamillary body was reported by Victor, Angevine, Mancall, and Fisher (1961). The patient survived for five years during which he showed a severe defect in recent memory and inability to learn new facts and skills. He also showed retrograde amnesia for the two years preceding the onset of his illness. Memory for remote events was virtually unaffected. There were mild behavioural changes such as persistent inactivity, indifference, and loss of initiative. By contrast general intellectual functions remained at a 'bright normal' level although mild and relatively inconspicuous abnormalities were disclosed by tests designed to measure concentration, shifting of mental set and abstract thinking. DeJong, Itabashi, and Olson (1969) reported severe memory impairment in a patient who survived the onset of the disorder for four months. There were discrete bilateral infarcts of the hippocampi greater in extent on the left side where the parahippocampal and fusiform gyri were involved along the collateral fissure. The infarcts extended into both occipital lobes to involve the inferior lip of the calcarine fissure, but these lesions were not clinically apparent and it was felt that they probably did not contribute to the memory disorder.

It was for some time a matter for debate whether unilateral lesions of the hippocampal formation could determine memory impairment. Fisher (1968) reported that in 60 cases of infarction in the territory of the posterior cerebral artery, memory loss and confusion were more common with lesions in the dominant hemisphere. They were present in 27 of 33 (82 per cent) with lesions on the dominant side and in only 5 of 27 (19 per cent) with lesions on the non dominant side. It was concluded that the

hippocampal 'region' in the hemisphere dominant for speech is dominant in the memory process. This applied not only to verbal-auditory memories but to visual, tactile, pain, olfactory, and gustatory memories as well. Escourolle and Gray (1975) reported 11 cases of unilateral infarction in the territory of the posterior cerebral artery. Eight involved the right side and in none was there a memory disorder. Three involved the left side and one resulted in right hemianopia and Korsakoff's psychosis. Neuropathological examination showed infarction of the posterior two-thirds of Ammon's horn and hippocampal gyrus with severe degeneration of the fimbria, fornix, and mamillary body. There was mild atrophy of the anterior nuclear complex of the thalamus. Benson, Marsden, and Meadows (1974) reported 4 cases in a series of 12 instances of posterior cerebral artery occlusion with apparently left sided occlusion and amnesia. Analysis of their cases and cases in the literature (including left temporal resections) led to the conclusion that lesions confined to the left side may cause temporary amnesia but that the evidence for permanent amnesia is inconclusive. Agitated delirium and dementia in relation to infarction of the hippocampal formation,

Some clarification has occurred in recent years about the frontal lobe syndrome (Meyer, 1974). The views of Luria (1969, 1970) are particularly noteworthy. Following Pavlov's concepts of separate analysers and second signal systems, Luria considers the precentral gyrus as the primary motor cortex, the premotor area as the secondary region in which movements are elaborated into motor skills, the prefrontal region as a tertiary system subserving planning and regulation of execution. Damage to frontal lobe results in slowness in mental activity, perseverations, impairment of analysis of sensory or language data, inability to carry out planned action, poor control of errors (Lhermitte, Derouesné, and Signoret, 1972). Such disorders are obviously reminiscent of symptoms and signs encountered in demented patients.

Binswanger encephalopathy

Binswanger (1894) described a particular chronic progressive subcortical encephalopathy

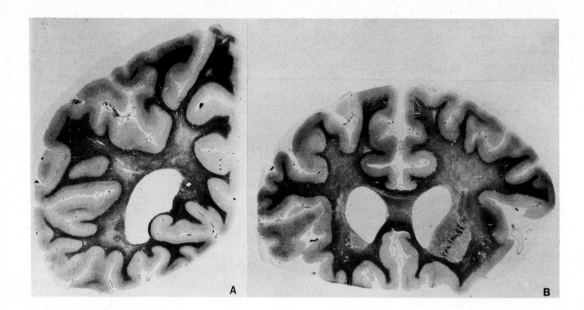

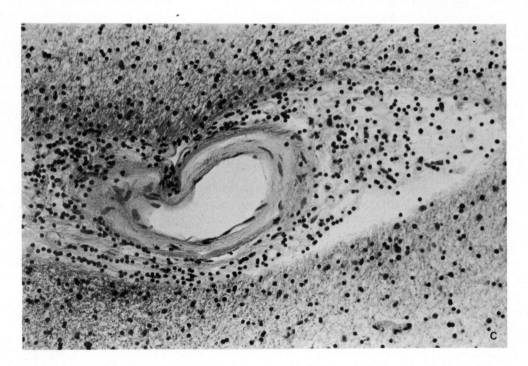

Fig. 10.16 Binswanger's encephalopathy.
A. Coronal section of left hemisphere just behind splenium of corpus callosum.
B. Coronal section of frontal lobes. Extensive demyelination. Celloidin. Loyez Stain.
C. Artery in white matter. Hyalinosis. H.E. × 120.

in hypertensive patients. Although he reported eight cases this is a very rare disease. Garcin, Lapresle, and Lyon (1960) reported three patients and found 20 reported cases. Mikol (1966) reported two additional patients. Clinical symptoms and signs appear generally between the ages of 50 and 60 and result in progressive pseudobulbar palsy and dementia in three to five years. Some cases, however, have a more protracted course. At neuropathological examination the brunt of the process falls on the white matter. Some of the regions of myelin destruction are sharply demarcated, some have less distinct contours. One or several convolutions may be affected. In most cases myelin lesions predominate in the occipital and temporal lobes. In severe cases nearly all the white matter of the brain is involved. The cortex and subacuate fibres are spared. Intracerebral arteries show extensive hyaline changes. Figures 10.16a, b, and c (unpublished case) are from a man who developed at age 66 disorders of memory and in the following years pseudobulbar palsy and dementia. At first examination blood pressure was recorded at 160/110 and on subsequent examination was often in the range of 200/100. At post-mortem, six years later, there was remarkably little atherosclerosis on the basal arteries.

The mechanisms of lesions in Binswanger's leucoencephalopathy are a riddle. Arterial lesions together with the sparing of the cortex have suggested a particular variety of distal ischaemic necrosis, somewhat similar to watershed infarction, but there is not much more than theoretical reasoning to support this view. Oedema of venous origin has been suspected by Stochdroph and Meesen (1958). Feigin and Popoff (1963) thought that in hypertensive individuals the changes in the white matter indicate that there is a tendency for cerebral oedema to develop around focal lesions or even in the absence of such detectable lesions, a view which is supported by present evidence. Feigin and Popoff (1963), however, go further and state that 'the basic change [i.e. arterial hyalinosis] is a late effect of cerebral oedema initiated by some aspects of hypertensive disease and that the vascular change is a secondary effect, secondary to the hypertensive disease itself, to the cerebral oedema and most likely to both'. There may obviously be some truth in these views but the role of each component of this rather elaborate hypothesis has yet to be determined.

Arteriopathic Parkinsonism

The term Parkinson's disease should be reserved for true paralysis agitans. According to all available evidence arterial disease is not an aetiological factor in this disease (Escourolle, de Recondo, and Gray, 1971). Parkinsonism is a syndrome, and several aetiological factors may cause the same clinical picture. Among the causes of Parkinsonism, arterial disease is a classical one; in a review of arteriosclerotic Parkinsonism Critchley (1936) stressed the clinical differences between it and paralysis agitans, in particular he aptly remarked that tremor is usually absent and that blood pressure is often high. He noted that in many cases of arteriosclerotic Parkinsonism there are 'bulbar' signs, emotional incontinence, and a variable dementia. Undoubtedly most of the cases which were in the scope of Critchley's paper could as well be classified as pseudobulbar palsy or *état lacunaire*. Their pathological basis may be assumed to be similar (i.e. occlusion of perforating arteries) and their preventive therapy should be treatment of arterial hypertension.

REFERENCES

Adams, C. W. M. (1967) *Vascular Histochemistry*, London: Lloyd-Luke.
Adams, R. D. (1955) Pathology of cerebral vascular disease. In *Princeton Conferences on Cerebrovascular Disease. Second Conference*, ed. Millikan, C. H. New York: Grune & Stratton.
Adams, R. D. & Fisher, C. M. (1961) Pathology of cerebral arterial occlusion. In *Pathogenesis and Treatment of Cerebrovascular Disease*, ed. Fields, W. S. Springfield, Illinois: Charles C. Thomas.

Alajouanine, T. & Hornet, T. (1939) L'oedème cérébral généralisé. Etude anatomique. *Annales d'Anatomie Pathologique*, **16**, 133.

Arab, A. (1954) Plaques séniles et artériosclérose cérébrale. *Revue Neurologique*, **91**, 22.

Arab, A. (1957) L'artériosclérose cérébrale scalariforme hypertensive. *Psychiatrie und Neurologie* (Basel), **134**, 175.

Baker, A. B. & Iannone, A. (1969a) Cerebrovascular disease. II. The smaller intracerebral arteries. *Neurology* (Minneap.), **9**, 391.

Baker, A. B. & Iannone, A. (1959b) Cerebrovascular disease. III. The intracerebral arterioles. *Neurology* (Minneap.), **9**, 441.

Baker, A. B., Resch, J. A. and Loewenson, R. B. (1969) Hypertension and Cerebral Atherosclerosis. *Circulation*, **39**, 701.

Bayliss, W. N. (1902) On the local reaction of the arterial wall to changes of internal pressure. *Journal of Physiology*, **28**, 220.

Beevers, D. G., Hamilton, M., Fairman, J. E. & Harpur, J. E. (1973) Antihypertensive treatment and the course of established cerebral vascular disease. *Lancet*, i, 1407.

Bell, J. A. & Hodgson, H. J. F. (1974) Coma after cardiac arrest. *Brain*, **97**, 361.

Benson, F. S., Marsden, C. D. & Meadows, J. C. (1974) The amnesic syndrome of posterior cerebral artery occlusion. *Acta Neurologica Scandinavica*, **50**, 133.

Binswanger, O. (1894) Die begrenzung der Allgemeinen progressiven paralysie. *Berliner Klinische Wochenschrift*, **31**, 1137.

Blackfan, K. D. (1926) Acute nephritis in children with special reference to the treatment of uremia. *Bulletin of the Johns Hopkins Hospital*, **39**, 69.

Bourgeois, M. & Blanc, M. (1966) Les séquelles neuro-psychiatriques des embolies graisseuses cérébrales post-traumatiques. *Encéphale*, **55**, 99.

Brain, Lord (1961) *Speech Disorders, Aphasia, Apraxia and Agnosia*. London: Butterworths.

Breckenridge, A., Dollery, C. T. & Parry, E. H. O. (1970) Prognosis of treated hypertension. *Quarterly Journal of Medicine*, **39**, 411.

Brierley, J. B. (1966) Article in *Amnesia*, ed. Whitty, C. W. M. & Zangwill, O. L. London: Butterworths.

Byrom, F. B. (1954) The pathogenesis of hypertensive encephalopathy and its relation to the malignant phase of hypertension: experimental evidence from the hypertensive rat. *Lancet*, ii, 201.

Byrom, F. B. (1969) *The Hypertensive Vascular Crisis*. London: Heinemann.

Cambier, J. & Gautier, J. C. (1965) Pronostic des accidents vasculaires cérébraux de nature ischémique. *Achter Internationaler Kongress für Lebenversicherungsmedizin*. Verlag, Basel, and Stuttgart: Schwaba and Co.

Castaigne, P., Lhermitte, F., Cambier, J. & Gautier, J. C. (1963) Obstruction bilatérale des carotides internes. Etude anatomo-clinique d'une observation avec survie prolongée. *Presse Médicale*, **71**, 757.

Castaigne, P., Buge, A., Cambier, J., Escourolle, R., Brunet, P. & Degos, J. D. (1966) Démence thalamique d'origine vasculaire par ramollissement bilatéral, limité au territoire du pédicule rétro-mamillaire (à propos de deux observations anatomo-cliniques). *Revue Neurologique*, **114**, 89.

Charcot, J. M. & Bouchard, C. (1868) Nouvelles recherches sur la pathogénie de l'hémorragie cérébrale. *Archives de Physiologie Normale et Pathologique*, **1**, 110; 643; 735.

Clarke, E. & Murphy, E. A. (1956) Neurological manifestations of malignant hypertension. *British Medical Journal*, **2**, 1319.

Cole, F. M. & Yates, P. O. (1967a) The occurrence and significance of intracerebral micro-aneurysms. *Journal of Pathology and Bacteriology*, **93**, 393.

Cole, F. M. & Yates, P. O. (1967b) Intracerebral micro-aneurysms and small cerebrovascular lesions. *Brain*, **90**, 759.

Cole, F. M. & Yates, P. O. (1968) Comparative incidence of cerebrovascular lesions in normotensive and hypertensive patients. *Neurology* (Minneap.), **18**, 225.

Comte, A. (1900) *Des Paralysies Pseudo-Bulbaire*. Paris: G. Steinheil.

Cook, T. A. & Yates, P. O. (1972) A histometric study of cerebral and renal arteries in normotensives and chronic hypertensives. *Journal of Pathology*, **108**, 129.

Critchley, M. (1936) Arteriosclerotic Parkinsonism. *Brain*, **52**, 23.

Dejerine, J. & Roussy, G. (1906) Le syndrome thalamique. *Revue Neurologique*, **12**, 521.

DeJong, R. N., Itabashi, H. H. & Olson, J. R. (1969) Memory loss due to hippocampal lesions. *Archives of Neurology*, **20**, 339.

Dinsdale, H. B., Robertson, D. M. & Haas, R. A. (1974) Cerebral blood flow in acute hypertension. *Archives of Neurology*, **31**, 80.

Divry, P. (1941–1942) De l'amyloidose vasculaire cérébrale et méningée (méningopathie amyloide) dans la démence sénile. *Journal Belge de Neurologie et de Psychiatrie*, **41–42**, 141.

Durant-Fardel, M. (1843) *Traité du ramollissement du cerveau*. Paris: J. B. Baillière; London: H. Baillière.

Duret, H. (1874) Recherches anatomiques sur la circulation de l'encéphale. *Archives de Physiologie*, **1**, 60; 316.

Earnest, M. P., Fahn, S., Karp, J. & Rowland, L. P. (1974) Normal pressure hydrocephalus and hypertensive cerebrovascular disease. *Archives of Neurology*, **31**, 262.

Escourolle, R., de Recondo, J. & Gray, F. (1971) Etude anatomopathologique des syndromes parkinsoniens. In *Monoamines, Noyaux Gris Centraux et Syndrome de Parkinson*. P. 173. Geneva: Georg and Cie; Paris: Masson et Cie.

Escourolle, R. & Gray, F. (1975) Les accidents vasculaires du système limbique. In *Seventh Congress of Neuropathology*, Budapest. 1–6 Sept. 1974. *Excerpta Medica*. Amsterdam: Elsevier.

Evans, H. (1933) Hypertensive encephalopathy in nephritis. *Lancet*, ii, 583.

Feigin, I. & Popoff, N. (1963) Neuropathological changes late in cerebral edema. The relationship to trauma, hypertensive disease and Binswanger encephalopathy. *Journal of Neuropathology and Experimental Neurology*, **22**, 500.

Ferrand, J. (1902) *Essai sur l'Hémiplégie des Vieillards. Les Lacunes de Désintégration Cérébrale.* Paris: J. Rousset.

Finnerty, F. A., Witkin, L. & Fazekas, J. F. (1954) Cerebral hemodynamics during ischemia induced by acute hypotension. *Journal of Clinical Investigations*, **33**, 1227.

Finnerty, Jr., F. A. (1972) Hypertensive encephalopathy. *American Journal of Medicine*, **52**, 672.

Fisher, C. M. (1961a) Clinical syndromes in cerebral arterial occlusion. In *Pathogenesis and Treatment of Cerebrovascular Disease*, Fields, W. S., ed. Springfield, Illinois: Charles C. Thomas.

Fisher, C. M. (1961b) The pathology and pathogenesis of intracerebral hemorrhage. In *Pathogenesis and Treatment of Cerebrovascular Disease*, ed. Fields, W. S. Springfield, Illinois: Charles C. Thomas.

Fisher, C. M. (1965a) Lacunes: small, deep cerebral infarcts. *Neurology* (Minneap.), **15**, 774.

Fisher, C. M. (1965b) Pure sensory stroke involving face arm and leg. *Neurology* (Minneap.), **15**, 76.

Fisher, C. M. (1967) Lacunar stroke. The dysarthria–clumsy hand syndrome. *Neurology* (Minneap.), **17**, 614.

Fisher, C. M. (1968) Dementia in cerebral vascular disease. In *Sixth Princeton Conference*. ed. Siekert, R. G. & Whisnant, J. P. New York and London: Grune & Stratton.

Fisher, C. M. (1969) The arterial lesions underlying lacunes. *Acta Neuropatholigica* (Berlin), **12**, 1.

Fisher, C. M. (1972) Cerebral miliary aneurysms in hypertension. *American Journal of Pathology*, **66**, 313.

Fisher, C. M. & Cole, M. (1965) Homolateral ataxia and crural paresis: a vascular syndrome. *Journal of Neurology. Neurosurgery and Psychiatry*, **28**, 48.

Fisher, C. M. & Curry, H. B. (1965) Pure motor hemiplegia of vascular origin. *Archives of Neurology*, **13**, 30.

Fisher, C. M., Gore, I., Okabe, N. & White, P. D. (1965a) Atherosclerosis of the carotid and vertebral arteries. Extracranial and intracranial. *Journal of Neuropathology and Experimental Neurology*, **24**, 455.

Fisher, C. M., Gore, I., Okabe, N. & White, P. D. (1965b) Calcification of the carotid syphon. *Circulation*, **32**, 538.

Fog, M. (1939) Cerebral circulation. II Reaction of pial arteries to increase in blood pressure. *Archives of Neurology and Psychiatry*, **41**, 260.

Foix, C. (1928) Aphasies. In *Nouveau Traité de Médecine*. P. 135. Paris: Masson et Cie.

Foix, C. & Hillemand, P. (1925) Les artères de l'axe encéphalique jusqu'au diencéphale inclusivement. *Revue Neurologique*, **2**, 705.

Foix, C., Chavany, A. & Marie, J. (1926) Diplégie facio-linguomasticatrice d'origine cortico sous corticale sans paralysie des membres. *Revue Neurologique*, **1**, 214.

Foix, C. & Lévy, M. (1927) Les ramollissements sylviens. Syndromes des lésions en foyer du territoire de l'artère sylvienne et de ses branches. *Revue Neurologique*, **2**, 1.

Folkow, B. (1971) The haemodynamic consequences of adaptive structural changes of the resistance vessels. *Clinical Science*, **41**, 1.

Garcin, R. & Lapresle, J. (1954) Syndrome sensitif de type thalamique et à topographie cheiro-orale par lésion localisée du thalamus. *Revue Neurologique*, **90**, 124.

Garcin, R. & Lapresle, J. (1960) Deuxième observation personnelle de syndrome sensitif de type thalamique et à topographie cheiro-orale par lésion localisée du thalamus. *Revue Neurologique*, **103**, 474.

Garcin, R., Lapresle, J. & Lyon, G. (1960) Encéphalopathie sous-corticale chronique de Binswanger. Etude anatomo-clinique de trois observations. *Revue Neurologique*, **102**, 423.

Garner, A. & Ashton, N. (1970) Ultrastructure of hypertensive retinopathy. *Excerpta Medica International Congress Series No. 222 Ophthalmology*.

Gautier, J. C. (1970) Histoire naturelle des accidents cérébraux dus à l'athérosclérose. *Encéphale*, **3**, 197.

Geshwind, N. (1965) Disconnexion syndromes in animals and man. *Brain*, **88**, 237; 585.

Giese, J. (1966) *The Pathogenesis of Hypertensive Vascular Disease.* Copenhagen: Munskgaard.

Graham, J. B. (1951) Pheochromocytoma and hypertension. An analysis of 207 cases. *International Abstracts of Surgery (Surgery Gynecology Obstetrics. Suppl.)*, **92**, 105.

Hachinski, V. C., Lassen, N. A. & Marshall, J. (1974) Multi-infarct dementia. A cause of mental deterioration in the elderly. *Lancet*, ii, 207.

Häggendahl, E. & Johansson, B. (1972) On the pathophysiology of the increased cerebrovascular permeability in acute arterial hypertension in cats. *Acta Neurologica Scandinavica*, **48**, 265.

Hamilton, M., Thompson, E. N. & Wisniewski, T. K. M. (1964) The role of blood pressure control in preventing complications of hypertension. *Lancet*, i, 235.

Harnish, A. & Pearce, M. L. (1973) Evolution of hypertensive retinal vascular disease. Correlations between clinical and post-mortem observations. *Medicine*, **52**, 483.

Hodge, J. V., McQueen, E. G. & Smirk, H. (1961) Results of hypotensive therapy in arterial hypertension. *British Medical Journal*, i, 1.

Hughes, W. H., Dodgson, M. C. H. & MacLennan, D. C. (1954) Chronic cerebral hypertensive disease. *Lancet*, ii, 770.

Jackson, J. H. (1874–1976; reprinted 1958) *Selected Writings*. Vol. 1., p. 265. London: Staples Press.

Jellinek, E. H., Painter, M., Prineas, J. & Ross Russell, R. (1964) Hypertensive encephalopathy with cortical disorders of vision. *Quarterly Journal of Medicine*, **33**, 239.

Jewett, J. F. (1973) Fatal intracranial edema from eclampsia. *New England Journal of Medicine*, **289**, 976.

Johansson, B. (1974) *Blood-Brain Barrier Dysfunction in Acute Arterial Hypertension*. Göteborg.

Johansson, B., Li, C. L., Olsonn, Y. & Klatzo, I. (1970) The effect of acute arterial hypertension on the blood brain barrier to protein tracers. *Acta Neuropathologica* (Berlin), **16**, 117.

Johansson, B., Strandgaard, S. & Lassen, N. A. (1974) On the pathogenesis of hypertensive encephalopathy. *Circulation Research*, **34**, 167.

Kannel, W. B. (1971) Current status of the epidemiology of brain infarction associated with occlusive arterial disease. *Stroke*, **2**, 295.

Kannel, W. B., Wolf, P. A., Verter, J. & McNamara, P. (1970) Epidemiologic assessment of the role of blood pressure in stroke. The Framingham Study. *Journal of the American Medical Association*, **214**, 301.

Kay, D. W. K., Beamish, P. & Roth, M. (1964) Old age mental disorders in Newcastle-upon-Tyne. I. A study of prevalence. *British Journal of Psychiatry*, **110**, 146.

Kernohan, J. W., Anderson, E. W. and Keith, N. M. (1929) Arterioles in cases of hypertension. *Archives of Internal Medicine*, **44**, 395.

Lassen, N. A. (1959) Cerebral blood flow and oxygen consumption in man. *Physiological Review*, **39**, 183.

Lassen, N. A. & Agnoli, A. (1972) The upper limit of autoregulation of cerebral blood flow. On the pathogenesis of hypertensive encephalopathy. *Scandinavian Journal of Clinical and Laboratory Investigation*, **30**, 113.

Leishman, A. W. D. (1959) Hypertension treated and untreated. A study of 400 cases. *British Medical Journal*, i, 1361.

Lhermitte, J. & Trelles, J. O. (1934) L'artériosclérose du tronc basilaire et ses conséquences anatomo-cliniques. *Jarhbücher für Psychiatrie und Neurologie*, **51**, 91.

Lhermitte, F., Gautier, J. C. & Derouesné, C. (1970) Nature of occlusions of the middle cerebral artery. *Neurology* (Minneap.) **20**, 82.

Lhermitte, F., Derouesné, J. & Signoret, J. L. (1972) Analyse neurologique du syndrome frontal. *Revue Neurologique*, **127**, 415.

Lhermitte, F. & Gautier, J. C. (1975) Sites of cerebral arterial occlusions. In *Modern Trends in Neurology*, **6**, London: Butterworth.

Low-Beer, T. & Phear, D. (1961) Cerebral infarction and hypertension. *Lancet*, i, 1303.

Luria, A. R. (1969) Frontal lobe syndromes. In *Handbook of Clinical Neurology*. Vol. II, ed. Vinken, P. J. & Bruyn, G. W. Amsterdam: North Holland.

Luria, A. R. (1970) *The Working Brain. An Introduction to Neuropsychology*, trans. Haigh, B. London: Penguin.

Marie, P. (1901) Des foyers lacunaires de désintégration et de différents autres états cavitaires du cerveau. *Revue de Médecine*, **31**, 281.

Marsden, C. D. & Harrison, M. J. G. (1972) Outcome of investigation of patients with presenile dementia. *British Medical Journal*, i, 249.

Marshall, J. (1964) A trial of long-term hypotensive therapy in cerebrovascular disease. *Lancet*, i, 10.

Marshall, J. & Kaeser, A. C. (1961) Survival after non-haemorrhagic cerebrovascular accidents. A prospective study. *British Medical Journal*, ii, 73.

McDonald, W. I. (1967) Recurrent cholesterol embolism as a cause of fluctuating cerebral symptoms. *Journal of Neurology, Neurosurgery and Psychiatry*, **30**, 489.

McMenemey, W. H. (1963) Article in *Greenfield's Neuropathology*, 2nd edn. London: Arnold.

Medina, J. L., Rubino, F. A. & Ross, E. (1974) Agitated delirium caused by infarctions of the hippocampal formation and fusiform and lingual gyri. *Neurology* (Minneap.),**24**, 1181.

Meyer, A. (1974) The frontal lobe syndrome, the aphasias and related conditions. A contribution to the history of cortical localisation. *Brain*, **97**, 565.

Meyer, J. S. (1961) The value of electroencephalography in diagnosis of cerebrovascular disease. In *Pathogenesis and Treatment of Cerebrovascular Disease*, ed. Fields, W. S. Springfield, Illinois: Charles C. Thomas.

Meyer, J. S., Waltz, A. G. & Gotoh, F. (1960a) Pathogenesis of cerebral vasospasm in hypertensive encephalopathy. I. Effects of acute pressure in intraluminal blood pressure on pial blood flow. *Neurology* (Minneap.), **10**, 735.

Meyer, J. S., Waltz, A. G. & Gotoh, F. (1960b) Pathogenesis of cerebral vasospasm in hypertensive encephalopathy. II. The nature of increased irritability of smooth muscle of pial arterioles in renal hypertension. *Neurology* (Minneap.), **10**, 859.

Mikol, J. (1966) *Contribution à l'Etude des Leucoencéphalopathies Artérioscléreuses: Maladie de Binswanger et Formes Apparentées*. Paris.

Milliez, P. (1943) *Accidents Cérébraux des Hypertendus et Oedème Méningo-Encéphalique*. Thèse Faculté Médecine. Paris: J. Peyronnet et Cie.

Nicolesco, J., Cretu, V. & Demetresco, L. (1932) Syndrome de l'artère cérébrale antérieure. Monoplégie crurale droite avec symptomatologie cérébelleuse prédominante. *Revue Neurologique*, **1**, 563.

Olesen, J. (1974) Cerebral blood flow: methods for measurement, regulation, effects of drugs and changes in disease. *Acta Neurologica Scandinavica.* Suppl. 57, **50**, 75.

Oppenheimer, B. S. & Fishberg, A. M. (1928) Hypertensive encephalopathy. *Archives of Internal Medicine*, **41**, 264.

Pal. J. (1905) *Die Gefässkrisen.* Leipzig: Hirzel.

Pantelakis, S. (1954) Un type particulier d'angiopathie sénile du système nerveux central: l'angiopathie congophile. Topographie et fréquence. *Monatschrift für Psychiatrie und Neurologie*, **12**, 219.

Rodda, R. & Denny-Brown, D. (1966a). The cerebral arteries in experimental hypertension. I. The nature of arteriolar constriction and its effects on the collateral circulation. *American Journal of Pathology*, **49**, 53.

Rodda, R. & Denny-Brown, D. (1966b) The cerebral arterioles in experimental hypertension. II. The development of arteriolonecrosis. *American Journal of Pathology*, **49**, 365.

Romanul, F. C. A. & Abramowicz, A. (1964) Changes in brain and pial vessels in arterial border zones. *Archives of Neurology*, **11**, 40.

Russell, R. W. R. (1963) Observations on intracerebral aneurysms. *Brain*, **86**, 425.

Russell, R. W. R. (1969) Cerebral embolism: pathogenesis and clinical features. In *Extracranial Cerebrovascular Disease and its Management*, ed. Gillespie, J. A. London: Butterworth.

Russell, R. W. R. (1973) Evidence for autoregulation in human retinal circulation. *Lancet*, ii, 1048.

Schuster, P. (1936–1937) Beiträge zur Pathologie des Thalamus Opticus. I–IV. *Archives für Psychiatrie und Nervenkrankheit*, **105**, 358; 550; **106**, 13; 201.

Sevitt, S. (1960) The significance and classification of fat embolism. *Lancet*, ii, 825.

Shekelle, R. B., Ostfeld, A. M. & Klawans, Jr., H. L. (1974) Hypertension and risk of stroke in an elderly population. *Stroke*, **5**, 71.

Simard, D., Olesen, J., Paulson, O. B., Lassen, N. A. & Skinhøj, E. (1971) Regional cerebral blood flow and its regulation in dementia. *Brain*, **94**, 273.

Stochdorpf, O. & Meesen, H. (1958) Article in *Handbuch der Speziellen Pathologischen Anatomie und Histologie*. Berlin: J. Springer.

Strandgaard, S., Olesen, J., Skinhøj, E. & Lassen, N. A. (1973) Autoregulation of brain circulation in severe arterial hypertension. *British Medical Journal*, i, 507.

Surbek, B. (1961) L'angiopathie dyshorique (Morel) de l'écorce cérébrale. Etude anatomo-clinique et statistique, aspect génétique. *Acta Neuropathologica* (Berlin), **1**, 168.

Thurel, R. (1929) *Les Pseudo-Bulbaires. Etude Clinique et Anatomo-Pathologique.* Paris: G. Doin.

Tissot, R. (1966) *Neuropsychopathologie de l'Aphasie.* Paris: Masson et Cie.

Tissot, R., Lhermitte, F. & Ducarne, B. (1963) Etat intellectuel des aphasiques. *Encéphale*, **4**, 285.

Tomlinson, B. E., Blessed, G. & Roth, M. (1968) Observations on the brains of non-demented old people. *Journal of the Neurological Sciences*, **7**, 331.

Tomlinson, B. E., Blessed, G. & Roth, M. (1970) Observations on the brains of demented old people. *Journal of the Neurological Sciences*, **11**, 205.

Torvik, A., Endresen, G. K. M., Abrahamsen, A. F. & Godal, H. C. (1971) Progressive dementia caused by an unusual type of generalised small vessel thrombosis. *Acta Neurologica Scandinavica*, **47**, 137.

Van Citters, R. L., Wagner, B. M. & Rushmer, R. F. (1962) Architecture of small arteries during vasoconstriction. *Circulation Research*, **10**, 668.

Vander Eecken, H. M. (1959) *The Anastomoses between the Leptomeningeal Arteries of the Brain.* Springfield, Illinois: Charles C. Thomas.

Veterans Administration Cooperative Study Group on Antihypertensive Agents (1967) Effects of treatment on morbidity in hypertension. *Journal of the American Medical Association*, **202**, 1028.

Victor, M., Angevine, J. B. Jr., Mancall, E. L. & Fisher, C. M. (1961) Memory loss with lesions of hippocampal formation. *Archives of Neurology*, **5**, 244.

Wang, H. S. (1969) Organic brain syndrome. In *Behavior and Adaptation in Later Life*, ed. Busse, E. W. & Pfeiffer, E. Boston: Little, Brown.

Whisnant, J. P. (1974) Epidemiology of stroke: emphasis on transient cerebral ischemic attacks and hypertension. *Stroke*, **5**, 68.

Wilson, C. (1963) Personal communication to Jellinek *et al.* (1964).

Wilson, C. (1969) Hypertension. In *Atherosclerosis, Pathology, Physiology, Aetiology, Diagnosis and Clinical Management*, ed. Schettler, F. G., Boyd, G. S. Amsterdam, London, New York: Elsevier.

Ziegler, D. K., Zosa, A. & Zileli, T. (1965) Hypertensive encephalopathy. *Archives of Neurology*, **12**, 472.

11. Spontaneous Intracerebral and Cerebellar Haemorrhage

Alan Richardson

SPONTANEOUS INTRACEREBRAL HAEMORRHAGE

Haemorrhage into the substance of the cerebral hemispheres may occur from a variety of causes but the type for discussion here is that associated with hypertensive disease or atherosclerosis, affecting the cerebral vessels. This group is commonly characterised by haemorrhage into the brain parenchyma in patients with known vascular disease who, at angiography, operation, or post-mortem, show no evidence of an associated vascular anomaly such as aneurysm, angioma, or tumour. The occurrence of minute angiomas or thrombosed aneurysms in similar cases has of course been described but these are outside the present context.

Pathology

Brief reference to the possible pathological sequence is necessary to understand the clinical and therapeutic problems. Most large clinical or post-mortem series indicate prevalence of hypertension of at least 50 per cent (Locksley, Sahs, and Sandler, 1966; Richardson and Einhorn, 1963), with a peak age incidence between 50 and 59 years (McKissock, Richardson, and Walsh, 1959). Though at first sight it may seem not unreasonable to expect haemorrhage from diseased vessels in hypertensive patients, the definition of the precise pathological substrate has excited much attention starting with Charcot and Bouchard in 1872 who postulated miliary aneurysms as the cause. This has been validated by Ross Russell (1963) who elegantly demonstrated microaneurysms on perforating vessels of 100 to 300 μm diameter, occurring almost exclusively in hypertensive patients. The fact that these were common on vessels at the usual

sites of primary haemorrhage was of great importance. It is naturally difficult to prove that such lesions are always the cause of such haemorrhage, and Fisher (1971) has suggested that the haemorrhage may arise from involvement sequentially of a number of small vessels. The microaneurysm hypothesis nevertheless seems the most attractive except that these lesions are relatively rare in normotensive patients under the age of 65 years (Cole and Yates, 1967) whereas primary brain haemorrhage in such patients at a younger age is not. Such haemorrhage most commonly seems to start in the putamenocapsular region or the thalamus and then may either arrest as a circumscribed haematoma or spread in various directions. It may suffuse to occupy predominantly the region of the external capsule or proceed further and by splitting along the planes of white matter form a substantial space occupying clot in the frontal, temporal, or parietal lobes or occasionally arise from the posterior capsular region and track into the occipital lobe. As an alternative the haemorrhage may remain confined to the ganglionic masses or rupture into the ventricular system. Such rupture may be massive and rapidly fatal or be a secondary event resulting in a communication between the haematoma cavity and the trigone of the lateral ventricle or less commonly between the haematoma and the frontal or temporal horns. Whether the haemorrhage is a single event or followed by further episodes of bleeding (Fisher, 1971) remains a matter for debate, but it is a surgical fact that clot of varying ages from within the cavity can only occasionally be confirmed. This brief pathological concept serves to highlight the three important clinical groups: firstly, the destructive massive ganglionic haemorrhages of a fatal character; secondly, more circumscribed

210

lesions in the same area causing maximal neurological deficit but with survival; thirdly, those cases in which the lobar component predominates and therefore present as a space occupying mass. Additionally one must consider the response of the brain to these sudden insults, and of paramount importance is the disruption of the normal vascular autoregulation in the region of the lesion to which is added the space occupying character of the lesion, resulting in rapid and often dramatic changes in intracranial pressure. It is well known that spontaneous intracranial bleeding may provoke rises in intracranial pressure approaching arterial systolic levels the persistence of which may cause arrest of the cerebral circulation and prevent its restitution even when the pressure falls. Lesser degrees of change may account for brief periods of unconsciousness at the moment of ictus, and slower but more persistent changes associated with brain oedema and loss of autoregulatory capacity must be responsible for the brain herniations and secondary brain stem haemorrhages so commonly seen in fatal cases. The origin of the haemorrhage, the vascular tonus at the time and the sequential pathological changes in the brain set the stage for the varied clinical presentation and courses and help to define the therapeutic aims as well as setting limits on their effectiveness.

Clinical features

Consideration of cerebral haemorrhage conjures the picture of sudden onset of severe headache with vomiting and the rapid evolution of a neurological deficit with depression of consciousness. This was the accepted classified description and less severe clinical events were regarded as thrombotic in aetiology. However, in a series of 244 cases of proven intracerebral haemorrhage (McKissock et al., 1959) it was possible to identify four major presenting groups:

1. Sudden onset without loss of consciousness (89 cases).
2. Sudden onset with loss of consciousness (117 cases).
3. Gradual onset without loss of consciousness (23 cases).
4. Gradual onset with later loss of consciousness (3 cases).

The exact mode of onset in the remaining 12 cases was unknown. Thus about half the patients did not lose consciousness at or soon after the ictus. If we follow the clinical course a little further it is noted that about one-third of those in the first group subsequently showed a depression of conscious level usually within two to five days, and a similar number of those in the second group regained consciousness in the same period of time. It therefore follows that consciousness will be preserved or regained in about half the cases of cerebral haemorrhage. The accurate assessment of neurological signs depends on the state of awareness of the patient. In this series of 244 cases, 86 were either in deep coma or simply capable of reflex protective responses. In the remainder hemiplegia or hemiparesis was the commonest sign with evidence of hemisensory disturbance in the more deeply placed lesions. Less than 10 per cent of the group were without an identifiable severe deficit, this most commonly amounting to severe confusion, disorientation, and often marked behaviour disturbance.

The more definitive clinical features have been described by Fisher (1961), and only brief reference needs to be made to them here. Severe headache was only a feature in 50 per cent of cases whereas vomiting was almost universal. Nuchal rigidity was not invariable and was usually mild in degree and slow of evolution.

PUTAMENOCAPSULAR HAEMORRHAGE

This produces the classical abrupt hemiplegic onset with an all-modality sensory disturbance, hemianopic defects and speech deficit in the dominant hemisphere. Loss of conjugate lateral gaze may be a prominent feature. Usually the motor deficit is more severe and persistent than the sensory, but even then may have a non-uniform distribution. Where the haemorrhage is more confined to the region of the caudate head the deficits may be less severe, transient, and associated with more obvious confusion. Alertness is commonly maintained. Rupture into the ventricular system is almost invariable.

THALAMIC HAEMORRHAGE

Vessel rupture in this region may produce a small haematoma or it may spread to involve the internal capsule or track into the cerebral peduncle. The clinical features will vary from abrupt coma proceeding to death, to less dramatic forms with global motor and sensory deficits often associated with marked ocular disturbances. There may be loss of upward gaze or downward deviation of the eyes. Skew deviation is common and pupillary inequality usual. Lateral gaze palsies were also noted in Fisher's cases (1961). He felt that these ocular defects were more common in such deeply placed haemorrhages but unfortunately they are also sometimes seen following aneurysmal rupture, acute subdural haematomas, and occasionally in lobar haematomas.

LOBAR HAEMATOMAS

These most commonly originate in the external capsule and split white matter to involve the appropriate lobe. Confusion and disorientation with more severe headache are common, the neurological signs being referable to the lobe involved, though the severity often seems to bear little relationship to the size of the haematomas unless it is truly massive. Epilepsy as an acute phenomenon is seen in these lesions, often generalised at the onset with a tendency to be focal later. Kaplan (1961) suggested a prevalence of 30 per cent for epilepsy in acute haemorrhage whereas our own experience would suggest a much lower prevalence.

Diagnosis

The occurrence of primary intracerebral haemorrhage is based on a combination of clinical suspicion aroused by the clinical characteristics, the nature of the onset, and the evolution of events, together with more definitive investigatory procedures designed directly or indirectly to demonstrate the haematoma and exclude the presence of an associated causal lesion. An abrupt onset with little preceding history, the absence of trauma, and with the other clinical features noted above is still the commonest starting point in the diagnostic procedure. In view of the known tendency for

blood to enter the ventricular system, examination of the CSF is usually considered the first step.

LUMBAR PUNCTURE

In the series of 244 cases (McKissock et al., 1959) this investigation had been performed in 201 patients. Evidence of recent haemorrhage was obvious in 161 of them but was absent in the remaining 40 cases. Forty-three patients did not have the lumbar CSF examined; of these the ventricular fluid was blood-stained and xanthochronic in 18 and in nine it was clear. In the remainder the time interval from the ictus was too long for valid conclusion. This study, therefore did not allow of any firm conclusion but suggested that in an appreciable proportion of cases the fluid showed no evidence of recent haemorrhage, therefore leaving some initial doubt between the diagnosis of haemorrhage and infarction. It was further interesting that in five cases the cerebrospinal fluid showed a marked pleocytosis such as to suggest the possibility of meningitis. This point had been earlier noted by Bedford (1958). The absence of blood from the CSF in a conscious patient may suggest vascular occlusion, whereas its presence simply indicates the entry of blood into the subarachnoid space and therefore does not exclude the possibility of an associated causal lesion. Further complicating the problem is the fact that diagnostic lumbar puncture may not be free from hazard. Certainly in a patient showing signs of mesencephalic embarrassment with depression of consciousness, hemiplegia and increasing pupillary inequality the hazards of lumbar puncture in accelerating a progressive haematoma will outweigh the advantage of the information so gained. In the unconscious patient following a deteriorating course the investigation should be employed only if a treatable alternative diagnosis presents itself.

ULTRASOUND

Harnessing transcephalic ultrasound transmission as an investigatory tool was first suggested by Leksell (1956). He described the registration of a characteristic mid-line echo pattern with pulsed ultrasound using a large transeiver applied to the intact skull with air excluded by using oil at the interface. Theoretically this benign, relatively simple investigation can be performed at the bedside and though the information it provides is limited it is still of value. Reflection takes place at interfaces of tissue density and thus the echo position of the midline can usually be identified. Similarly the walls of the lateral ventricles may be delimited and occasionally surface brain haematomas indicated by unusual echo patterns. Achar, Coe, and Marshall (1966) made the case for its use in differentiating haemorrhage from infarction on the basis that displacement of the 'mid-line' echo was an early event in haemorrhage and either absent or late in development and slight in degree in cases of vascular occlusion.

Whilst this is quite clearly so in differentiating small infarcts from large haematomas there is considerable overlap in the smaller clots and larger infarcts. Developments in more precise and more informative methods of investigation have diminished the use of this benign, non-invasive technique.

RADIOACTIVE BRAIN SCANNING

Rectilinear brain scanning in neurological diagnosis using various radioisotopes is a well established procedure in many acute brain lesions, particularly brain tumours. Its usefulness in the diagnosis of primary intracerebral haematomas has been less well validated though some authors have suggested that it will demonstrate the lesion in nearly three-quarters of cases. (Ojemann, 1973). Extensive experience in our own department does not really substantiate this claim throughout the varied range of such cases. The uptake and retention of isotope in the compressed tissue surrounding such a haematoma is remarkably variable, depending on the site, size, configuration, and most importantly on the age of the lesion. It is more common to demonstrate a zone of increased uptake in relation to a chronic lesion than to an acute one and even then differentiation from other types of pathology may be difficult. In the general context of acute cerebral lesions it may be useful in excluding other lesions such as massive infarction, tumour, abscess, or the occasional acute spontaneous subdural haematoma (Tallala and McKissock, 1971).

EMI SCANNING

In 1961 Oldendorf devised a system for displaying anatomical structures as a complex demonstration of their radiodensity. This idea was brought to fruition by Hounsfield in 1969, who evolved the radiological system and computer programme to represent the skull and its contents in serial axial slices in relation to their X-ray density. The technique has been fully described (Hounsfield, Ambrose, Perry, and Bridger, 1973) and needs no amplification except to stress that it is a benign, non-invasive method of investigation uniquely relevant to the accurate diagnosis of intracerebral haematomas. Clotted blood, partly due to its calcium has an X-ray density in striking contrast to that of the surrounding brain and much greater than that of the fluid filled ventricular system. It therefore allows of accurate assessment of the size, situation, and configuration of the haematoma (high density—represented as white), as well as indicating the degree of displacement or distortion of the ventricular system and the presence of any associated oedema in the brain parenchyma (diminished density—represented by black or dark grey areas).

A series of 66 intracerebral haematomas all verified by operation or autopsy were investigated in this way and reported by Paxton and Ambrose (1974). In each case the haematoma was accurately diagnosed and its precise configuration, extent, and relationship to the cerebral structures and the ventricular system demonstrated. The overwhelming majority of the lesions were seen as high density areas, with some increase in density noted in those cases subjected to serial examination. This was thought to be due to subsequent clot retraction, loss of fluid and therefore relative increase in calcium ion content. Figure 11.1 shows a typical high density clot in the region of the external capsule with a medial margin of oedema (black), and clearly shows the compression and displacement of the body and part of the frontal horn of the lateral ventricle. A much larger haematoma with more marked ventricular

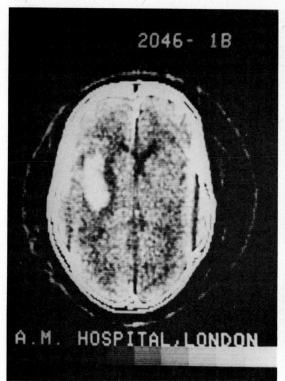

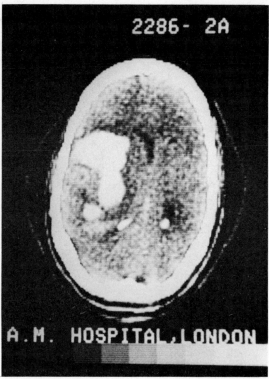

Fig. 11.1   Scan orientation achieved by viewing slice from above. The scan index number is anterior. Right and left sides are as viewed from above.

   Typical haematoma (dense white) in external capsule of left hemisphere. Frontal horn displacement obvious. Medial margin of oedema (black).

Fig. 11.2   More extensive dissection by haematoma (white) to a superficial position in left temporal lobe. Frontal horn markedly displaced and compressed.

displacement is shown in Figure 11.2, with the lesion dissecting towards a more superficial position in the temporal lobe but also extending far posteriorly. In contrast Figure 11.3 shows a small sub-ependymal haematoma as a small white area in the region of the caudate head on the left side at the junction of the frontal horn and the body of the ventricle. A haemorrhage into the right thalamus in a restless patient is shown in Figure 11.4. This clearly demonstrates the dilatation of the ventricular system and the distortion of the third ventricle which is almost obliterated. Finally Figure 11.5 shows a large haemorrhage dissecting towards the fronto-temporal operculum, arising from the region of the internal capsule and showing clear evidence of marked ventricular distortion with actual

rupture into the ventricular system. In the collected series of Paxton and Ambrose (1974) further examples are shown including primary massive intraventricular rupture.

There is no doubt that this form of scanning has revolutionised not only the ease of diagnosis of intracerebral haemorrhage but has also provided vital information in relation to associated pathology necessary to the formulation of a logical treatment policy.

ANGIOGRAPHY

Whilst this remains the most commonly available method of investigation it is an invasive procedure not without hazard. It is therefore necessary to assess the timing of the procedure in order that the potential hazards shall not outweigh the possible therapeutic benefit. In general it should be employed when the pat-

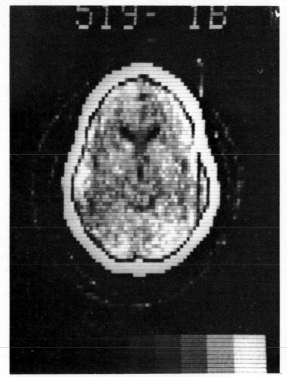

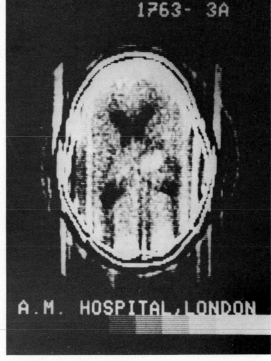

Fig. 11.3 Small, spherical haematoma (white) at point of junction of anterior horn and body of lateral ventricle. Subependymal in position. Virtually no ventricular distortion and certainly no displacement.

Fig. 11.4 Typical right thalamic haemorrhage. The patient was restless and confused causing some artefact. This did not preclude accurate lesion diagnosis and delineation.

ient's vegetative and neurological state has stabilised, the delay period being kept as short as is practicable in view of the diagnostic doubt. Persisting deep coma is never an indication for angiography in an abrupt cerebral episode with subarachnoid bleeding since surgical treatment at that stage is unrewarding. It is always preferable to await the attainment of the patient's most satisfactory state unless after a period of improvement there is evidence of neurological decline. Under these circumstances the hazard of angiography must be accepted as the prognosis otherwise becomes poor.

The clinician requires positive and negative information from the angiogram which is usually designed to show both carotid circulations; it is only rarely necessary to perform a vertebral angiogram. The examination must exclude a causal lesion by adequate visualisa-

tion of the vessels and indirectly by showing the absence of arterial spasm such as might indicate a non-filling aneurysm. Delineation of the clot which is successful in about 75 per cent of cases is by indirect means of large vessel displacement, perforating vessel distortion, or displacement or angulation of the deep venous system. The size of the lesion and its location together with its destructive or space occupying nature set limits on the degree of disturbance of the normal angiographic vascular pattern and therefore account for the shortfall in diagnostic accuracy. A recent study by Benes, Kouholik and Obroski (1972) has attempted to equate the site and type of haemorrhage with prognosis. Their findings will be discussed later, but it is relevant here that they further the suggestion that the ganglionic destructive haemorrhages, i.e. those less easily demonstrated by angio-

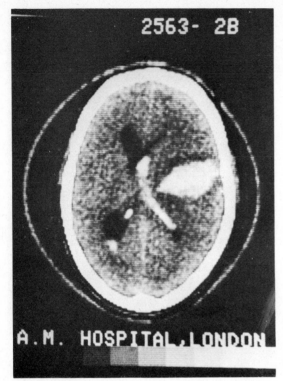

Fig. 11.5 Dissection of haematoma to a superficial position. Rupture into the right lateral ventricle is clearly seen.

graphy, may be in the most lethal group and that the definitive diagnosis may be of little consequence. This paper suffers the disadvantage of being based solely on post-mortem material so that the situation in the survivors is not known. Unless or until the EMI scanner becomes more readily available, most clinicians will still require recourse to angiography as soon as the patient's general and neurological condition permits.

PNEUMOENCEPHALOGRAPHY

Visualisation of the ventricular system by the direct injection of air via a burrhole or indirectly by air encephalography is rarely indicated in the diagnostic evaluation of cerebral haemorrhage. That it is dangerous in the acute phase is not questioned for it not only causes an acute upset in intracranial pressure dynamics but it may increase brain shifts or cause rupture of the haematomas into the ventricular system with its attendant complications of aseptic ependymitis or mechanical ventricular obstruction by clot. The use of air as a contrast study should be reserved for chronic cases in which there is diagnostic doubt or in cases wherein a late complication of haemorrhage, such as hydrocephalus, is suspected.

Initial management

All authors are agreed that of all the factors affecting prognosis, the level of consciousness is the most significant and that any factor influencing this will affect the outcome. Whilst it is true that initial and unremitting coma carries a mortality risk approaching 100 per cent and preservation of consciousness may reduce this to 20 per cent (McKissock et al., 1959), the conscious state may vary for differing reasons and it is therefore logical initially to take all possible medical measures to improve the patient's state optimally before embarking on invasive investigation or contemplating surgical evacuation.

Sudden depression of consciousness associated with a space taking mass and consequent elevation of intracranial pressure has a number of abnormal pathological concomitants. Foremost is depression or alteration of the respiratory cycle with diminution of cough reflex and the usual pattern of intermittent sighing which aerates the lungs and is characteristic of the normal state. Reduction of coughing leads to retention of normal pulmonary secretion, and this is made worse if there is increased secretion engendered by high intracranial pressure or by a markedly elevated systemic arterial pressure. Cardiac failure may prove rapidly fatal under these circumstances. Total pulmonary care is required utilising expert physiotherapy and skilled suction with meticulous maintainance of the airway. Intubation with an endotracheal tube may be necessary as a temporary expedient with adequate humidification and optimal oxygen concentration. Tracheostomy is best avoided as it may simply prolong a chronic vegetative state in the severely obtunded.

Hypertension is a common causally related

problem and demands careful treatment in its own right; Meyer *et al* (1960) showed that brain swelling usually increased at pressures above 180 mm systolic when the filtration pressure may well exceed the colloid osmotic pressure. More recent studies (Strandgaard *et al.*, 1973) have shown that autoregulation in hypertensive patients may be more complex with a shift of the whole autoregulatory range to a higher level. Above this range the resistance vessels react passively and below the range they fail to respond to a falling inflow pressure. The balance must therefore be achieved with caution but without undue delay to effect a steady and stable blood pressure within the physiological limits appropriate to the patient's previous vascular status. Without the benefit of cerebral blood flow studies this usually means gradual reduction of blood pressure to levels consistent with the patient's age or known previous levels, modified always by the clinical response. The acute hypertensive response ascribed to cerebral haemorrhage is rare in previously normotensive patients and if it occurs is relatively transient and therefore requires no treatment.

The biochemical changes following spontaneous subarachnoid haemorrhage have also been studied (Buckell, Richardson, and Sarner, 1966) and highlight the importance of rapid fluid depletion and occasional electrolyte disturbance as a result of ADH secretion or pathological sodium redistribution. Where clouding of consciousness dulls thirst or reduces the ability to satisfy it, dehydration rapidly ensues. If this is complicated by hyperventilation or excessive sweating, significant fluid loss can occur in 24 to 48 hours leading to hypovolaemia and impaired cerebral perfusion. This state may not be obvious clinically but is usually suggested by plasma electrolyte and urea levels and confirmed by estimating simultaneously the osmolality of blood and urine. Correction of dehydration must be accurate but unhurried as sudden transfusion of fluid in a previously hyperosmolar situation may aggravate brain swelling.

These concepts are also important in using osmotherapy, as the objective of such treatment is to withdraw fluid from the brain and not to dehydrate the whole patient. Intravenous mannitol as a 20 per cent solution in a quantity of of 250 to 500 ml is occasionally advocated as a short term measure to induce reduction of intracranial pressure. The small risk of provoking further haemorrhage by such a manoeuvre must be accepted. It is certainly a minor hazard particularly if the treatment is reserved for those cases showing early deterioration in whom it is desired to produce a temporary amelioration prior to some more elective form of management.

There has been no conclusive study on the effectiveness of large doses of mineralocorticoids either to diminish the oedema associated with such lesions, or to improve the efficiency of small vessel perfusion. Dramatic improvements may follow their use in patients obtunded by brain tumours but their effects in cerebral haemorrhage seem less predictable. Personal clinical studies (Richardson, 1969) have not shown any convincing beneficial effects, though it is the increasing impression of many surgeons that such treatment is helpful.

Surgical management

The presence of a potentially removable space occupying lesion in a possibly fatal condition has naturally attracted much surgical interest. Over the years operative enthusiasm has waxed and waned and controversy still exists in relation to the benefits and particularly the timing of surgery. Our own early studies were reported fully in relation to a controlled trial of treatment (McKissock, Richardson, and Taylor, 1961). This compared active medical treatment with global application of surgery performed immediately after diagnosis, wherein surgery was employed within two hours of the ictus. No superiority for surgery thus randomly applied *early* was forthcoming but suggested that delayed operation might have some benefit. Some important points emerged from the study and deserve brief comment.

CONSCIOUS LEVEL

An assessment of conscious level and neurological deficit at 24 hours from the ictus was a good prognostic guide, showing a mortality of

30 per cent for medical treatment in the non-comatose as judged at a six month follow-up. Acute surgical results were similar. Patients in coma however suffered a 75 per cent death rate mostly in the first week.

SEX

The incidence of haemorrhage in men and women was similar but females sustained the lesion with a lower death rate when treated medically. In general they fared less well than men when subjected to early surgery.

ARTERIAL TENSION

Hypertension seemed to improve the natural history as compared with the small number of normotensive patients, but surgery had the reverse effect having a higher death rate in hypertensive cases and a lower mortality in normotensive patients.

ANGIOGRAPHIC FINDINGS

For simplicity these were divided into two groups—those with mid-line displacement suggesting a significant space taking mass and those without, indicating a smaller strategic lesion. Absence of mid-line disturbance carried a better natural prognosis (49 per cent survived) as opposed to a natural death rate of 58 per cent where significant displacement was seen. Surgery increased the death rate in the group with no displacement largely from the complications of attempting to remove deeply placed lesions. An attempt was made to correlate these various factors in hypertensive patients. This showed no striking difference in the cross section of conscious levels in the two angiographic groups, but again confirmed the relatively good prognosis in untreated females with little angiographic displacement. In the remaining subgroups early surgery appeared to offer little advantage over energetic medical treatment. This study which has been subject to some valid criticism did, however, establish some prognostic criteria for the medically treated group with a global six month mortality of 51 per cent, a figure much lower than that generally accepted at the time. It also demonstrated that the random application of very early surgery produced little overall benefit whilst suggesting that delayed surgery might be more helpful. In such a study the diagnostic accuracy has been held in question in the conservative group. A recent review by Paillas and Alliéz (1973) returns to the contention that the natural death rate is of the order of 80 per cent, at the same time expressing their belief that many patients who survive after unverified cerebral haemorrhage were in fact afflicted by brain softening. Such an argument is retrograde and will be refuted totally in the future in studies using the EMI scanner as the diagnostic method. For the present our own study must suffice. The trial structure was so designed that the presumptive diagnosis was established and the possibility of surgery confirmed *before* inclusion in the study and therefore preceding the random allocation to surgery or conservative treatment. One could therefore postulate that the rate of diagnostic error in the surgical group should approximate that of the non-surgically treated. Of the 89 cases allocated to surgery the diagnosis was incorrect in 4 cases, an error rate of 4.5 per cent. There was a subsequently verified error rate of 5.5 per cent in the group of 91 patients allocated to non-surgical treatment. Since the diagnostic criteria were established prior to treatment allocation, and any cases of diagnostic doubt excluded, any gross discrepancy in diagnostic accuracy in the two treatment groups seems unlikely.

Luessenhop *et al.* (1967) in a review of the literature and detailed analysis of 64 cases concluded that patients in a non-comatose condition showing a clear-cut arterial phase demonstration of the clot could have their natural mortality reduced to approximately one-third by the use of surgery. They divided their cases into three groups. Group 1 (seven patients) were fully alert, with minimal or resolving signs clearly destined to make a good recovery. None were subjected to surgery and all survived. Group 3 (24 patients) were the obverse of group 1 as most were in extremis and death seemed almost certain. In these surgery was performed in 13 cases with a total management mortality of 86 per cent. This group probably may be compared with our control group (McKissock *et al.*, 1961) designated as stupor/coma wherein the natural mortality was 76 per cent and the global surgical mortality was 79 per cent. In this group therefore there seems little difference between medical treatment, early surgery, or selective surgery.

Their group 2 cases are the most interesting. These 33 cases apparently had major neurological deficits and focal signs with conscious levels ranging from drowsiness to deep stupor — the breakdown is unfortunately not further analysed. Craniotomy was performed within 24 hours on 24 patients with two deaths, a mortality of 8 per cent. Operation was not performed in the remaining nine cases of whom one, a man of 90, died. Thus the untreated mortality in this group treated conservatively was only 12 per cent. This suggested the possibility of a rather skew population in this limited study as our own much larger group in a similar category had a natural death rate of 40 per cent.

Their study does confirm earlier views that early surgery in haematomas largely confined to the capsular or immediate paracapsular regions is unrewarding, whilst at the same time suggesting that the mortality for such lesions was of the order of 92 per cent. This is clearly fallacious for they removed from consideration the presumed capsular lesion in group 2 treated non-surgically with a death rate of only one in nine cases. Confusion of this order is common in published series and highlights the value of the work of Benés et al. (1972) who simply differentiated between destructive and limited haemorrhage. They made the important points that destructive haemorrhage much more frequently presents with immediate coma whereas limited haemorrhage, whether capsular or not, is accompanied by less neurological disturbance initially though not precluding subsequent deterioration in some. Thus they differentiate destructive bleeding with massive hemisphere or ganglionic involvement proceeding to rapid brain stem embarrassment or death as opposed to lesions of a more limited character in the basal ganglion or cerebral hemisphere which may be amenable to surgery or may have a good natural history.

A more recent presentation by Paillas and Alliéz (1973) reviews the literature and gives the results in 250 cases of intracerebral haemorrhage treated by surgery but without reference to cases excluded. The number of males was twice that of females in contrast to most other studies and carrying a definite augury for more favourable surgical results. The age range was average, diagnosis was by angiography, and air studies were not employed in the acute stage. Conscious level is only divided into subnormal and coma without further definition or indication as to the stage at which the conscious level was assessed. A mortality of 24 per cent at one month was achieved in the subnormal group of 58 patients as opposed to a death rate of 63 per cent of 79 patients in 'coma'. Three time groupings for surgery were used, the first being of 61 patients who survived for two to five days and were subjected to clot evacuation. Fifty-four per cent of these died. In the second time scale surgery took place from 5 to 10 days from the ictus with a death rate of 30 per cent of 75 cases. The largest single group of 114 received surgery at an interval of more than 10 days with a mortality of 29 per cent. Though this represents a very mixed series the size of the groups demands attention and suggests that delayed surgery may be optimal even allowing for the inevitable death rate in the interval. They also detail the quality of survival and subsequent death. Of a group of 132 survivors followed for one year it was found that 11 had died and of the remainder about one-third were with minimal defects, one-third had major deficits, and the remaining third had severe deficits. In the more prolonged follow-up the number of deaths due to further haemorrhage was 11 out of 121 cases. This compares reasonably with our own late death rate in 102 survivors followed for 1 to 10 years in whom five died from a further cerebrovascular accident.

Consideration of our own controlled studies and the reviews and reports of Luessenhop et al. (1967) and Paillas and Alliéz (1973), whilst confusing, strongly suggested a selective approach to the surgery of intracerebral haemorrhage both in terms of the patient's clinical status and the timing of surgery, having satisfied the potential necessity of surgery by demonstrating a significant accessible haematoma. A trial of treatment regime reported by Richardson (1969) helped to clarify some of the problems raised by earlier studies and is not refuted by subsequent series. This study concerned the management of 138 cases of intracerebral haemorrhage diagnosed by the usual criteria between 1961 and 1964. Patients who were admitted in coma and remained in that state were excluded as all previous evidence suggested that surgery was of little benefit. By the same token patients in whom the neurological deficit was mild and consciousness was preserved were not considered as surgical intervention was never indicated. These two groups were totally excluded from the study design.

The regime adopted for the trial was that after diagnosis of a potentially removable haematoma a decision relating to immediate therapy was taken. Almost always the primary choice was for active medical management aimed at improving ventilatory function, restoring normal fluid and electrolyte status, and managing raised intracranial pressure. Treatment of any complicating medical disease was also immediately commenced. During the next 7 to 10 days careful neurological and general medical assessments were made at the end of which time a decision regarding further treatment was made. In some cases during this interval pre-existing disease such as severe hypertension, renal failure, diabetes became exacerbated and often sufficiently severe to preclude serious consideration of surgery. These together with pulmonary complications were the commonest causes of death in the non-surgical group. Approximately 10 days after the ictus a decision was taken regarding surgery. If at this time the patient had only a mild deficit or was still improving, the decision against surgery was automatic. Where the deficit remained severe but the conscious level was satisfactory, craniotomy evacua-tion was undertaken within 48 hours. In a small group, some deterioration occurred in the waiting period and these were operated upon as the 'Immediate Operation' group. As will be seen they were small in number and occurred early in the series. Subsequent experience suggested that early deterioration was equally well managed by energetic conservative measures to correct hypoxia, abnormal hydration or raised intracranial pressure.

Table 11.1 shows the overall results as assessed six months following admission. It must be stressed that the treatment groups are not to be compared with each other. The conservative group represents those dying from other causes or recovering to a point where surgery was not thought indicated. Delayed surgery implies a persisting severe deficit at a ten-day interval from the ictus wherein surgical evacuation was designed to reduce the disability. The 'Immediate Operation' group has been explained and though small has a reasonable mortality and acceptable morbidity when compared to the whole series. A global mortality of 20 per cent for this regime may best be compared with the results in the previous controlled study wherein the natural mortality of cases in the combined alert and drowsy categories was 38 per cent and for the same group treated by early surgery was nearly 55 per cent. To draw many conclusions from such a retrospective comparison may be less than valid but sampling of some of the variables is instructive. In the controlled study group the 'alert/drowsy' mortality for patients admitted within three days of the ictus was $20/52$ in the untreated group compared with $16/96$ in the treatment trial study. This is lower than the total case mortality, this being explained by the higher mortality in patients referred more than

Table 11.1   Quality of survival at six months

	Total	Full recovery	Partial disability	Total disability	Dead
Conservative	60	33	13	1	13 = 21%
Delayed surgery	69	19	31	6	13 = 19%
Immediate operation	9	3	3	1	2 = 22%
	138	55	47	8	28 = 20%

seven days after the ictus as the reason for referral was often that of late but untreated deterioration. Reviewing the admission conscious status in more detail shows a natural mortality in the controlled study (1961) of 16 per cent for alert patients and 38 per cent for those drowsy or stuporose, whereas in the treatment trial (1969) of the 37 alert patients only four died (11 per cent) and of the 101 drowsy patients 24 died, a mortality of 24 per cent. A comparison of the timing of operation is excluded by definition as one study was concerned with early surgery and the other with delayed operation.

Many authors have stressed the improved surgical prognosis if the haematoma is predominantly lobar. We were unable to show this in our controlled studies as many of these represented the lobar extension of a destructive medially placed haemorrhage, and therefore the global lobar mortality was only 20 per cent, less than that for capsular lesions (McKissock *et al.*, 1961). In the treatment trial study (1969) the non-destructive lobar haematomas had a combined mortality of $12/88$ or 14 per cent whereas capsular haematomas had a death rate of $16/50$ or 32 per cent, this being increased to $7/14$ or 50 per cent if the thalamus was involved. It is interesting that the lobar haematomas were equally distributed between the groups making a good recovery medically and the group subjected to delayed surgery, the latter, however, by definition containing those cases remaining with a severe deficit. Clearly this indicates a fundamental good natural history for this type of haematoma with surgery only being indicated if deterioration occurs or a severe deficit persists after clinical stabilisation. Surgery at this time can confer benefit in about one-third of the cases. Similarly the distribution of ganglionic or paraganglionic haemorrhage was equal in the

two major treatment categories, suggesting that if they do not produce coma, though their mortality may be higher, their capacity for recovery may be good (Table 11.2). This certainly conflicts with the view of King (1973), who suggested that quality of survival depends on the site of the haematoma, being good if lobar, but stating that capsular haematomas always leave severe disabilities. It may be that some of the discrepancy is a matter of definition.

The present position of surgery is clear in that it cannot alter the course of unremitting coma nor will it further improve the natural recovery of mild cases tending towards resolution. Regardless of site of the lesion the proper place of surgery is in relation to lesions of significant size and in accessible situations where the clinical course is of subsequent deterioration from a previous satisfactory level or where a severe deficit exists after clinical stabilisation. With increasing knowledge of abnormal cerebral physiology and of methods for its correction, together with more urgent and intensive medical treatment the prognosis may be further improved. Techniques such as EMI scanning will resolve the previous diagnosis difficulties with its capacity not only to delineate the haematoma accurately but also to show associated cerebral pathology and brain displacements. With this more precise diagnostic tool and improved preoperative and postoperative care it may be necessary once again to compare earlier surgical regimes with later methods.

SPONTANEOUS CEREBELLAR HAEMORRHAGE

Non-traumatic spontaneous haemorrhage into the cerebellum represents approximately 10 per cent of all massive brain haemorrhage, this

Table 11.2   Quality of survival by haematoma site

	Total	Dead	Survivors	Full recovery	Partial disability	Total disability
Lobar	88	12	76	40	35	1
Putamenocapsular	36	9	27	13	8	6
Thalamic	14	7	7	2	4	1

proportion reflecting the relative weights of the cerebellum and cerebral hemispheres. In a post-mortem series of 40000 cases Courville (1950) described 117 cases of haemorrhage of the cerebellum in a total of 1487 cases of intra-cerebral bleeding. A similar prevalence was found in the clinical series of McKissock, Richardson, and Walsh (1960) wherein 344 cases were analysed in which 34 affected the cerebellum. In a more recent study by McCor-mick and Rosenfield all cases of massive brain haemorrhage were subject to detailed examina-tion and in the total series of 144 cases no less than 15 involved the cerebellum. This close correspondence of prevalence in clinical and post-mortem series suggests that the mortality of the two conditions is not dissimilar.

Aetiology

Most authors seem in general agreement that hypertension is the commonest causally related process in patients in whom no other pathologi-cal entity is identified. Hyland and Levy (1964) made this point but also suggested that blood dyscrasias were more common than generally supposed, finding five such cases in a series of 32 patients. Ransohoff, Derby, and Kricheff (1971), however, suggested that when other aetiological factors are excluded hypertension is present in 90 per cent of cases. In a careful review of the literature and an extensive prospective study of 144 cases, McCormick and Rosenfield (1973) made a strong case of hypertension being a coincidental factor, other lesions being pre-dominantly responsible. Their arguments were more strongly put in relation to lesions of the cerebral hemispheres but in their 15 cases involving the cerebellum a definitive lesion such as aneurysm, angioma, or brain tumour were present in 10, with hypertensive vascular disease as a possible cause in four of the remain-der. From the practical point of view one need not consider tumour haemorrhage further. Angiomas tend to occur in the age range of 0 to 40 years whereas the hypertensive vasculo-pathies occur most frequently in the fifth, sixth, and seventh decades. Aneurysms, particularly of the posterior inferior cerebellar arteries, are relatively rarely associated with massive cere-bellar haemorrhage with survival, though the possibility of such a lesion may influence the decisions relating to investigation.

Pathology

The vasculopathy most commonly associated with hypertension is of a degenerative process affecting the small perforating brain arteries giving rise to microaneurysms similar in genesis to the more common berry aneurysms of the Circle of Willis. Coles and Yates (1967) reported the incidence of these lesions in a series of 200 cases subject to detailed study. The basis of the study was to exclude cases subject to natural or surgical trauma and only to include those in which the examination could be performed with-in 24 hours of death. For the purpose of com-parison half the studies were in previously hypertensive patients and in the remainder there was no such evidence of pre-existing high blood pressure. Vessel lesions were more common in the pons and brain stem than in the cerebellum, but multiplicity of the lesion in the cereberal and cerebellar hemispheres was common. It was interesting, however, that these small aneurysms were seven times more common in hypertensive patients than they were in normo-tensive subjects and in this particular series there were no instances of haemorrhage from the lesions in patients with normal blood pres-sure. A point of surgical interest is that these lesions were noted most frequently in branches of the superior cerebellar artery in the region of the dentate nucleus, this explaining the common situation of the more circumscribed haematomas in elderly patients. Lesions were rare in the vermis vessels, whereas, as will be seen, this is a not uncommon situation for angiomas in the younger age groups. Angiomas are usually of arteriovenous type. In a large review article McCormick and Nofzinger (1966) analysed 308 small arteriovenous anomalies of the brain and showed that no less than 44 were situated in the cerebellar hemispheres. The collected series from the literature and their own cases include those that had and had not bled, and so conclusions in relation to responsibility for haemorrhage are tenuous. Nevertheless the relative incidence in the different parts of the brain correlates with the clinical impression of the high proportion of angiomas in clinical cerebellar haemorrhage in the younger age groups.

Venous angiomas have also been described by Wolf *et al*. (1967), which were labelled as cryptic due to the difficulty of radiological demonstration. Such terms cannot be regarded as synonymous as it is not uncommon to fail to visualise the more usual arteriovenous lesion, particularly when it was initially small and its rupture has resulted in a large compressing parenchymatous haematoma. Many reports describe small angiomas which have been virtually destroyed by the haemorrhage and remnants of which are found during the course of surgical removal of the consequent haematoma. Again it must be stressed that the majority of such cases occur below the age of 40 years with only an occasional incidence in the later decades.

Haemorrhage, therefore, most commonly occurs within the white matter or nuclear masses of the cerebellar hemisphere and may be so confined. Some communication with the fourth ventricle is common and accounts for the presence of blood in the subarachnoid space. More massive haemorrhage may involve the fourth ventricle and in severely hypertensive patients may pass in retrograde fashion into the third and lateral ventricles. Direct rupture of the haematoma into the pons or medulla is rare.

Secondary pathological effects may then follow as a result of swelling of the cerebellar white matter causing local compression of the brain stem which may rapidly proceed to obstruction to the ventricular outlet. Obstruction is more likely and more rapid if complicated by solid blood clot in the ventricular system. As the majority of such sequences in older people are on the basis of vasculopathy it is not uncommon to find evidence of previous or at times co-existent haemorrhage in the cerebral hemispheres or internal capsule.

Clinical features

In view of these variable basic pathological events the mode of presentation, evolution, and outcome are protean, but certain features can be identified to give clues to the probable diagnosis. In a series of 34 cases treated surgically (McKissock *et al*., 1960) there were three basic patterns. Approximately 20 per cent declared dramatically with rapid and progressive deterioration into coma with death ensuing within 48 hours. A small group presented a very slowly evolving pattern in whom the onset was gradual or apparently episodic and in which the course and neurological features were consistent with an expanding cerebellar lesion. In more than half the cases an intermediate onset and course was noted and as these are the most important from the diagnostic and prognostic viewpoint they require more detailed consideration. The original series (McKissock *et al*., 1960) and a later review by Richardson (1972) stressed the relative infrequency of convincing cerebellar signs in this group, particularly where the conscious level was markedly disturbed. Signs of brain stem embarrassment were, however, common with constricted or assymetrical pupils and lateral conjugate gaze palsies. Periodic respiration was often detected at some stage in the illness. A true hemiplegia contralateral to the lesion was noted in more than half the more obtunded cases; this should not be confused with the paucity of movement that may typify a cerebellar deficit. Thus in this group presenting as a moderately rapidly or episodically evolving lesion the triad of constricted but reacting pupils with a gaze palsy to the side of the lesion and periodic respiration often raised the diagnostic suspicion.

Fisher *et al*. (1965) presented a detailed review of the literature to which they added their own cases. Their objective was to analyse the clinical course and to differentiate cerebellar lesions from haemorrhage involving the brain stem, cerebral hemispheres and those arising from ruptured saccular aneurysms. Symptom analysis showed vomiting as a consistent early feature with headache as less prominent and true vertigo as infrequent. Consciousness, in their series was rarely lost early but ataxia often of gross degree was a marked feature. Various permutations of mutism with transient or progressive quadriparesis or paraparesis were noted with evidence of disturbance of ocular movement. It is very relevant that of their 21 personal cases, 13 arrived at the hospital within two hours of the ictus and eight within eight hours of onset. This very early assessment may explain the rather different clinical features in surgical series as the time interval from ictus to admission to a specialised neurosurgical department may be longer and some of the important initial neurological data may be lost. It is therefore necessary to examine these early cases in some detail. Of the 21 cases only 14 were sufficiently alert to assist in the examination. Greatest diagnostic importance was placed on the presence of dysarthria; dysphagia was rare. Ocular signs consisted of normal or constricted pupils with disturbance of conjugate gaze to the side of the lesion in 60 per cent, usually a paralysis but in two cases associated with forced deviation of gaze to the opposite side. Forced downward deviation was not seen and vertical eye movements were usually preserved. Nystagmus was only seen in 5 of 12 patients and was virtually confined to the horizontal plane. They suggest that monoplegia or hemiplegia was not seen unless due to an old stroke. Instead cerebellar ataxia is reported initially in four cases and became apparent in a further three patients as the picture evolved, with a marked tendency for truncal ataxia and instability of gait to be more prominent than individual cerebellar signs. With the onset of stupour an ipsilateral facial palsy became apparent in 8 of 13 cases but again hemiparesis was not found. Summarising the situation they stress the relative retention of power and sensation in contradistinction to pontine or capsular lesions with small pupils, gaze palsy, cerebellar ataxia, and a peripheral facial palsy. Consciousness, they felt, was often preserved initially but supervention of stupour was usually accompanied by marked increase in the neurological deficits.

In a detailed study of 56 cases Ott, Kase, Ojemann, and Mohr (1974) agreed that hypertension was the commonest cause but mention the use of anticoagulants in eight cases. The fifth, sixth, and seventh decades represented the usual age incidence and there was a slight preponderance of males. Good clinical details were available in 44 of the cases and the presenting symptoms in order of frequency are detailed. Nausea and vomiting, 'dizziness'—i.e. not necessarily true vertigo—ataxia, and headache were most common with vomiting occurring in 42 of the patients. Early loss of consciousness was uncommon but dysarthria or mutism was apparent in one-third of the cases. Of the patients examined within 24 hours, 14 were alert, 22 were drowsy, 5 stuporose, and 15 comatose. In the non-comatose patients ataxia was noted in nearly three-quarters with facial palsy in 60 per cent and an obvious gaze palsy in more than half, with horizontal nystagmus in a similar proportion. They suggest that an abrupt onset with preservation of consciousness with vomiting as a prominent feature and the presence of limb ataxia, gaze palsy, and a peripheral facial weakness must arouse the strong suspicion of a cerebellar haemorrhage. On these grounds they suggest that the diagnosis was considered in 34 of 53 patients admitted soon after the ictus in a non-comatose state.

Differential diagnosis

In spite of the apparent discrepancies in varying series the clinical differentiation from other types of haemorrhage is important since the alternative method of radiological assessment is not without hazard, may be inconclusive and may delay urgent surgical treatment. The patient, due to direct pressure on brain stem structures or due to the onset of hydrocephalus, may deteriorate dramatically and without warning and place himself beyond the possibility of recovery. Fisher et al. (1965) stressed the motor signs in putaminal or capsular haemorrhage with heminaopia and sensory disturbance. In such lesions gaze paresis is contralateral to the lesion and may be reversed by contralateral caloric stimulation. They admit however that the ocular and pupillary changes may be confusing. Pontine haemorrhage is dismissed as a devastating event typified by severe motor deficits but occasionally cerebellar signs and ocular disorder may predominate. The forced downward deviation of the eyes or at least loss of vertical gaze is not specified but is in fact common in upper brain stem and thalamic lesions.

It is conceded that frontal haematomas and ruptured aneurysms cause the greatest difficulty but the presence of hemisphere signs or the absence of obvious brain stem embarrassment may be helpful.

Such detailed clinical analyses are helpful in pointing the guidelines to a high degree of clinical suspicion particularly, in those cases in whom consciousness is preserved, and are thus potential candidates for successful treatment.

Investigations

In the general context of cerebrovascular accidents or acute neurological disturbances the common first investigation is a diagnostic lumbar puncture. The presence of blood in the sub-arachnoid space indicates the pathological basis and will determine the urgency of further diagnostic procedures. Blood-stained cerebrospinal fluid is likely to be found in about 80 per cent of cases with cerebellar haemorrhage, due to egress of blood into the fourth ventricle or rarely to direct rupture on to the cerebellar surface in cases of angioma or aneurysm. However, in the remainder the clot may be confined to the cerebellar hemisphere, particularly in the more slowly evolving cases presenting a more classical cerebellar syndrome. In these the fluid may be completely uncontaminated or contain a slight excess of protein or white cells allowing for confusion with infarction or encephalitis. The dangers of lumbar puncture in a compressing posterior fossa lesion need no emphasis and the possible value of this procedure must be considered in each case. Presenting features, rapid evolution, and evidence of brain stem embarrassment may preclude its use and suggest alternative diagnostic measures or in some cases be sufficiently convincing to lead to surgical exploration on clinical grounds alone.

EMI SCANNING

In the routine elective radiology pride of place must now be taken by the use of computerised transverse axial tomography (CAT scan) by the apparatus devised by EMI. Numerous publications have recently described the technique and its application in detail (Ambrose 1973, 1974), and its relevance to the diagnosis of intracranial haematomas (Paxton and Ambrose, 1974). Basically the method which is entirely benign and non-invasive and utilises a rotating X-ray tube on a common arm with a sensitive detector. Movement of both is biplanar in that the tube rotates through 1° arcs to a total traverse of 180° and at each 1° point traverses vertically a distance of 1.3 cm. Each linear traverse produces 160 transmission readings; thus at the end of the examination, 28 000 readings of transmission or absorption are available for computer analysis. This absorption data is transmitted to an appropriately programmed computer to produce a print-out of absorption figures on a predetermined matrix having 80×80 cells or more recently 160×160 cells, the volume of each matrix cell being determined by the matrix size and the thickness of the cranial slice, usually 1.3 cm. For pictorial representation this data is transferred to a fluoroscope screen in the configuration corresponding to the shape of the head with the density of the intracranial contents shown on a 'grey scale' from white for dense bone to black for air, water, or fat. Most cerebral tissues occupy the lower grey ranges but haematoma invariably shows as a white zone of much higher density than the surrounding brain. Serial slices are necessary to demonstrate the entire intracranial contents.

Preliminary investigation of cerebrovascular accidents of all types has been facilitated by this means (Paxton and Ambrose, 1974) for it not only demonstrates the presence of haematomas or infarcts but will show dilatation, distortion, or displacement of the ventricular system. Figure 11.6 shows a basal brain slice in which the bony skull is white and the brain greyish black. An obvious white almost circular area is seen in the position of the left cerebellar hemisphere clearly separate from the petrous ridge. The small dark square on its right side represents the distorted displaced fourth ventricle. Figure 11.7 A is the scan of a restless patient, this producing some artefact but not detracting from the diagnosis. A definite haematoma is seen in the region of the right cerebellar hemisphere with the blood filled fourth ventricle distorted and displaced to the left. Figure 11.7B is a higher level slice showing blood in the lateral and third ventricles and also in the temporal horns. The degree of reliability of this benign procedure is so high that further investigative procedures are unnecessary unless the clinical presentation, patient's age, or atypical appearance of the haematoma or surrounding brain suggest the presence of a vascular anomaly of importance to surgical management. Increasing availability of this diagnostic method will diminish the need for any other investigation.

ECHOENCEPHALOGRAPHY

In an earlier publication (Richardson, 1972) the use of the simple 'A' mode ultrasonic method was discussed. The investigation requires skill and training but can be performed at the bedside to provide limited but useful information. Ambrose and McKissock (1969) defined the technique for estimating ventricular size and showed that the normal ratio between the width of the

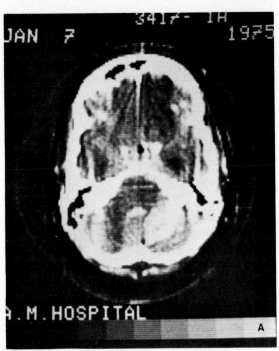

Fig. 11.7A Right cerebellar haematoma with adjacent blood-filled fourth ventricle.

lateral ventricle to that of half the brain was one-fifth to one-sixth and that ratios of one-third indicated significant ventricular dilatation. Such enlargement occurs rapidly in most cases of cerebellar haematoma being recorded as early as four to six hours by Dinsdale (1964). To summarise the uses of ultra sound in stroke patients with neurological deficit, the finding of a normal mid-line with the absence of ventricular dilatation would suggest infarction, the presence of a mid-line displacement would suggest a supra-tentorial lesion, whereas no displacement but the presence of ventricular dilatation would raise the possibility of a posterior fossa lesion. This simplistic view has, however, to be tempered with the knowledge that a dilated third ventricle may so distort the mid-line echo as to suggest a displacement; furthermore clot in the ventricular system may so disturb the echo pattern as to make interpretation very difficult. Finally a cerebellar haemorrhage can exist in the absence of significant ventricular dilatation.

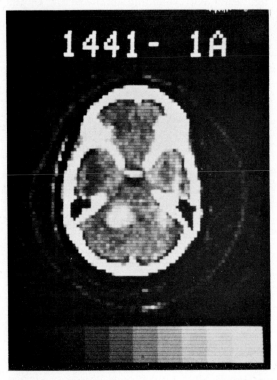

Fig. 11.6 Cerebellar haematoma on left side showing as spherical region of increased density separate from petrous ridge.

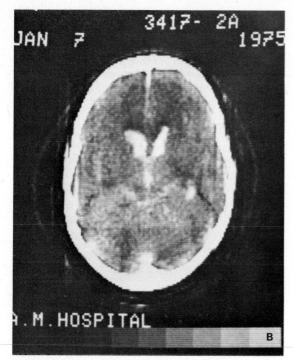

Fig. 11.7B Haematoma (white) in the lateral ventricles, third ventricle, and the right temporal horn.

ANGIOGRAPHY

Carotid angiography would be used in patients in whom a ruptured aneurysm of the anterior Circle of Willis could not be excluded clinically. This angiogram should not only exclude such a causal lesion but also indicate ventricular dilatation by virtue of the exaggerated sweep of the callosal arteries and the displaced course of the thalamostriate veins in the antero-posterior projections. Visualisation of the vertebral system by any technique has advanced since the earlier review by McKissock et al. (1960) and the publication of Spatz and Bull (1957) and Odom et al. (1961). The latter, in small series of cases felt, that the demonstration of a haematoma by itself by this technique was doubtful. More recently Bull and Kotlowski (1970) suggested that a study of the venous system is helpful in at least lateralising a lesion and may indicate its situation. Nornes and Hauge (1972) in a series of five patients with cerebellar haemorrhage demonstrated the presence of an expanding lesion by dislocation of the posterior inferior cerebellar artery. A similar high diagnostic rate is suggested by Ott et al., (1974). They described seven patients in whom retrospective reinterpretation resulted in the correct diagnosis of a cerebellar mass lesion in five.

AIR STUDIES

The experience of most surgeons is strongly against the use of air studies in the acutely evolving haemorrhage causing, as they do, considerable disturbance in intracranial dynamics and necessitating turning the patient into the prone position for radiography. Both lumbar air encephalography and ventriculography often result in significant deterioration of the patient's condition, this being irreversible in a small number. In our earlier studies reliance was placed on this examination (McKissock et al., 1960) but subsequently (Richardson, 1972) it was substantially avoided and much reliance placed on clinical assessment with careful ultrasound investigation and if necessary vertebral angiography or more commonly elective surgical exploration. The advent of CAT scanning has largely solved this problem but where it is not available a combination of careful clinical assessment with minimal radiological investigation and a willingness for surgical exploration must suffice.

Treatment

Prompt surgical evacuation of the haematoma whilst the patient is still responsive seems to be the accepted method of management. Detailed study of the natural history has been precluded previously by diagnostic failures, complications of investigation and urgent surgery. The series of 67 cases analysed by Richardson (1972) and the 56 patients detailed by Ott et al. (1974) show that spontaneous and often unpredictable deterioration in the early stages is very common, this risk only diminishing after complete stabilisation at a high conscious level after 8 to 10 days. Against this must be weighed the unheralded lapses into stupor and coma from a previously alert state and the fact that the major prognostic factor for recovery after surgery is strongly correlated with the conscious state prior to operation. Thus surgical mortality in patients previously responsive is of the order of 20 per cent rising to 75 per cent when stupor or coma supervene. Analysis of the cause of death most commonly shows tonsillar impaction with brain stem distortion and secondary haemorrhage but rarely direct implication of brain stem structures by the presenting ictus. More significantly the reaccumulation of clot is recorded in a number of cases, usually in those comatose prior to surgery whose condition remained unchanged and therefore gave no indication of this complication. The absence of primary intrinsic brain stem damage in such patients and the fact that occasionally surgery will enable such previously comatose patients to survive suggests that in some, minor recurrence of haemorrhage may tip the balance. In most of the comatose cases, however, the secondary brain stem vascular lesions have occurred before operation.

The method of surgical evacuation has varied in reported small series but in the larger quoted analyses, formal suboccipital craniectomy and removal of the haematoma with meticulous haemastosis produces the best results. Temporising measures such as ventricular drainage or simple burrhole evacuation of the clot are not to be recommended.

If surgery is undertaken promptly and the patient survives, the quality of survival is usually gratifying. There were 20 survivors in a total surgical series of 32 patients (Richardson, 1972) observed for periods of 2 to 10 years with an average of 4.5 years. Of these 11 have returned to their normal life, five have minor disabilities due to cerebellar deficits, and the remaining four have some limits on their activities and should be regarded as partially disabled. Three patients died subsequently, one from a further cerebrovascular accident, one from coronary occlusion, and the last from a brain tumour in the cerebral hemisphere. All deaths were remote from the cerebellar ictus. Thus 75 per cent made an excellent recovery this agreeing with the series by Ott *et al.* (1974) wherein two-thirds of 12 survivors were either well or minimally disabled and able to resume full activity. Only one could be regarded as totally disabled.

Conclusions

The natural history of cerebellar haemorrhage in patients who initially retain consciousness is one of unpredictable and grave deterioration in the majority, with no clear-cut prognostic criteria to allow identification of patients maximally at risk. Whilst natural recovery can occur, the diagnostic criteria in such untreated and uninvestigated patients must be less than firm when compared with surgical series wherein the nature of the lesion is established absolutely. In most studies spontaneous survival depended on a process of natural selection with the patients remaining untreated by virtue of delayed referral and clear evidence of a progressive recovery. Such patients would almost certainly have a small surgical risk which must be accepted if the general principle of early surgical intervention is followed. The capacity to establish the precise diagnosis, the exact configuration of the haematoma, its direct effects on the brainstem and fourth ventricle and the complication of hydrocephalus by the use of benign CAT scanning will not only allow a prompt surgical decision but may help to delineate by sequential examination those cases likely to survive spontaneously. At present it is still necessary to place reliance on careful preliminary clinical examination with a view to early surgery after the minimum investigation in order that early elective formal surgical evacuation may proceed. This holds the greatest promise for a greater percentage of survival with an excellent prospect of good quality life for those thus saved.

REFERENCES

Archar, V. S., Coe, P. K. & Marshall, J. (1966) Echoencephalography in the differential diagnosis of cerebral haemorrhage and infarction. *Lancet*, i, 161.
Ambrose, J. (1973) Computerised transverse axial scanning (tomography). Part II. Clinical application. *British Journal of Radiology*, **46**, 1023.

Ambrose, J. (1974) Computerised X-ray scanning of the brain. *Journal of Neurosurgery*, **40**, 679.

Ambrose, J. & McKissock, W. (1969) The use of pulsed ultrasound in the detection of space occupying intracranial lesions. In *Measurement and precision in Surgery*. Oxford: Blackwell.

Bedford, P. D. (1958) Intracranial haemorrhage, diagnosis and treatment. *Proceedings of the Royal Society of Medicine*, **51**, 209.

Benés, M., Koukolik, F. & Obrovski, D. (1972) Spontaneous intracerebral haemorrhage due to hypertension. *Journal of Neurosurgery*, **37**, 509.

Buckell, M., Richardson, A. & Sarner, M. (1966) Biochemical changes after spontaneous subarachnoid haemorrhage. *Journal of Neurology, Neurosurgery and Psychiatry*, **29**, 291.

Bull, J. & Kotlowski, P. (1970) The angiographic pattern of the petrosal veins in the normal and pathological. *Neuroradiology*, **1**, 20.

Cole, F. M. & Yates, P. O. (1967) The occurrence and significance of intracerebral microaneurysms. *Journal of Pathology and Bacteriology*, **93**, 393.

Courville, C. B. (1950) *Pathology of the Central Nervous System*. 3rd ed. Mountain View, California: Pacific Press.

Dinsdale, H. B. (1964) Spontaneous haemorrhage in the posterior fossa. *Archives of Neurology* (Chicago), **10**, 200.

Fisher, C. M. (1961) Clinical syndromes in cerebral haemorrhage. In *Pathogenesis and Treatment of Cerebrovascular Disease*, ed. Fields, W. S. Ch. 13, p. 318. Springfield, Illinois: Charles C. Thomas.

Fisher, C. M. (1971) Radiological observations in hypertensive cerebral haemorrhage. *Journal of Neuropathology and Experimental Neurology*, **30**, 536.

Fisher, C. M., Pickard, E. H., Polak, A., Dalal, P. & Ojemann, R. G. (1965) Acute hypertensive cerebellar haemorrhage. Diagnosis and surgical treatment. *Journal of Nervous and Mental Diseases*, **140**, 38.

Hounsfield, G., Ambrose, J., Perry, J. & Bridger, C. (1973) Computerised transverse axial scanning. *British Journal of Radiology*, **46**, 1016.

Hyland, H. H. & Levy, D. (1964) Spontaneous cerebellar haemorrhage. *Canadian Medical Association Journal*, **71**, 315.

Kaplan, H. (1961) Clinical syndromes in cerebral haemorrhage. In *Pathogenesis and Treatment of Cerebrovascular Disease*, ed. Fields, W. S. Springfield, Illinois: Charles C. Thomas.

King, T. T. (1973) Cerebral haemorrhage. *British Journal of Hospital Medicine*, **10**, 250.

Leksell, L. (1956) Detection of intracranial complications following head injury. *Acta Chirurgica Scandinavica*, **110**, 301.

Locksley, H. B., Sahs, A. L. & Sandler, R. (1966) Report on the cooperative study of intracranial aneurysms and subarachnoid haemorrhage. *Journal of Neurosurgery*, **24**, 1034.

Luessenhop, A. J., Shevlin, W. A., Ferrero, A. A., McCullough, D. C. & Barone, B. (1967) Surgical management of primary intracerebral haemorrhage. *Journal of Neurosurgery*, **27**, 419.

McCormick, W. F. & Nofzinger, J. D. (1966) Cryptic vascular malformations of the central nervous system. *Journal of Neurosurgery*, **24**, 892.

McCormick, W. F. & Rosenfield, D. B. (1973) Massive brain haemorrhage. A review of 144 cases and an examination of their causes. *Stroke*, **4**, 946.

McKissock, W., Richardson, A. & Taylor, J. (1961) Primary intracerebral haemorrhage. A controlled trial of surgical and medical treatment in 180 unselected cases. *Lancet*, ii, 221.

McKissock, W., Richardson, A. & Walsh, L. S. (1959) Primary intracerebral haemorrhage. *Lancet*, ii, 683.

McKissock, W., Richardson, A. & Walsh, L. S. (1960) Spontaneous cerebellar haemorrhage. A study of 34 consecutive cases treated surgically. *Brain*, **83**, 1.

Meyer, J. & Bauer, R. (1962) Medical treatment of spontaneous intracranial haemorrhage by the use of hypotensive drugs. *Neurology*, **12**, 36.

Nornes, H., & Hauge, T. (1972) Spontaneous intracerebellar haemorrhage. *Acta Neurologica Scandinavica*, Suppl. 51, 253.

Odom, G. L., Tindall, G. T. & Dukes, H. T. (1961) Cerebellar Haematoma caused by angiomatous malformation. *Journal of Neurosurgery*, **18**, 777.

Ojemann, R. G. (1973) Intracerebral and cerebellar haemorrhage. In *Neurological Surgery*. Vol. 2, ch. 38, p. 844. Philadelphia: Saunders.

Oldendorf, D. (1961) Isolated flying spot detection of radiodensity discontinuities. *I.R.E. Transactions on Biomedical Electronics*, **8**, 68.

Ott, K. H., Kase, C. S., Ojemann, R. G. & Mohr, J. P. (1974) Cerebellar haemorrhage. Diagnosis and treatment. *Archives of Neurology*, **31**, 160.

Paillas, J. E. & Alliéz, B. (1973) Surgical treatment of spontaneous intracerebral haemorrhage. *Journal of Neurosurgery*, **39**, 145.

Paxton, R. & Ambrose, J., (1974) The E.M.I. Scanner. A brief review of the first 650 patients. *British Journal of Radiology*, **47**, 530.

Ransohoff, J., Derby, B. & Kricheff, I. (1971) Spontaneous intracerebral haemorrhage. *Clinical Neurosurgery*, **18**, 247.

Richardson, A. (1969) Surgical therapy of spontaneous intracerebral haemorrhage. In *Progress in Neurological Surgery*, Vol. 3, p. 397. Chicago: Karger Basle and Year Book.

Richardson, A. (1972) Spontaneous cerebellar haemorrhage. In *Handbook of Clinical Neurology*, ed. Venken, P. J. & Bruyn, G. W. Amsterdam: North Holland Publishing Co.

Richardson, J. C. & Einhorn, R. W. (1963) Primary intracerebral haemorrhage. *Clinical Neurosurgery*, **9**, 114.

Ross Russell, R. W. (1963) Observations on intracerebral aneurysms. *Brain*, **86**, 425.

Spatz, E. L. & Bull, J. W. D. (1957) Vertebral arteriography in the study of subarachnoid haemorrhage. *Journal of Neuro-surgery*, **14**, 543.

Strandgaard, S., Olesen, J., Skinhøj, E. & Lassen, N. A. (1973) Autoregulation of brain circulation in severe arterial hyper-tension. *British Medical Journal*, i, 507.

Tallala, A. & McKissock, W. (1971) Acute spontaneous subdural haemorrhage. *Neurology*, **21**, 19.

Wolf, P. A., Rosman, P. N. & New, P. F. J. (1967) Multiple small cryptic venous angiomas of the brain mimicking cerebral metastases. *Neurology* (Minneapolis), **17**, 491.

12. Subarachnoid Haemorrhage from Intracranial Aneurysm and Angioma

Lindsay Symon

In most Western countries, vascular disease of the brain ranks third in the causes of death at the present time. Analysis of the stroke problem reveals that between 5 and 10 per cent of strokes are more properly classified as subarachnoid haemorrhage (SAH), and in this group two of the main causes of pathology are potentially surgically treatable lesions. In the extensive cooperative review of SAH undertaken in America some years ago, Locksley (1966) demonstrated that in over 5000 cases of SAH studied with angiography or at autopsy, 51 per cent had as their origin an intracranial aneurysm or aneurysms. Arteriovenous malformations (AVM) with an incidence of 6 per cent were much less common. Even in this careful and exhaustive study, just over 20 per cent of cases showed no proven aetiology. It is apparent, however, that in general neurosurgical practice, especially in the middle decades of life, aneurysm is the most probable cause of SAH. In the decade 40 to 49 its frequency is nearly twice that of other causes, and over 25 times that of AVM. The frequency of AVM as a cause of SAH, however, equals that of aneurysms in the second decade; over the age of 70 'other' causes of SAH outweigh both aneurysm and AVM appreciably. The high preponderance of aneurysms as the cause of SAH, and the operative and physiopathological problems which still exist in their management, render them of relatively greater importance in neurosurgical management of SAH. AVMs constitute another and, in some respects, a simpler problem.

THE NATURAL HISTORY OF SUBARACHNOID HAEMORRHAGE FROM RUPTURED INTRACRANIAL ANEURYSM

Although excellent accounts of SAH have appeared in the standard medical literature since Gull's description in 1859, and occasional descriptions date back to the early eighteenth century, it was not until the development of cerebral angiography by Moniz (1927), and more particularly its widespread use in neurological and neurosurgical clinics throughout the world after the Second World War, that a true appreciation of SAH emerged. Thus, it was generally assumed in pre-angiographic days that aneurysmal SAH was predominantly a disease of the young. We now know this to be untrue. It is now certain that while a congenital factor may have a part to play in the origin of intracranial aneurysm (Hassler, 1965), the factors of arteriosclerosis and raised blood pressure in later life play a clear role in the development of aneurysms, and most neurosurgeons have experience of patients with one aneurysm who, in subsequent years, have bled from a second which was either not present or very small at the time of the first study.

While neurosurgery as a whole has operative mortality statistics of acceptably low proportions, in the treatment of intracranial aneurysms the cooperative study from 24 centres suggested that a 30 to 35 per cent overall operative mortality rate might be taken as a guideline. This could in no way be regarded as acceptable. It was already apparent from the publications of McKissock, Paine, and Walsh (1960) that the prognosis of SAH varied very considerably according to the condition of the patient at the time of admission to hospital, and much study has been devoted to the identification of factors which determine surgical risk. It has emerged that the two most important factors determining surgical mortality are the condition of the patient at the time of surgery, and the time which has elapsed from SAH. The earlier operation is undertaken, the more dangerous it is, and the sicker the patient when operation is advised, the higher the risks of surgery.

Perhaps not surprisingly, analysis of the

mortality rates of cases treated medically shows that these same criteria indicate risks also in medical treatment. Figure 12.1, which is taken from Locksley's study, shows an attempt to establish graphical analysis of the regression curve of survival. The determination of such curves is based on the assumption that the number of patients dying during any given period of time is proportional to the number of patients alive at the beginning of this interval. The early portion of this curve in the first few days following the onset of SAH has a steep and constantly changing slope, which after six weeks becomes a slow, almost linear, decline. Using the type of exponential stripping familiar to blood flow analysts, the slow tail of the exponential may be stripped from the first portion to reveal three populations at risk. The slow component describes the behaviour of about 43 per cent of cases of SAH who may be expected to survive beyond the first six weeks. The behaviour of the other 57 per cent can be visualised by subtracting the slow component from the main curve, and this second or slowly decaying curve — K2 in the figure of Locksley — describes the behaviour of about 47 per cent of the initial cases. A third, steeply decaying slope K3, describes about 9 per cent of patients who died very rapidly within the first few days of SAH. This third group represents patients who are probably moribund on arrival in hospital or who die in their homes, and who are at the moment impossible to treat by any method. It is the second group, about 47 per cent of the total cases, whose numbers decline by about 6.6 per cent per day, who constitute the challenge to neurosurgical treatment. The average survival of this group after the first SAH is about two weeks, and in the absence of treatment designed to improve their survival, few will remain alive at the end of three months.

A careful study by Alvord *et al.* (1972), employing material from the cooperative study and also material in an earlier study by Pakarinen (1967) in Finland, has created even more detailed survival probability graphs, taking into account the time of presentation of the patient with SAH in hospital. It will be apparent from Locksley's graph (Fig. 12.1) that if a clinic

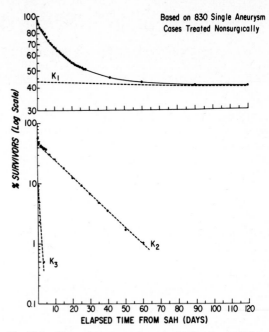

Fig. 12.1   Regression curve of survival following SAH from aneurysm. (Reproduced by kind permission of the *Journal of Neurosurgery* and of H. B. Locksley, from his article (1966) Report on the cooperative study of intracranial aneurysms and subarachnoid haemorrhage. Section V, Part 1: Natural history of subarachnoid haemorrhage, intracranial aneurysms and arteriovenous malformations. *Journal of Neurosurgery*, **25**, 219.)

admits cases only after the rapidly decaying K3 group have died, its expected natural mortality should be very much lower than the grouped mortality of SAH as a whole. Alvord *et al.*, from their own and other data, constructed the graph shown in Figure 12.2, once again reaching the conclusion that at the end of two months after a SAH only some 40 per cent of cases would be alive, provided the population could include cases studied immediately from the time of the bleeding. If the clinic's admission policy delayed the average time of admission to one day following the haemorrhage, then at the two-month interval nearly 60 per cent of cases would survive. It is therefore apparent that were one to consider the extreme example of a neurosurgical unit operating on all cases presented to it immediately after SAH, a mortality rate of anything better than 60 per cent would constitute

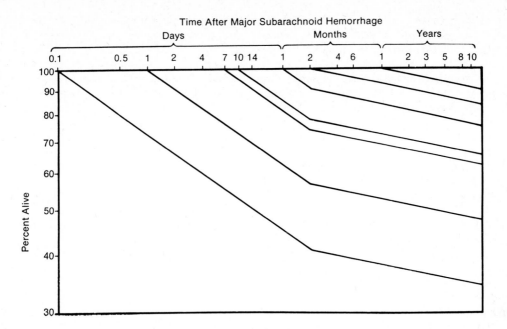

Fig. 12.2   Survival rates of patients admitted to study at particular times after their initial major subarachnoid haemorrhage. (Reproduced by kind permission of *Archives of Neurology* and of Alvord *et al.*, from their article (1972) Subarachnoid haemorrhage due to ruptured aneurysms. *Archives of Neurology*, **27**, 273.)

an improvement on natural mortality. On the other hand, if the unit admitted only one day after SAH, a mortality rate at operation of greater than 40 per cent would be worse than the natural survival, and the patient would be better left unoperated. In the same way, a study of Alvord's graph shows that cases presenting one month after SAH will have a natural survival at two months of very nearly 90 per cent, and to operate on aneurysms presenting as late as this, therefore, the surgeon must offer a negligible mortality.

THE NATURAL HISTORY OF ARTERIOVENOUS MALFORMATIONS

Despite large numbers of neurosurgical publications on the subject of cerebral angiomas, the exact risk which these lesions present is far from clear. There is no doubt that the early re-bleeding rate of angiomas is very much lower than that of aneurysms. Thus, in the cooperative study, only 10 per cent of patients who had survived a single haemorrhage from AVM bled again within six weeks, whereas in survivors from an initial aneurysmal SAH the figure for re-bleeding within six weeks was 30 per cent. The initial mortality rate from haemorrhage from AVM was also appreciably lower. Thus, in the cooperative study, 281 bleeding supratentorial AVMs had a mortality rate from the initial haemorrhage of 10 per cent, whereas of 830 cases of first bleeding single aneurysm patients treated conservatively, 68 per cent had died by the time the study was completed, 93 per cent of them by the end of one year (Graaf, 1971). The cause of death in AVM is almost invariably haemorrhage within the substance of the brain. Indeed, it has been pointed out in more than one series (Perret and Nishioka, 1966; Paterson and McKissock, 1956; Henderson and Gomez, 1967; Morello and Borghi, 1973) that the small angioma is more likely than the large one to be associated with a large haematoma. This has been common surgical experience, perhaps related to the fact that the smaller angiomas tend to lie within the depths of the sulci and therefore to bleed naturally into the white matter rather than on to the surface and into the subarachnoid space. Each centre managing SAH, however, rapidly becomes aware that many cases with AVM re-bleed relatively infrequently, and some patients survive for many years following several haemorrhages. Kelly *et al.* (1969) followed 33 patients for an average of 15.5 years after an initial haemorrhage from AVM, at which time there had been a mortality rate of 28 per cent, and half the patients had little, if any, disability. In Olivecrona and Ladenheim's (1957) series, 55 per cent of 44 cases which had not been radically operated on, had either complete disability or had died. Pool and Potts (1965), making a retrospective study of cases of angioma, found that 56 per cent of cases conservatively managed either died or were completely incapacitated. Troupp (1965), on the other hand, following 60 patients conservatively managed found that 37 (60 per cent) were in good health and at full work, and 11 were partially disabled, in a follow-up between 17 months and 16 years (mean 5 years) after the diagnosis of angioma had been made.

Where epilepsy alone is the presenting symptom, the management may be somewhat easier, although the enthusiastic aggression of such as Kunc (1965, 1973) indicates that the radical excision of even critically placed AVMs may be attended with success. Where, however, an AVM has presented with haemorrhage, it is likely that further haemorrhage will occur, though probably over a period of years, and the common practice in Britain at any rate is to remove the lesion if it is at all surgically accessible, whatever its size. Figures 12.3 and 12.4 indicate two AVMs of considerable size, one supra- and the other infratentorial, successfully excised without increase in neurological deficit. There is no convincing evidence that infratentorial AVMs are associated with a significantly worse prognosis than those placed supratentorially.

THE CLINICAL PRESENTATION OF SUBARACHNOID HAEMORRHAGE

The onset of classical SAH presents few diagnostic difficulties. The sudden severe headache, of an intensity such as the patient has never suffered before and sometimes accom-

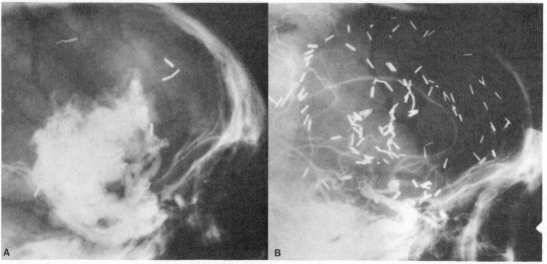

Figs. 12.3A and 12.3B   A large supratentorial, arteriovenous malformation before and after surgery. The patient had moderate hemiparesis and was intellectually impaired prior to surgery. He made a good though protracted postoperative recovery. (Photographs reproduced by kind permission of Professor Valentine Logue.)

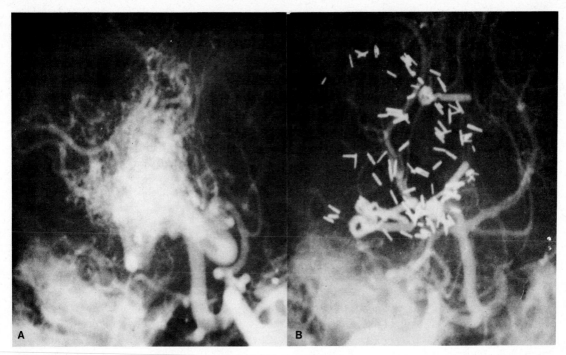

Figs. 12.4A and 12.4B   A large, subtentorial, arteriovenous malformation which had presented with four subarachnoid haemorrhages over a period of four-and-a-half years, accompanied by progressive cerebellar deficit. The patient, an 18-year-old boy, showed appreciable neurological improvement postoperatively. Preoperative angiograms are shown in Fig. 12.4A. Postoperative angiograms are shown in Fig. 12.4B.

panied by the feeling of something snapping inside the head, is a description so clear and so striking that it is not usually overlooked. A number of factors have been thought to predispose to SAH, but the most clearly related of these appears to be the episodic increase in blood pressure, related particularly to coitus or to defaecation. Thus, in the combined study (Locksley, 1966), SAH occurred during coitus in 3.8 per cent of patients who bled from intracranial aneurysms, and in 4.1 per cent of patients who bled from AVM. In a rather nondescript group of 'other' SAH, this was the predisposing factor in 2.2 per cent. Lifting or bending was associated with rupture in 12 per cent of aneurysms, and with the onset of haemorrhage in 14 per cent of AVMs. It seems likely that transient severe rises in blood pressure are responsible for this predisposition. The progress after the onset of headache depends a good deal upon the severity of the haemorrhage. Thus, a severe

haemorrhage either from aneurysm or AVM will be associated with a rapid loss of consciousness, deep coma, and death within a few hours, usually as the result of extensive intracerebral bleeding. More commonly, a transient loss of consciousness succeeds the sudden severe headache, but the onset is normally recalled with great clarity by the patient on recovering from the short period of unconsciousness. Fits as a presenting feature in association with the haemorrhage are not common, although in cases of AVM a preceding history of epilepsy is present in a number of cases (see below). After the initial onset, the patient may return to full consciousness or may pass through a phase of extreme irritability or with evident focal neurological signs, which may give a clue as to the situation of the lesion which has bled. Sometimes immediately, and at any rate within a few hours, evident neck stiffness and signs of meningeal irritation, such as a positive Kernig's sign, become apparent and are detectable in due course even though the patient remains unconscious. Other detectable abnormalities include transient disturbance of vegetative functions manifested by an increase in blood glucose, the development of perhaps severe glycosuria, sometimes albuminuria and, not infrequently, abnormalities in the electrocardiogram which may suggest associated ischaemia and which have been attributed to high concentration of circulating catecholamines as a result of the stress induced by haemorrhage. The pattern of any focal neurological deficit may give a clue to the site of the offending lesion. Thus, the complaint by the patient that the onset of the headache was associated with a severe feeling of weakness in the legs may be a clue to the haemorrhage having arisen from anterior communicating complex, while the development of a facio-brachial weakness might suggest an origin of the haemorrhage within the distribution of the middle cerebral artery. Sudden dense hemiplegia is uncommon in SAH unless the lesion has resulted in bleeding into the deep nuclei in the region of the internal capsule, and this may occur of course either with the deep AVMs or with upward rupture of aneurysms in the region of the posterior communicating artery or in the middle cerebral complex. While a long period of confusion and irrationality may occur in SAH of any origin, it is often seen in lesions involving di-encephalic structures, of which anterior communicating aneurysms and aneurysms at the top of the basilar artery are perhaps the most specific. A focal neurological deficit may be of some clinical value in potential localisation of the lesion, but its value is slight in comparison with the necessary subsequent angiography. Of even less value is any focally sited headache, with the possible exception of the aching peri-orbital or the forehead headache which, preceding sudden rupture, may betoken an aneurysm in the region of the terminal carotid artery particularly close to the origin of the posterior communicating complex (Okawara, 1973). These aneurysms more than any other may manifest their presence very clearly by progressive enlargement over some days or weeks prior to subsequent rupture and, if this

is so, then the associated third nerve palsy is of absolute diagnostic significance. Less commonly, aneurysms on the proximal portion of the posterior cerebral artery may also involve the third nerve, but the relative infrequency of this last group renders a third nerve palsy almost diagnostic of posterior communicating aneurysm. Involvement of the fifth nerve, while it may occur in aneurysms which subsequently bleed into the subarachnoid space, is much more associated with aneurysms of the internal carotid within the cavernous sinus and, as a rule, these do not produce SAH.

Particular features of the presentation of arteriovenous malformations

AVMs differ from intracranial aneurysms in that a substantial proportion of these lesions present not with SAH but with epilepsy. SAH may appear at any stage later in the development of the lesion, although there is a tendency for each AVM to run true to type, that is, more lesions which develop epilepsy continue with epilepsy as their only symptom than subsequently develop haemorrhage. This may be, as pointed out by Morello and Borghi (1973), because epilepsy occurs in its major form particularly with very large lesions, and there is a slight but definite preponderance for subarachnoid or intracerebral haemorrhage to occur with rather smaller lesions. However, a clear history of epilepsy followed by the development of SAH is a valuable diagnostic point, and since the prognosis for SAH following rupture of AVMs and of aneurysms is very different—the latter having a much more serious outlook— the differentiation is worthwhile from the point of view of management of relatives, even at an early stage before angiography has made confirmation of the nature of the lesion absolute.

The particular presenting features of intracranial AVM in six recent large series (Paterson and McKissock, 1956; Mackenzie, 1953; Olivecrona and Riives, 1948; Kelly et al., 1969; Perret and Nishioka, 1966; Morello and Borghi, 1973) are shown in Table 12.1. There is a fairly general agreement that between 30 and 60 per cent of these lesions present with haemor-

Table 12.1   Initial symptoms of intracranial arteriovenous malformations

Symptoms	Paterson & McKissock 110 cases (1956	Mackenzie 50 cases (1953)	Olivecrona 43 cases (1948)	Kelly et al. 70 cases (1969)	Perret & Nishioka 453 cases (1966)	Morello & Borghi 154 cases (1973)
Haemorrhage	46 (42%)	15 (30%)	17 (40%)	36 (51%)	307 (68%)	86 (56%)
Epilepsy	29 (26%)	16 (32%)	17 (40%)	26 (37%)	119 (28%)	31 (20%)
Progressive hemianopia	16 (15%)	12 (24%)	—	2 (3%)	Uncertain	—
Migraine or other headache, and other neurological symptoms	8 (7%)	6 (12%)	—	6 (9%)	44 (10%)	14 (9%)

rhage as their first sign, and somewhere between 25 and 40 per cent present with epileptic seizures. Rather less frequently, progressive neurological deficit is the mode of presentation, while such features as recurrent migraine or other non-specific headache, or curious neurological signs such as those of the cerebello-pontine angle, may betoken AVMs in unusual sites.

While the classical features of SAH render diagnosis fairly straightforward, occasional cases may be missed, and this is of particular regret where a small so-called 'warning leak' from an intracranial aneurysm is disregarded, only to be followed within some weeks by a second disastrous or even fatal haemorrhage. As will be discussed in the section under management, surgery for the average supratentorial aneurysm has reached such a stage of development that the warning leak should now be followed by prompt surgical obliteration of the aneurysm. In a small but significant group of cases, the headache is relatively less intense or is disregarded by the patient, and the main complaint which the patient presents is that of back pain and sciatica. This results from the collection of blood in the subarachnoid space about the lumbar nerve roots, and has even been followed by the excision of an entirely blameless lumbar disc.

Later features associated with subarachnoid haemorrhage

One of the most interesting complicating features of massive SAH either from intracranial aneurysm or angioma, results from the extensive blockage of the absorptive mechanisms of the cerebrospinal fluid by breakdown products of blood or by direct adhesions induced in the subarachnoid space by the breakdown products of the haemorrhage (Gallera and Greitz, 1970; Shulman et al. (1963). Thus, in a recent series presented by Yasargil et al. (1973), 10 per cent of the 280 cases with intracranial aneurysm developed communicating hydrocephalus. This complication usually occurs within one to three weeks following the haemorrhage, and it may occur when the patient is managed conservatively or following craniotomy for the aneurysm. Although it has been recorded following AVM, the relative infrequency of this lesion has led to its occurrence there being noted only in an incidental fashion. The usual picture is for the patient apparently recovering from severe SAH to become increasingly obtunded. Gradual confusion, disorientation, memory impairment, and a decrease in mental and physical activity are early symptoms, and the condition, although progressing no further, may yet thereby mar an otherwise reasonable recovery. Bilateral pyramidal and extrapyramidal signs may then appear, there is quite commonly increasing neck stiffness, increasing papilloedema, and a gradual descent, at the worst, into akinetic mutism. Where the SAH has been severe, the coma associated with the original haemorrhage —perhaps with focal hypothalamic damage as in the case of an anterior communicating artery aneurysm, in its own turn producing akinesia and mutism—may merge imperceptibly into the

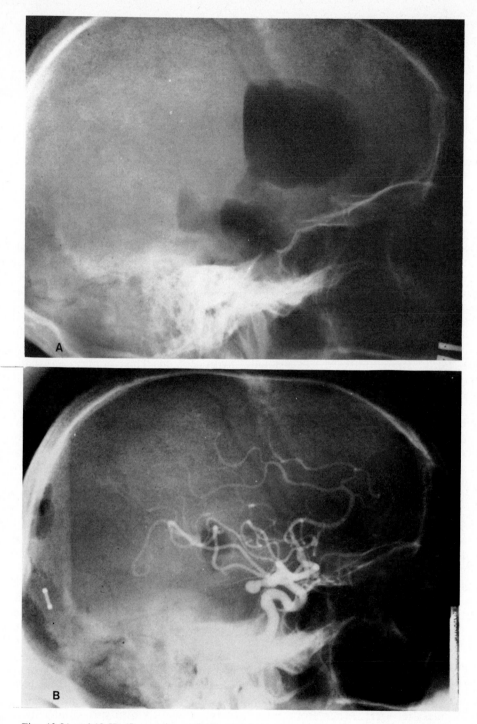

Figs. 12.5A and 12.5B. (See caption on facing page.)

prolonged unconsciousness and severely raised intracranial pressure of communicating hydrocephalus (Fig. 12.5). In these cases, the development of severe and persistent papilloedema may be the only sign giving the clue to the nature of the progressive and continuing pathology. This form of communicating hydrocephalus responds particularly well to ventriculo-atrial shunt procedures and the diagnosis should, therefore, be considered in all cases of SAH where the level of consciousness shows an unexpected decline some weeks after haemorrhage, or where prolonged unconsciousness is associated with papilloedema.

Less commonly, the communicating hydrocephalus may prove of the 'normal pressure' or, more properly, infrequently raised pressure type, when its recognition may prove less easy, demanding careful continuous pressure measurement over some days to detect the abnormal

pressure wave phenomena (Symon, Dorsch, and Stephens, 1972; Symon and Dorsch, 1975). Treatment by bypass shunt operation is no less necessary in such cases, and is often equally rewarding.

Grading of patients with subarachnoid haemorrhage from aneurysm

The accumulated experience over almost 30 years from the Second World War has produced general agreement among neurosurgeons that the risks of operation on patients with SAH from intracranial aneurysm are closely related to the condition of the patient at the time of surgery. The first serious attempt to codify the condition of patients suffering from SAH was made by Botterell *et al.* (1956), and it is a modification of this original classification developed by Hunt and Hess (1968) which has been

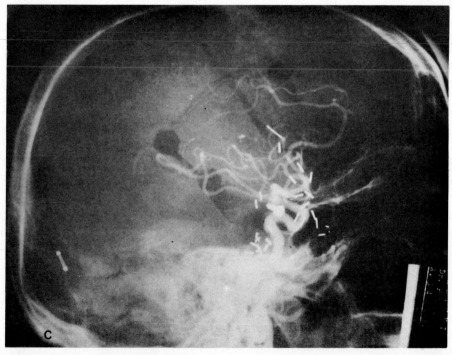

Figs. 12.5A, 12.5B, and 12.5C   A 60-year-old general practitioner who became akinetic and mute after a severe subarachnoid haemorrhage. Figure 12.5A shows the evident communicating hydrocephalus on air encephalogram, Figure 12.5B, the reduction in size of the ventricles following shunt surgery and the continued presence of the posterior communicating aneurysm which became active again about five weeks following the first haemorrhage when a complete third nerve palsy developed. The aneurysm was then satisfactorily occluded, as shown in Figure 12.5C.

adopted in most neurosurgical units to describe a patient's condition either on admission or at surgery. The adoption of this simple classification has been one of the most useful aspects of aneurysm study in recent years, since it has enabled the comparison of data from one clinic to another and, if stated in association with the time of operation from the time of SAH, enables calculation of surgical contribution to survival in comparison with natural mortality, as Alvord *et al.* (1972) have made clear. The classification which in most features approximates to that used by Nishioka (1966) in the combined study is expressed in Table 12.2 from Hunt and Hess's original work. Their suggestion that 'serious systemic disease such as hypertension, diabetes, severe arteriosclerosis, chronic

Table 12.2   The grading of patients with subarachnoid haemorrhage

Grade 1	Asymptomatic, or minimal headache, and slight neck stiffness.
Grade 2	Moderate to severe headache, neck stiffness, no neurological deficit other than cranial nerve palsy.
Grade 3	Drowsiness, confusion, or mild focal deficit.
Grade 4	Stupor, moderate to severe hemiparesis, possible early decerebrate rigidity and vegetative disturbances.
Grade 5	Deep coma, decerebrate rigidity, moribund appearance.

(*After* Hunt and Hess (1968) Surgical risk as related to time of intervention in the repair of intracranial aneurysms. *Journal of Neurosurgery*, **28**, 14. By kind permission of the authors and publishers.)

pulmonary disease and severe vasospasm seen in arteriography, results in placement of the patient in the next less favourable category' is less uniformly applied, and if this amendment to the grading of patients is employed it is advisable that it be stated in the breakdown of patient data. Analysing 275 cases of their own, Hunt and Hess showed that the overall mortality from the time of admission varied from 11 per cent in Grade 1 patients to 100 per cent in Grade 5 patients, giving a total mortality rate of 35 per cent. Separating off those patients whom they were able to submit to surgery, the mortality figures of a group of 156 cases subjected to

operation ranged from 1.4 per cent in Grade 1 to 43 per cent in Grade 4. They operated on no patients in Grade 5, and their total operative mortality was 16 per cent.

The objection is often raised, however, that in the usual surgical series a number of cases have died in the interval between admission and surgery. These being abstracted from the surgical mortality inevitably favour the surgical results in relation to natural mortality. This frequent criticism of surgically analysed series led Alvord *et al.* (1972) to create a matrix of probability in relation to clinical grade, in which they combined the time after the last SAH with the clinical grade (Table 12.3). Their analysis had previously indicated that there was little difference in the natural decay curves for aneurysm cases, whether one constructed the tables in relation to either the first or the last SAH. This related to two factors: firstly, each SAH rendered the prognosis worse; secondly, recurrence of bleeding took place in only about 25 to 30 per cent of patients. This impressive work has enabled us to relate surgical results corrected for time following haemorrhage and grade at operation to Alvord *et al.*'s predictions of natural mortality, and has enabled for example the analysis of 108 personal cases treated by intracranial operation following SAH, shown in Table 12.4. It appears from this table that the surgical mortality has improved on natural mortality significantly in Grades 1, 2, and 3, most particularly in Grade 3. Evidence of improvement in relation to surgery is less impressive in Grade 4, and operation is now rarely undertaken on such patients. A recent remarkable series from Krayenbühl *et al.* (1972) reported an overall mortality rate in 250 operations for intracranial aneurysm of 5 per cent. The mortality rate for operations on Grades 1, 2, and 3 patients was 1.6 per cent, and there were no deaths in 112 patients operated on in Grades 1 and 2. Twenty-four per cent of the cases were operated on within one week of haemorrhage and 52 per cent within two weeks. Although it is impossible to place this series in relation to Alvord *et al.*'s criteria without the data, the remarkably low mortality rate in good-risk patients is clearly superior to natural mortality.

Table 12.3   (Reproduced by kind permission of the *Archives of Neurology* and of Alvord *et al.*, from their article (1972) Subarachnoid haemorrhage due to ruptured aneurysms. *Archives of Neurology*, **27**, 283.)

	Probabilities Days after subarachnoid haemorrhage						
Clinical grade	0 to 1	1 to 3	3 to 7	7 to 21	21 to 60	60+	All intervals
1	65	80	90	95	95	95	90
2	55	70	75	90	95	95	75
3	45	55	65	75	85	95	65
4	30	40	45	50	60	70	45
5	5	5	5	5	5	5	5
All grades	45	55	65	75	85	95	65

Assessment of the comparative morbidity of conservative and surgical treatment is less easy, largely because of inadequate information concerning the natural morbidity. It is, however, regrettably true that a proportion of surgical survivors are intellectually or physically handicapped (Logue *et al.*, 1968), but once again the general surgical experience has been that unsatisfactory results are, like deaths, commoner in bad-risk cases.

Table 12.4   Per cent probability of survival after SAH

Clinical grade	Days post-haemorrhage									
	0–1		2–3		4–7		8–21		22–60	
2	65	70	70	75	75	80	90	90	95	100
	(0)		(2)	100	(12)	91.5	(17)	88	(3)	100
3	45	50	55	60	65	70	75	80	85	90
	(0)		(9)	100	(12)	100	(16)	100	(2)	100
4	30	40	40	45	45	50	50	55	60	
	(4)	75	(7)	71	(8)	75	(13)	70	0	
5			5							
			(1) 0							

A comparison of predicted mortality in terms of grade and age compared with the actual mortality of surgery under the same conditions of age and grade. The matrix is prepared by Alvord's criteria using 108 personal intracranial aneurysm operations of the author's. The two figures in the top line in each box are the percentage probability of natural survival at two years and at two months following subarachnoid haemorrhage. The lower line in each box contains two figures. The one in parentheses is the total number of cases in each group: the other is the percentage of survivors at 12 months following surgery.

(*After* Alvord *et al.* (1972) Subarachnoid haemorrhage due to ruptured aneurysms. *Archives of Neurology*, **27**, 283.)

TIMING OF INVESTIGATION AND OPERATION IN CASES OF ANEURYSMAL SUBARACHNOID HAEMORRHAGE

From the careful analytical work of the Co-Operative Study and other authors, it is clear that operation on intracranial aneurysms following SAH cannot be undertaken in all cases immediately the patient presents in the clinic. It follows, therefore, that if immediate operation in all cases is not to be undertaken, one must first make a decision about the propriety and extent of angiographic investigation. Complete angiographic investigation in our hands, particularly in the unconscious or restless patient, almost invariably requires general anaesthesia. Provided that the patient is in a condition fit to sustain a general anaesthetic lasting perhaps one-and-a-half to two hours, immediate angiography is recommended. Only in this way will the information as to the site and accessibility of the aneurysm be available, the presence or absence of intracranial haematomata be defined, and detailed planning of any surgical intervention put on a rational basis. Much has been written about delayed angiography with the caveat that immediate angiography soon after SAH increases the risk, but, in these terms, this has not been the author's experience. Careful angiography performed by skilled radiologists early after SAH has not contributed significantly to morbidity or mortality.

Having established the site and accessibility of the aneurysm responsible for the SAH, the question of the timing of operation arises. It is apparent from numerous studies that there is nothing to be said for intervention in cases of Grade 4 or Grade 5 early after haemorrhage, unless an intracranial haematoma appears to threaten life when a judicious burrhole with evacuation of the clot may enable the patient's condition to be sufficiently improved to warrant further surgery at a later date. A word of caution is necessary here, however. The mere presence of an intracranial haematoma does not demand its immediate evacuation. The work of Löfgren and Zwetnow (1972) and perhaps that of Nornes (1973) also has indicated that marked induced changes in intracranial pressure may provoke further rupture from aneurysms, so that if the patient's life is not threatened by the intracranial haematoma and the condition appears to be improving, then the haematoma is best left. The presence of a haematoma of moderate size may well enhance the accessibility of an aneurysm at the time of definitive surgery and make the whole procedure very much easier. Thus patients of Grade 5 should not be subjected to surgery at all unless a life-threatening haematoma is present, patients of Grade 4 should not be operated on within the first week unless a life-threatening haematoma is present, and operation after the first week should be undertaken only advisedly in such cases as, for example, in younger patients with a reasonable prospect of a worthwhile long-term neurological recovery. Patients in this grade over the age of 60 are probably best left unoperated.

The decision for or against surgery reaches its maximum difficulty in patients of Grade 3. Here, the rewards for success are high and, conversely, the sharp postoperative deterioration of a patient apparently improving in Grade 3 is a burden which every neurosurgeon carries. The author's view, which has gradually hardened over the years, is that patients who are stable over a period of 48 hours in Grade 2 or who show signs of improvement from Grade 3, merit surgery as soon as may be. Circumstances which may alter this decision are the presence of marked hypertension or extreme neck stiffness in association with drowsiness or hemispheral signs, since there is a strong clinical impression, not backed by any significant statistical analyses, that these patients are more likely than others to develop extensive vasospasm following surgery. Operation is delayed, therefore, on Grade 3 cases associated with very marked neck stiffness and very heavy blood staining in the CSF.

In patients of Grades 1 or 2, there can be little justification for delay. The probability is only that such patients will get worse if bleeding should recur, and there is little doubt that in skilled hands at this time the mortality of surgery in these grades is appreciably lower than the risk which these patients run of recurrent haemorrhage. The careful work of Drake (1968a) some years ago, which proposed that surgery even in good-risk patients be deferred to the end of the first week, has been so at variance with the author's and other colleagues' practice that early surgery in good-risk patients has continued. The mortality rate may be somewhat higher than after delay, but this increased mortality rate is compensated for by the absence of re-bleeding in these patients over the week of delay.

Some recent advances in general techniques of management

TECHNICAL SURGICAL CHANGES

There have been two principal changes in surgical technique in recent years. The first of these has been the development of the torsion bar clip, in which the clip is applied to the neck of the aneurysm, not with the surgeon's musculature under active contraction, but with a relaxing grip. The likelihood of the neck of the aneurysm being torn by the vibration of muscular effort, even avoiding any suggestion of tremor, is markedly reduced by this development. Figure 12.6 shows the EMG recorded from the author's adductor pollicis applying a straightforward MacKenzie clip in one instance and releasing a Scoville clip in the other. The comparison in muscular effort is quite striking and justifies the complete abandonment of clips which are not applied by relaxation of the surgeon's hand.

The second great technical advance has been the increased use of the operating microscope.

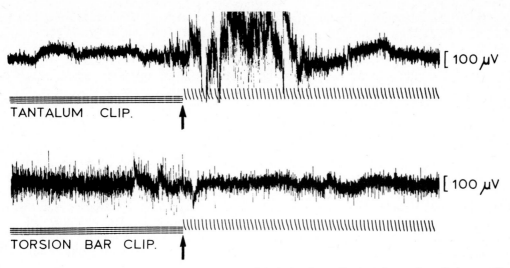

Fig. 12.6 The electromyogram of the author's adductor pollicis during the application of a tantalum clip (*top panel*) and a torsion bar clip (*bottom panel*) (under test conditions).

To this neurosurgeons owe a great debt to Professor Yasargil of Zurich, who popularised the neurosurgical applications of Jacobson's original work in Burlington, Vermont, taken up locally by Dr Peardon Donaghy. Yasargil's immense enthusiasm and fertile mind enabled the creation of a full range of neurosurgical instruments suitable for use under the microscope and the development of operating microscopes more particularly designed for neurosurgical use. Yasargil's own views of the advantages of the microscopic technique are, firstly, the production of excellent illumination; secondly, the early recognition of field detail and the accurate delineation of blood vessels; thirdly, increased safety in clip placement because of clear vision and dissecting ease; and, fourthly, minimal retraction necessary for satisfactory completion of the operation.

Personal experience has fully borne out these contentions. The decreased retraction associated with aneurysmal surgery under the microscope is one of the main advantages of the method. Self-retaining retractors with constant and gentle pressure enable dissection even of such difficult sites as the anterior communicating complex under direct vision, with minimal distortion of neuraxial structures, and there is no doubt that the magnification and intensity of illumination enable the recognition of blood vessel detail behind covering arachnoid, so that accurate dissection through the arachnoid results, rather than the previous tentative opening hoping to avoid important underlying vessels. No young surgeon who proposes taking up aneurysmal surgery can today omit the development of microscopic techniques.

PATHOPHYSIOLOGICAL DEVELOPMENTS CONCERNED WITH SUBARACHNOID HAEMORRHAGE IN RECENT YEARS

The past two decades have seen a vast increase in the knowledge and understanding of the cerebral circulation and its reactions. A series of international meetings since the first meetings in Lund and Copenhagen in 1965 have resulted in a wealth of physiological detail culled from both the experimental laboratory and the clinic, associated with the development of increasingly accurate techniques for regional and quantitative measurement of cerebral blood flow. Recent work in clinics both in North America and in Europe has indicated the generalised depression in hemispheral blood flow associated with recent SAH and the focal reduction in blood flow in areas supplied by spastic arteries (Heil-

brun, Olesen, and Lassen, 1972; Symon, Ackerman *et al.*, 1972). The realisation that these
problems are open to physiological analysis
has encouraged others to take up analytical
techniques. As a result of greater understanding
of the cerebral circulation and its reactivity,
assisted ventilation in anaesthesia has become
the norm in surgery of intracranial aneurysms,
and hypotensive anaesthesia has become safer
with the understanding of the diminished
autoregulatory capacity of areas of the circulation already exposed to stress, such as vasospasm or swelling.

Also, in the past decade, the increased use of
steroids such as dexamethasone, which protect
the blood brain barrier and diminish the tendency for oedema to follow transient vascular
occlusion, brain retraction, or the vascular
occlusion encouraged by vasospasm, has resulted in a decreased incidence of the much
swollen brain with which many of us were
familiar in operating on SAHs early after
haemorrhage in past years.

THE USE OF ANTI-FIBRINOLYTIC AND HYPOTENSIVE
AGENTS IN CONSERVATIVE MANAGEMENT, OR AS
AN ADJUNCT TO SURGERY

In recent years, a number of authors have
reported experiences with drugs designed to
prevent clot lysis, which it is presumed is
responsible for re-bleeding from aneurysms.
The bleeding tendency is known to rise to a
maximum around the end of the first week, and
thereafter to fall to a relatively low level after the
third week, although the exact distribution of
re-bleeds in time varies from one particular
aneurysm to another. There is, thus, evidence
that aneurysms of the internal carotid artery
show a tendency to remain active longer, for
example, than other intracranial aneurysms,
but on the whole the incidence of re-bleeding
after three months has fallen to very low levels.
The rationale of antifibrinolytic drugs is to
protect the aneurysm from re-bleeding during
the early posthaemorrhagic period when other
circulatory disturbances are at their maximum,
and when experience has shown the operation
carries a much higher mortality than later.

In 1967, Norlén and Thulin reported experiences with epsilon aminocaproic acid (EACA)
in neurosurgery. This drug acts principally by
competitive inhibition of the activator substances converting plasminogen into the pro-
teolytic enzyme plasmin, and also to a lesser
extent by direct plasmin inhibition. Since the
initial report, therapeutic trials have been
published by Mullan and Dawley (1968), with
the encouraging suggestion that a re-bleed rate
of 2 out of 35 patients constituted an improvement on natural re-bleeding rate, although the
design of their trial was not a standard one and
the duration of the treatment varied from periods of several days to six weeks. A further trial,
reported by Ransohoff, Goodgold, and Vallo
Benjamin (1972), combined antifibrinolytic
drugs (again EACA) with hypotension for two
weeks following the period of haemorrhage, and
concluded that both ancillary methods were
probably of value, since in 50 cases in which the
two techniques were used together there were
only six re-bleeding incidents, the latest occurring on the twenty-fifth day of treatment in one
case. A more recent brief report of the use of
tranexamic acid (AMCA) in 182 patients with
SAH (Uttley and Richardson, 1974) indicated
that the re-bleeding rate in the first 14 days from
the original ictus was 12.1 per cent. It is a matter
of regret that, although the drug has been
widely used since the initial encouraging reports
in 1968, there is as yet no conclusive evidence
that its use significantly diminishes the re-
bleeding rate, and there have been isolated
reports of toxic reactions (Charytan and Purtilo,
1969; Naeye, 1962). These have included peripheral gangrene, vascular thrombosis and pulmonary embolism, although not in neurosurgical patients, and angiographic appearances
suggesting arteritis or thrombosis in association with a deteriorating clinical course in
patients treated with the drug following SAH
(Sonntag and Stein, 1974). In Norlén and Thulin's initial report of 14 cases, one death occurred
due to bilateral thrombosis of the anterior cerebral arteries 10 days after surgery. It is of course
not certain that this could be attributed to the
use of the drug, but it is certainly a most unusual
postoperative complication. The standard regime for the use of EACA is an oral dose of 4 g

four-hourly. The closely related drug tranexamic acid (AMCA), which appears to act in the same way although in a much lower concentration, is usually given in divided doses to a total of 12 g in 24 hours.

The use of hypotensive agents in the management of subarachnoid cases early after the ictus was suggested by Slosberg (1973), but there is as yet no firm statistical evidence of a significant protective effect. In 109 cases of aneurysmal bleeding treated with hypotension alone in the cooperative aneurysm study (Sahs, 1966), there was a 48 per cent mortality rate and no clear evidence of protective effect of the treatment. In addition, the maintenance of a steady level of blood pressure in the course of treatment with antihypertensive drugs may prove difficult. As a rule, therefore, the conservative management of SAH cases is, in most centres, restricted to supportive treatment of the chest and respiration in comatose cases and the maintenance of strict bed rest for a period of four to six weeks following the ictus. Many would take the view that bed rest should not exclude the patient arising for toilet purposes.

THE SPECIFIC TECHNICAL APPROACH TO ANEURYSMS IN VARIOUS SITUATIONS

The great majority of intracranial aneurysms —95 per cent in the combined series—are in the anterior part of the Circle of Willis, affecting either the region of the anterior communicating complex, the middle cerebral artery, or the terminal carotid artery in the region of the origin of the posterior communicating artery. The distribution of aneurysms in the combined study and in a personal series is shown in Table 12.5.

It is generally agreed now that the approach to anterior circle aneurysms is best made by a small fronto-temporal craniotomy, with excision of the outer part of the sphenoidal wing. This approach, used by many surgeons and most specifically advocated in recent years by Yasargil, has the considerable merit that the surgeon, who may deal with a relatively small number of

Table 12.5 Distribution of 120 aneurysms in 116 personal cases of subarachnoid haemorrhage, compared with the distribution in the combined study (Locksley, 1966) in 2672 cases.

	Combined series (%)	Personal series (%)
Anterior communicating complex	39.1	28.0
Distal anterior cerebral artery	1.6	2.6
Middle cerebral artery	18.3	20.0
Posterior communicating artery	32.5	25.0
Terminal carotid artery	5.0	9.0
Posterior circulation	3.3	3.5

these cases in the course of a year, makes what is essentially the same initial approach to the common aneurysms. Dissection, under the operating microscope assisted by appropriate self-retaining retractors, is pursued down to the terminal carotid artery, and the branches of the internal carotid followed to the aneurysm-bearing area.

Anterior communicating artery aneurysms

While the common approach now, following the initial stages common to all aneurysms, is to excise a portion of the gyrus rectus just above and in front of the optic nerve and to dissect into the anterior communicating complex through the gyrus rectus, some surgeons still find merit in the interhemispheric approach, with excision of the medial portion of the frontal pole, popular a number of years ago. The use of this approach is particularly favoured by some in aneurysms lying above and behind the plane of the anterior communicating artery. The gyrus rectus approach, however, although it is certainly more difficult in such cases, is still satisfactory for them and lends the continued great advantage of familiarity of approach, which the interhemispheric approach does not possess. An example of an aneurysm attacked by the subfrontal approach is shown in Figure 12.7, while Figure 12.8 shows a large aneurysm above the level of the complex attacked by the interhemispheric route. Both are satisfactory, but the simplicity of surgery in the former route along the sphenoidal wing renders it the most suitable at the present time, in the author's experience.

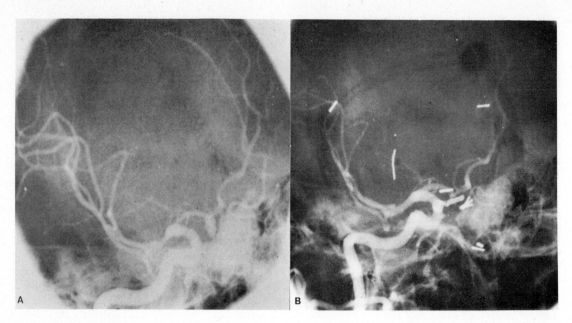

Figs. 12.7A and 12.7B   Pre- and postoperative views of an anterior communicating artery aneurysm clipped by an approach along the sphenoidal wing.

Posterior communicating artery aneurysms and aneurysms on the terminal carotid artery

Here there is little debate. The direct access along the wing brings the terminal carotid artery closer than any other approach, and the exact siting of the flap may be varied a little according to whether one wishes to approach the aneurysm more from anteriorly or from laterally. It is the author's current practice to divide, if necessary, the polar temporal veins to enable self-retaining retraction of the tip of the temporal lobe, assisting in the opening of the Sylvian fissure in aneurysms of the posterior communicating complex which are directed downwards and backwards so that the fundus of the aneurysm lies entirely behind the tentorium. By this method, excellent visualisation of the origin of the neck, of the anterior choroidal artery, and of the posterior communicating artery, may be assured. The anterior choroidal artery, if it is clearly visualised on angiography and is demonstrably some distance from the origin of the aneurysm, need not be visualised at surgery; the minimum of dissection in the region of

aneurysms necessary to ensure satisfactory clipping is the ideal. The posterior communicating artery need not necessarily be preserved, the artery itself usually being a 'no-flow' vessel, but if careful angiography has demonstrated that the artery is in fact a fetal posterior cerebral artery with the ipsilateral posterior cerebral filling preferentially or entirely from the carotid, great care must be taken to preserve the posterior communicating artery itself. Extreme care is necessary also in those instances where, either from the size or multiplicity of aneurysms, the exact relationship of the neck to the anterior choroidal artery is in doubt (Drake, Vanderlinden, and Amacher, 1968).

Terminal carotid aneurysms present problems in proportion to their association with the perforating branches of the proximal middle cerebral artery. The terminal carotid itself and the region of the first centimetre of its main branches are, as pointed out by Shellshear (1920) many years ago, commonly entirely devoid of branches, but the situation of the fundus of an aneurysm arising from the terminal carotid in relation to the perforating vessels determines not only the

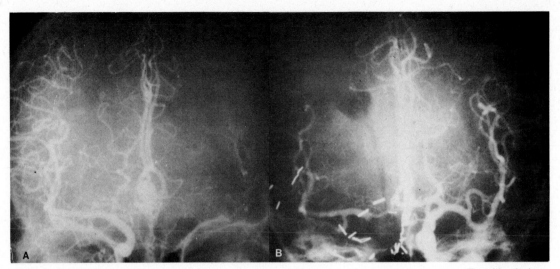

Figs. 12.8A and 12.8B   Pre- and postoperative views of an anterior communicating artery aneurysm clipped by the interhemispheric route.

degree of deficit which the SAH may produce, but also the operative difficulty of exposure of the aneurysm. If, however, the neck can be shown angiographically to be free from perforating vessels, then dissection of the parent artery and the neck alone may prevent disturbance and distortion of the perforating vessels in attempted dissection of the fundus. The greatest degrees of difficulty arise where the neck itself is in close relation to perforating vessels, and here the great advantages of illumination and magnification afforded by the operating microscope have their greatest reward.

Middle cerebral artery aneurysms

The aneurysms of the region of the middle cerebral artery commonly have their origin at the first bifurcation of the vessel. They are there in close relationship with the major insular branches, frequently being embraced by them as Figure 12.9 shows; and even now with the advantages of the operating microscope and its illumination, the surgeon may feel it unwise to dissect these vessels with sharp dissection from the fundus of the aneurysm to enable a clipable neck to be created. In this aneurysm there is still a place for gauze or gauze reinforced

with acrylic applied as an investment to the whole complex. There is no doubt, however, that the proportion of aneurysms invested, in the author's own experience, has declined since microscopic techniques have been employed, but the ease and safety of the investment technique should not be entirely abandoned. More proximal aneurysms of the middle cerebral artery are certainly most easily approached by following the main vessel out along the sphenoidal wing from the terminal carotid artery. Peripheral aneurysms, as for example in a very lateral trifurcation of the vessel, may still be approached by dissection through the superior temporal gyrus. This is particularly so if a temporal haematoma is present; dissection through the haematoma will often bring the surgeon directly on to the aneurysm without the necessity of disturbing the perforating-bearing area of the middle cerebral complex. It does, of course, carry the disadvantage of approaching the fundus of the aneurysm first, and each individual approach and aneurysm must be considered on its own merits in this sometimes most difficult technical dissection.

Less common anterior circle aneurysms lie distally on the branches of the carotid. Of these, perhaps the commonest is the distal anterior

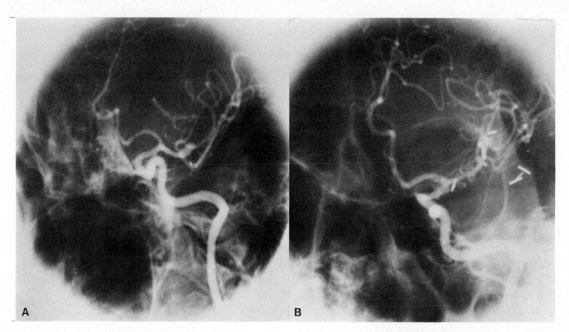

Figs. 12.9A and 12.9B   Pre- and postoperative views of a typical middle cerebral trifurcation aneurysm clipped by an approach through the superior temporal gyrus.

cerebral artery aneurysm, which is often associated with congenital anomalies of the anterior communicating complex such as a single anterior cerebral artery bifurcating at the level of the genu of the corpus callosum (Fig. 12.10). This aneurysm has a sinister reputation, so that although the approach to it is straightforward and easy, clipping of the aneurysm is not infrequently followed by intense spasm of the distal pericallosal vessels and considerable damage to the medial aspect of both motor strips. Indeed, some experienced surgeons regard this aneurysm with such misgiving that they invariably wrap the region with gauze or gauze and acrylic rather than attempt to clip it. Yasargil and Carter (1974) recently published a group of distal communicating aneurysms clipped with excellent results, and no doubt this will encourage the majority of surgeons to attempt the standard obliteration techniques even with this less common and widely feared lesion.

Aneurysms of the vertebro-basilar system

These aneurysms have a sinister surgical reputation arising in part from the fact that, being relatively uncommon, the majority of surgeons have a limited experience of their management. Aneurysms of the vertebro-basilar trunk, indeed, were very commonly regarded as inoperable lesions until the work of Drake (1961, 1965, 1968b), in which he showed that, while the results were far from satisfactory, it was possible to approach these lesions with careful technique, and in a certain number of instances to occlude them. His vast experience has now encouraged him in this belief, and surgeons throughout the world are less inclined to treat such conditions as vertebro-basilar aneurysms invariably by conservative methods. There is, however, no doubt that the lesions in the upper end of the basilar artery or in the basilar trunk lower in its course represent formidable technical dissections. There are few who would consider it feasible to attack them in the conditions of patient grade at which surgery would now be thought feasible in anterior circle aneurysms; for example, few would consider operation on vertebro-basilar aneurysms in Grade 3. The question, therefore, arises whether the surgeon is accomplishing more than con-

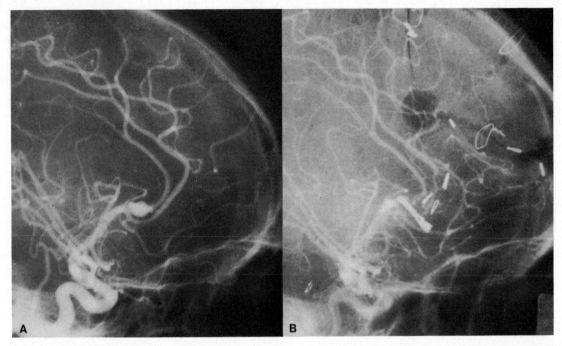

Figs. 12.10A and 12.10B   Pre- and postoperative views of a pericallosal artery aneurysm clipped by the interhemispheric approach.

servative management, although the rate of late re-bleeding in untreated vertebrobasilar aneurysms has been suspected to be greater than that of the more common sites.

Figures 12.11 and 12.12 show that even the 'occasional vertebro-basilar surgeon' will have success from time to time, but against this must be set the disasters which vertebro-basilar surgery, even in careful and experienced hands, will continue to present.

The problem of the giant aneurysm

Giant aneurysms may present either in association with SAH or as space occupying lesions in their own right. In the second group, of course, they fall outside the review scope of the present article, but the technical problems are no less severe when they present with SAH. Indeed, the question of patient condition is superimposed on the technical difficulty of the separation of a large sac from its parent vessel. Possibly the main hazard of which the surgeon should be aware is that the angiographic visualisation of

the sac may fall far short of its true mass. Distortion of the surrounding vessels apparently round a circular and non-opacified region should arouse suspicion; as Figure 12.13 shows, the true size of the sac may well exceed the central area opacified by dye. Since these lesions commonly take many years to reach the presenting size, dissection of vessels from their close attachment to a thickly fibrous sac presents enormous problems and is really technically feasible only with magnification and excellent lighting. In the author's experience with direct approach to some six giant aneurysms, the essential feature in their approach is the capacity to occlude temporarily the aneurysm-bearing artery proximal to the neck of the aneurysm.

It is perhaps surprising that even the proximal middle cerebral artery may be occluded for some appreciable time—in one of the author's own cases a period of 20 minutes—without infarction of the peripheral distribution of the vessel, the reason being given by the angiographic appearances. For example, in the case

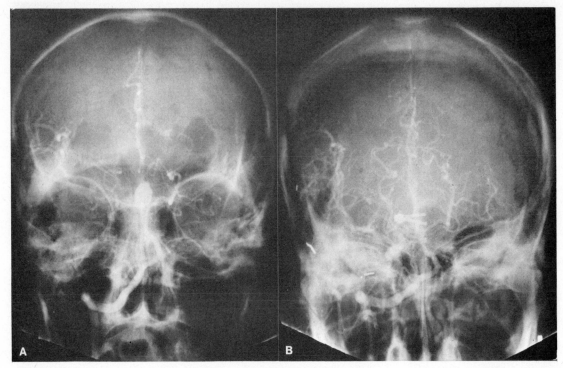

Figs. 12.11A and 12.11B   Pre- and postoperative views of a terminal basilar artery aneurysm approached along the petrous ridge by the mid-temporal approach of Drake.

shown in Figure 12.14 the distal distribution of the middle cerebral artery was seen to be filling very much more slowly, partly by delayed forward flow from the middle cerebral branches and partly by backward reflux from peripheral anastomoses. The territory had therefore been accustomed to hypoperfusion from its main trunk for some little time and had established some degree of leptomeningeal collateral circulation elsewhere. Yasargil, indeed, used this fact in a case some years ago to justify implantation of the superficial temporal artery to the distal middle cerebral distribution, since the symptoms of the patient appeared more related to ischaemia in the distal middle cerebral distribution than to the aneurysm itself. Figure 12.14 shows that occlusion of the parent vessel for some 20 minutes may be followed by successful ligation of the aneurysm, facilitated by direct opening of the aneurysm and the clearance of contained clot. The application of a circumferential

ligature is often difficult in the presence of contained clot, but much easier when the aneurysmal sac has been collapsed. While this is technically feasible in middle cerebral aneurysms and no doubt in aneurysms of the anterior cerebral complex, the difficulties and dangers of such techniques in the vertebro-basilar situation makes the giant vertebrobasilar aneurysm still usually an inoperable lesion.

Multiple aneurysms

In the cooperative study on aneurysms, Perret and Nishioka (1966) reported an autopsy study of 888 cases in which single aneurysms had been found in 78 per cent, a second aneurysm in 17 per cent, and three or more aneurysms in the remaining 5 per cent of cases. The data from a very much larger angiographic series of over 3000 cases showed a very similar distribution, although single aneurysms were detected in 81

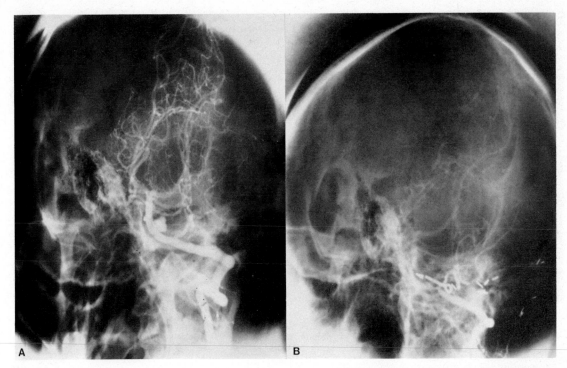

Figs. 12.12A and 12.12B   Pre- and postoperative views of an aneurysm at the junction of vertebral and basilar arteries in the pre-pontine cistern. This aneurysm was clipped by a lateral posterior fossa approach.

per cent, suggesting that unless careful angiography is carried out a second aneurysm may occasionally be missed. The problem of management of cases with multiple aneurysms, therefore, is a very real one. Sometimes there is no doubt from the clinical features as to the origin of the haemorrhage. On occasions, although the clinical features are non-specific, the angiographic appearances may give a strong indication. Thus, irregularity in the shape of one aneurysm, the presence of focal associated vascular spasm near one of the aneurysms, or the presence of small vascular displacements suggesting the presence of a perivascular haematoma may provide an adequate guide. Where there is neither angiographic nor clinical clue, the difficulties of management are maximal.

Other special investigations may assist in the decision as to which aneurysm has bled. Some days after SAH focal disturbances in the EEG may assist at least in lateralising the hemisphere most affected by the bleeding, and

recent experience with the EMI-scanner has indicated that small, intra-Sylvian haematomata scarcely detectable by angiography, or changes in brain density suggestive of the presence of focal oedema, may assist in the attribution of haemorrhage to one particular aneurysm.

The author's practice is to operate only on the aneurysm which has bled, but if several aneurysms may be reached comfortably in one craniotomy, then all may be clipped at the same time. It is probably bad practice, however, to prolong aneurysm surgery where the management of the bleeding aneurysm has proved technically difficult. In a recent series (Heiskanen and Martila, 1970), a six-year follow-up of 76 patients with a known unoperated second aneurysm showed that over this period of time there was a 5 per cent mortality. This, of course, represents a similar mortality to that of the majority of centres in the management of aneurysmal SAH in grades 1 and 2 cases, and it

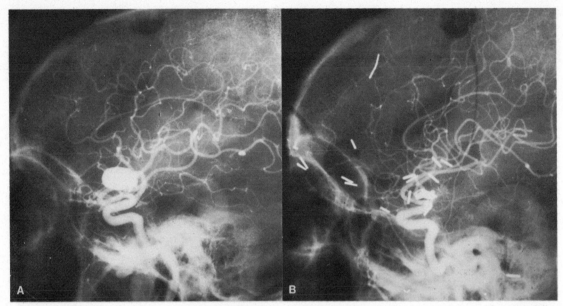

Figs. 12.13A and 12.13B   Pre- and postoperative views of a giant anterior communicating artery aneurysm. The upward displacement of the proximal anterior cerebral artery (Fig.12.13A) is a clue to the fact that only a portion of the sac is opacified, the sac itself extending into close contact with the planum sphenoidale. The displacement of the proximal portion of the artery has disappeared following excision of the sac (Fig. 12.13B).

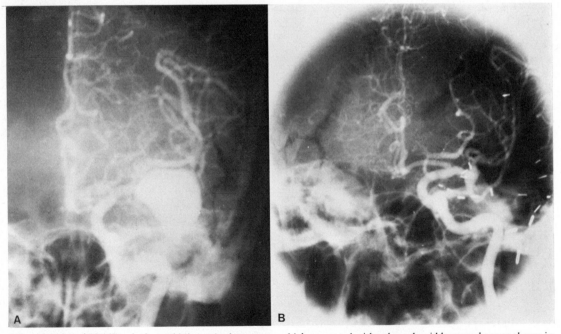

Figs. 12.14A and 12.14B   A giant middle cerebral aneurysm which presented with subarachnoid haemorrhage as shown in Figure 12.14A, with postoperative view (Fig. 12.14B) following successful ligation and excision of the sac.

is clear that serious consideration should now be given to operations on aneurysms which are demonstrated either incidentally at angiography or are known to be present in patients who have had SAH from a successfully operated aneurysm. Studies recently reported demonstrating an appreciable late mortality in unoperated single aneurysms (Winn, Richardson, and Jane, 1973) tend to support this decision, although there is as yet no clear evidence that the behaviour of an aneurysm which is known to have bled on one occasion is necessarily the same as that of an aneurysm present which has never occasioned SAH. The decision will clearly remain a highly personal one and will probably continue to be influenced mainly by the accessibility of the second aneurysm and the age and clinical state of the patient.

Other possible surgical manoeuvres in the treatment of intracranial aneurysms

In past years, the procedure of carotid ligation was widely practiced, particularly for treatment of aneurysms of the terminal carotid artery, and the series presented by McKissock, Paine, and Walsh (1960) demonstrated beyond question, in a randomised clinical trial, that this reduced mortality in single bleeding aneurysms as compared with the expected natural survival. Most surgeons, however, have experience of re-bleeding in subsequent years from aneurysms in the region of the posterior communicating artery, which had remained patent and re-bled through collateral supply either from the verte-bro-basilar system or from the opposite carotid. Figure 12.15 shows such a case. The increasing experience with intracranial surgery, particularly the very low mortality rate reported by Paterson (1968) in a series of posterior communicating aneurysms directly attacked, has encouraged the majority of centres to pursue direct attack on these aneurysms and to reserve carotid ligation solely for aneurysms in the region of the terminal carotid artery closely involved with perforating vessels, where the technical difficulties of surgery are likely to be great and the risks of surgical morbidity appreciable. The technique of proximal ligation of the anterior cerebral artery for aneurysms of the anterior communicating complex, which was originally described by Logue (1956), was practiced by the author and his colleagues for a number of years, but with the introduction of microscopic techniques it is now little used.

Other techniques which have been used are piloinjection —the injection of bristles by a special apparatus (Gallagher, 1964) —at craniotomy, particularly in the treatment of very large aneurysms, and endo-aneurysmorrhaphy by fine copper needles (Mullan et al., 1965), or the obliteration of the aneurysm by the injection of iron filings, whose position is maintained by a magnet. This technique (Alksne, 1971) can be performed either by direct puncture of the aneurysm or by injection of the filings through a catheter introduced into a proximal artery. Perhaps not surprisingly, none of these methods has obtained widespread favour, and Drake's experience (1968b) would suggest that permanent occlusion of giant aneurysms by the pilojection method cannot be relied upon.

Continuing problems in the management of aneurysmal subarachnoid haemorrhage

It will be apparent from this review that accepted technical advances have now made the surgery of anterior circle aneurysms relatively routine. The results in good-risk cases are excellent, and although the technical complexities of operations on the posterior circle means that surgical results here will continue to lag behind until a greater body of surgeons have achieved widespread experience in the surgery of these dangerous lesions, there is no reason to suppose that technical problems in the posterior circle lesions will prove any more insurmountable than in the more common lesions in the anterior part of the circle. The unsatisfactory results in patients in poor clinical grades, however, leaves the surgeon in no doubt that the major problem still to be solved in the surgery of SAH is the effect of the haemorrhage on the cerebral circulation, with the attendant problems of brain swelling and infarction secondary to reduced perfusion.

The reason for the unsatisfactory state of the

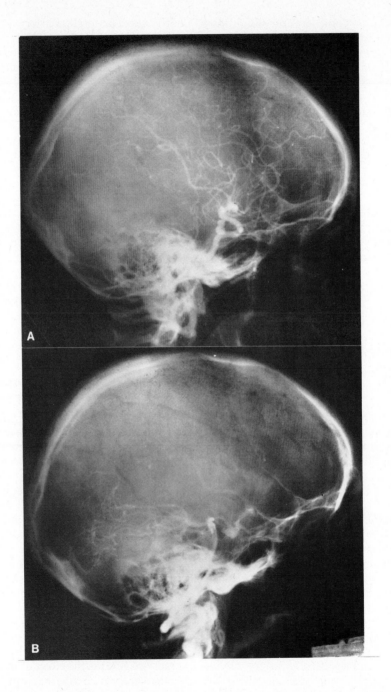

Figs. 12.15A and 12.15B   A posterior communicating aneurysm (Fig. 12.15A) was treated by carotid ligation. Seven years later (Fig. 12.15B) recurrent subarachnoid haemorrhage from the same aneurysm occurred, and filling from the vertebro-basilar circulation with enlargement of the posterior communicating artery is shown.

brain in patients after recent SAH is still not certain. The concept of intracranial vasospasm has been brought forward to explain reduction in peripheral perfusion in the territory of an aneurysm-bearing artery, and neurosurgeons in general are familiar with the angiographic appearances of marked vascular narrowing in the immediate area of intracranial aneurysms at some time following SAH (Symon, 1971). The association of vasospasm with the severity of the patient's illness has varied, however; Allcock and Drake (1963), in the analysis of post-operative vasospasm, noted that 27 per cent of patients with satisfactory recovery showed evidence of vasospasm, but that vasospasm was present postoperatively in 71 per cent of patients with unsatisfactory results. In a series analysed by the author (Symon, 1966), it has appeared that vasospasm is commoner in patients who are severely ill. Of 33 patients who died, 14 showed significant vasospasm; of 53 patients who survived, only 17 showed vasospasm. In individual cases, however, the fairly frequent failure to establish correlation between the severity of vasospasm and the severity of the patient's illness has made it clear that factors other than the actual apparent luminal reduction in afferent arteries must be playing a part. Some patients with quite severe vasospasm are clinically alert and without neurological deficit others with severe neurological deficit have little or no vasospasm. In recent years, however, there has been a considerable amount of work to show that vasospasm has an influence upon the state of perfusion of the brain distal to the vasospastic vessels. Thus, Symon, et al. (1972) showed in an analysis of postoperative angiograms and blood flow good correlation between angiographic demonstration of vasospasm and focal reduction in blood flow in brain supplied by the spastic segments. Similar conclusions were reported by Heilbrun, Olesen, and Lassen (1972), and have also been confirmed by Overgaard (1973). All these authors have commented upon the state of hemispheral perfusion, and it has been clear that hemispheral blood flow has correlated more clearly with the level of consciousness than with the presence or absence of vasospasm. Possible complicating factors here

are the presence or absence of an adequate collateral circulation, since the perfusion pressure distal to a vasospastic segment may remain almost unchanged if the vasospasm, though focally intense, has no effect on adequate collateral circulation. If, however, the collateral vessels are also involved, a much lesser degree of vasospasm may induce considerable fall in hemispheral perfusion, with the production of clinical symptomatology.

Once perfusion has fallen, there may be prompt damage to the blood brain barrier, with the development of vasogenic oedema and locally raised tissue pressure. If the area involved is sufficiently large, secondary gradual rises in intracranial pressure will result, maximal first in the supratentorial compartment involved in the initial swelling. This will further reduce the available perfusion pressure and lead to sequential changes in blood brain barrier, with further swelling and circulatory obstruction. As a consequence of the fall of perfusion to critical levels, local tissue acidosis will result, with focal vasodilatation (vasoparalysis) and global loss of autoregulation (Lassen, 1966). The way becomes open to the development of 'intracerebral steals', and the full pattern of circulatory abnormality demonstrated in experimental infarction. Heilbrun et al. (1972) recently demonstrated such global loss of autoregulation in patients who had deteriorated following SAH, suggesting that while angiographic and CBF correlations are best on a focal level, the general effects of tissue acidosis and dimunition of perfusion are much more widespread.

Current investigations as to the aetiology of vasospasm

Experimental production of vasospasm, either by trauma to cerebral arteries (Echlin, 1965; Symon, 1967; Simeoni, Ryan, and Kotter, 1968) or by the infusion of blood into the subarachnoid space (Ogata, Marshall, and Lougheed, 1973; Crompton, 1964), have led analyses of vasospasm to concentrate either on direct vascular damage or upon the effects of vaso-active material released into the CSF from effused blood. Damage to vessels in the area of SAH has been well documented (Crompton, 1964; Conway and McDonald, 1972). Direct damage to basal cerebral vessels in the experimental situation induces marked vasoconstriction indistinguishable angiographically from the appearances of clinical vasospasm, although it is a much more transient phenomenon lasting, in an intense form, as a rule less than half-an-hour.

A possible biphasic type of spasm (Brawley, Strandness, and Kelly, 1968) suggested that later secondary phenomena may superimpose upon the initial vasospasm induced by trauma to the blood vessel. The appearances of experimental vasospasm strongly suggest the local release of vaso-active material, possibly from the wall of the damaged artery, possibly from effused blood, and the potential nature of this material has been subjected to a great deal of investigation (Arutiunov, Baron, and Majarova, 1970; Kapp, Mahaley, and Odom, 1968a,b; Wilkins et al., 1967; Landau and Ransohoff, 1968; Weir et al., 1970). Serotonin (Raynor, McMurty, and Pool, 1961) or some serotonin-like factor (Wilkins, Silver, and Odom, 1966) was at first a common suggestion but, more recently, the potential role of prostaglandins (Yamamoto et al., 1972) has been advanced, since these substances have been found to be present in effused blood and to reduce the calibre of epicerebral vessels in the experimental situation. Recent work in North America (Rice-Edwards, 1973) has suggested that the role of the platelet aggregation on vessel walls deserves further investigation, while degeneration of the catecholamine plexus has been put forward on the basis of Nielsen and Owman (1971), and elaborated in the form of a hypothesis by Symon (1971) and du Boulay et al. (1972), with the suggestion that the initial SAH produced degeneration of catecholamine-containing nerve endings, which subsequently became sensitive to normal levels of adrenergic amine in the familiar delayed pharmacological hypersensitivity.

What seems clear, however, is that vasospasm is more likely to occur where the SAH has been massive, and re-analysis of the role of blood constituents on cerebral vasoconstriction is under way in several centres in Europe and the United States at the present time. This is particularly welcome in view of the disappointing results obtained by alpha blockade. A further potential link between tissue damage and muscular contraction has been the work of Peterson et al. (1973), who have demonstrated that certain adenosine compounds dilate vessels in states of vasospasm induced by effused blood. They suggested that disorder of the endogenous myogenic metabolism of the spastic vessel had been induced by ischaemia, and that re-supply of exogenous adenosine compounds resulted in the resolution of this abnormality.

There can be few neurosurgeons concerned with the treatment of SAH who will not agree that the problems of the technical approach to aneurysms have largely been solved at this time. Clear guidelines to the preservation of the cerebral circulation by pharmacological techniques, particularly during anaesthesia, have emerged in the past 10 years, and it would not be too optimistic to say that the clear recognition of the salient remaining problem—the unspecified origin of impaired cerebral perfusion consequent upon SAH—has focused the attention of both pharmacologists and neurosurgeons on this major continuing problem. Within the next 10 years or so, we have good grounds to expect further encouraging improvements in the prognosis of this most serious disease.

THE TREATMENT OF SUBARACHNOID HAEMORRHAGE FROM ARTERIOVENOUS MALFORMATION

Although at this time there can be no conclusive proof that the surgical management of haemorrhage from arteriovenous malformation is associated with a lesser mortality than the death rate by natural re-bleeding, the experience of several large series (Olivecrona and Ladenheim, 1957; Morello and Borghi, 1973; Pool and Potts, 1965) would suggest that this is so. Indeed, it would now appear that complete excision of the AVM is the most satisfactory treatment following the presentation of such a lesion with subarachnoid or intracerebral haemorrhage. It is clear, however, that this conclusion cannot be applied in all cases, since the location of the lesion involving brain stem or inaccessible in deep structures will make surgical treatment impossible. Figure 12.16 shows such a lesion which, although it had not in fact presented with SAH, clearly would have been technically inoperable however it had presented. Careful angiography, however, may demonstrate that even in infratentorial lesions which at first sight appear to involve important arteries supplying the brain stem, the AVM may be entirely extracerebral and removable by meticulous dissection under the microscope. Figure 12.4 shows such a case, which had been deemed technically inoperable after angiography some five years before the final presentation, during which time the young man had suffered four recurrent haemorrhages and developed a progressive cerebellar deficit. Angiography indicated that although the lesion was fed by branches of the anterior inferior cerebellar artery, the brain stem distribution of this vessel was uninvolved, and the lesion was successfully and totally removed. A group of such cases of posterior fossa AVM demonstrably extracerebral on careful angiography has been reported by Drake (1973).

Even where AVMs are in close relation to major vessels so that extensive feeding arteries pass straight into the malformation from major portions, for example, of the middle cerebral artery, careful dissection under the operating microscope in association with hypotensive anaesthesia will result in these lesions being accessible to dissection in an increasing proportion of cases, with an acceptable mortality. Thus, Moody and Poppen (1970) radically removed 51 angiomas, with a mortality rate of 12 per cent; Müller, Köller, and Titgemeyer (1970) operated on 88 mixed supra- and infratentorial AVMs, with a mortality rate of 20.5 per cent; Maspes and Marini (1970) excised 60 cases, with an 8 per cent mortality; Krayenbühl's mortality (Wegmann, 1970) for the resection of 69 angiomas was 8.7 per cent; Morello and Borghi (1973) completely excised 88 angiomas in their series of 150, with an operative mortality of 9 per cent. Comparing their own mortality with those of conservatively treated cases, this was approximately half the death rate from recurrent haemorrhage in 44 conservatively managed cases.

While, of course, this would appear impressive and convincing, surgical series on the whole tend to divide themselves into those cases which are considered operable by the surgeon and those which are not, and it is scarcely fair to

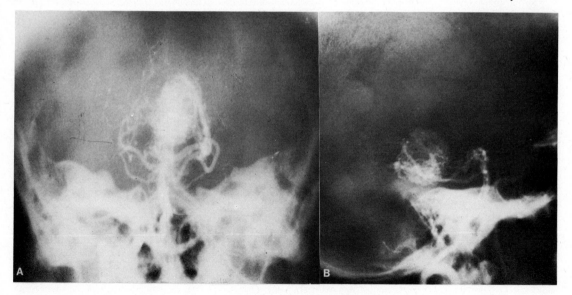

Figs. 12.16A and 12.16B   An arteriovenous malformation of the upper brain stem which presented as aqueduct stenosis. The location of such an AVM renders surgery impossible.

compare the two groups in order to indicate a superior mortality for surgery when such favourable selection has already been applied. As Moody and Poppen (1970) commented, however, it is in general good judgement to avoid surgery for the asymptomatic malformation, or where the symptoms are those of the occasional convulsion which may be adequately controlled by anticonvulsants. Otherwise, in the case of haemorrhage as a presenting feature, surgery should certainly be considered, provided adequate anaesthesia and meticulous technique is used.

There is general agreement in the management of AVMs that, with the rare exception of occasional deep lesions feeding from single vessels, ligation of the feeding vessels has nothing to offer (Pool, 1968). This is almost invariably followed within a short time by the refilling of the angioma from feeding vessels which were not visualised at the time of the original angiography; similar restrictions apply to the previously used practice of carotid ligation.

More recently, embolisation of portions of AVMs (Luessenhop and Spence, 1960; Luessenhop et al., 1965; Kusske and Kelly, 1974), themocoagulation by stereotactic techniques, or operative excision after partial obliteration of the lesion by cryosurgical means have been recommended. These techniques must be regarded as under trial, and have so far yielded acceptable results only in the hands of their developers.

REFERENCES

Alksne, J. F. (1971) Stereotactic thrombosis of intracranial aneurysms. *New England Journal of Medicine*, **284**, 171.
Allock, J. M. & Drake, C. G. (1963) Post-operative angiography in cases of ruptured intracranial aneurysm. *Journal of Neurosrugery*, **20**, 752.
Alvord, E. C., Loeser, J. D., Bailey, W. L. & Compass, M. K. (1972) Subarachnoid haemorrhage due to ruptured aneurysms. *Archives of Neurology*, **27**, 273.
Arutiunov, A. J., Baron, M. A. & Majarova, N. A. (1970) Experimental and clinical study of the development of spasm of the cerebral arteries related to subarachnoid haemorrhage. *Journal of Neurosurgery*, **32**, 617.
Botterell, E. H., Lougheed, W. M. Scott, J. W. & Vandewater, S. L. (1956) Hypothermia, and interruption of carotid or carotid and vertebral circulation, in the surgical management of intracranial aneurysms. *Journal of Neurosurgery*, **13**, 1.
Brawley, B. W., Strandness, D. E. & Kelly, W. A. (1968) The biphasic response of cerebral vasospasm in experimental subarachnoid hemorrhage. *Journal of Neurosurgery*, **28**, 1.
Charytan, C. & Purtilo, D. (1969) Glomerular capillary thrombosis and acute renal failure after Epsilon-aminocaproic acid. *New England Journal of Medicine*, **280**, 1102.
Conway, L. W. & McDonald, L. W. (1972) Structural changes of the intradural arteries following subarachnoid hemorrhage *Journal of Neurosurgery*, **37**, 715.
Crompton, M. R. (1964) The pathogenesis of cerebral infarction following the rupture of cerebral berry aneurysms. *Brain*, **87**, 491.
Drake, C. G. (1961) Bleeding aneurysms of the basilar artery: Direct surgical management in four cases. *Journal of Neurosurgery*, **18**, 230.
Drake, C. G. (1965) Surgical treatment of ruptured aneurysms of the basilar artery: Experience with 14 cases. *Journal of Surgery*, **23** 457.
Drake, C. G. (1968a) Discussion of the paper by Junt and Hess. *Journal of Neurosurgery*, **28**, 19.
Drake, C. G. (1968b) Further experience with surgical treatment of aneurysms of the basilar artery. *Journal of Neurosurgery*, **29**, 372.
Drake, C. G. (1973) Cerebello-pontine angle arteriovenous malformations. In *Advances in Neurosurgery*, ed. by Schürmann, K., Broch, M., Reulen, H.-J. & Voth, D. Berlin: Springer-Verlag.
Drake, C. G., Vanderlinden, R. G. & Amacher, A. L. (1968) Carotid-choroidal aneurysms. *Journal of Neurosurgery*, **29**, 32.
Du Boulay, G., Symon, L., Shah, S., Dorsch, N. & Ackerman, R. (1972) Cerebral arterial reactivity and spasm after subarachnoid haemorrhage. *Proceedings of the Royal Society of Medicine*, **65**, 80.
Echlin, F. A. (1965) Spasm of basilar and vertebral arteries caused by experimental subarachnoid hemorrhage. *Journal of Neurosurgery*, **23**, 1.
Gallagher, J. P. (1964) Pilojection for intracranial aneurysms. Report of progress. *Journal of Neurosurgery*, **21**, 129.
Gallera, R. G. & Greitz, T. (1970) Hydrocephalus in the adult secondary to the rupture of intracranial arterial aneurysms. *Journal of Neurosurgery*, **32**, 634.

Graaf, C. J. (1971) Prognosis for patients with non-surgically treated aneurysms. Analysis of the cooperative study of aneurysms and subarachnoid hemorrhage. *Journal of Neurosurgery*, **35**, 438.

Gull, W. (1859) Cases of aneurysm of the cerebral vessels. *Guy's Hospital Report* (S3), **5**, 281.

Hassler, O. (1965) On the etiology of intracranial aneurysms. In *Intracranial Aneurysms and Subarachnoid Hemorrhage*, ed. Fields, W. S. & Sahs, A. L. Springfield, Illinois: Charles C. Thomas.

Heilbrun, M. P., Olesen, J. & Lassen, N. A. (1972) Regional cerebral blood flow studies in subarachnoid hemorrhage. *Journal of Neurosurgery*, **27**, 36.

Heiskanen, O. & Martila, I. (1970) Risk of rupture of a second aneurysm in patients with multiple aneurysms. *Journal of Neurosurgery*, **32**, 295.

Henderson, W. R. & Gomez, R. L. (1967) Natural history of cerebral angiomas. *British Medical Journal*, iv, 571.

Hunt, W. E. & Hess, R. M. (1968) Surgical risk as related to time of intervention in the repair of intracranial aneurysms. *Journal of Neurosurgery*, **28**, 14.

Kapp, J., Mahaley, M. S. Jr. & Odom, G. L. (1968a) Cerebral arterial spasm. Part 2: Experimental evaluation of mechanical and humoral factors in pathogenesis. *Journal of Neurosurgery*, **29**, 339.

Kapp, J., Mahaley, M. S. Jr. & Odom, G. L. (1968b) Cerebral arterial spasm. Part 3: Partial purification and characterization of a spasmogenic substance in feline platelets. *Journal of Neurosurgery*, **29**, 350.

Kelly, D. L., Alexander, E., Davis, C. H. & Maynard, D. C. (1969) Intracranial arteriovenous malformations. Clinical review and evaluation of brain scans. *Journal of Neurosurgery*, **31**, 422.

Krayenbuhl, H. A., Yasargil, M. G., Flamm, E. S. & Tew, J. M. (1972) Microsurgical treatment of intracranial saccular aneurysms. *Journal of Neurosurgery*, **37**, 678.

Kunc, Z. (1965) The possibility of surgical treatment of arteriovenous malformations in anatomically important cortical regions of the brain. *Acta Neurochirurgica*, **13**, 361.

Kunc, Z. (1973) Surgery of arteriovenous malformations in the speech and motor sensory regions. *Journal of Neurosurgery*, **40**, 293.

Kusske, J. A. & Kelly, W. A. (1974) Embolisation and reduction of the steal syndrome in cerebral arteriovenous malformations. *Journal of Neurosurgery*, **40**, 313.

Landau, B. & Ransohoff, J. (1968) Prolonged cerebral vasospasm in experimental subarachnoid hemorrhage. *Neurology* (Minneap.), **18**, 1056.

Lassen, N. A. (1966) The luxury perfusion syndrome and its possible relation to acute metabolic acidosis localised within the brain. *Lancet*, ii, 1113.

Locksley, H. B. (1966) Report on the cooperative study of intracranial aneurysms and subarachnoid hemorrhage. Section V, Part 1: Natural history of subarachnoid hemorrhage, intracranial aneurysms and arteriovenous malformations. *Journal of Neurosurgery*, **25**, 219.

Löfgren, J. & Zwetnow, N. N. (1972) Kinetics of arterial and venous haemorrhage in the skull cavity. In *Intracranial Pressure*, ed. Brock, M. & Dietz, H. Berlin: Springer-Verlag.

Logue, V. (1956) Surgery in spontaneous subarachnoid haemorrhage. *British Medical Journal*, i, 473.

Logue, V., Durward, Marjorie, Pratt, R. T. C., Piercy, M. & Nixon, W. L. B. (1968) The quality of survival after rupture of an anterior cerebral aneurysm. *British Journal of Psychiatry*, **114**, 137.

Luessenhop, A. J., Kochman, R. Jnr., Shevlin, W. *et al.* (1965) Clinical evaluation of artificial embolisation in the management of large cerebral arteriovenous malformations. *Journal of Neurosurgery*, **23**, 400.

Luessenhop, A. J. & Spence, W. T. (1960) Artificial embolisation of cerebral arteries. Report of use in a case of arteriovenous malformation. *Journal of American Medical Association*, **172**, 1153.

Mackenzie, I. (1953) The clinical presentation of a cerebral angioma. Review of 50 cases. *Brain*, **76**, 184.

McKissock, W., Paine, K. W. E. & Walsh, L. S. (1960) An analysis of the results of treatment of ruptured intracranial aneurysms. *Journal of Neurosurgery*, **17**, 762.

Maspes, P. E. & Marini, G. (1970) Results of the surgical treatment of intracranial arteriovenous malformations. *Vascular Surgery*, **4**, 164.

Moniz, E. (1927) L'encéphalographie artérielle, son importance dans la localisation des tumeurs cérébrales. *Revue Neurologique*, **2**, 72.

Moody, R. A. & Poppen, J. L. (1970) Arteriovenous malformations. *Journal of Neurosurgery*, **32**, 503.

Morello, G. & Borghi, G. P. (1973) Cerebral angiomas. A report of 154 personal cases and a comparison between the results of surgical excision and conservative management. *Acta Neurochirurgica*, **28**, 135.

Mullan, S. & Dawley, J. (1968) Antifibrolynitic therapy for intracranial aneurysms. *Journal of Neurosurgery*, **28**, 21.

Müller, N. L., Köller, L. & Titgemeyer, A. (1970) Katamnestische Untersuchungen nach Operation eines intrakraniellen Rankenangiomas. *Acta Neurochirurgica*, **22**, 53.

Naeye, R. L. (1962) Thrombotic state after haemorrhagic diathesis; a possible complication of therapy with Epsilon-aminocaproic acid. *Blood*, **19**, 694.

Nielsen, K. C. & Owman, C. (1971) Adrenergic innervation of pial arteries related to the Circle of Willis. *Brain Research*, **27**, 25.

Nishioka, H. (1966) Evaluation of conservative management of ruptured intracranial aneurysms. *Journal of Neurosurgery*, **25**, 574.

Norlén, G. & Thulin, C. A. (1967) Experiences with Epsilon-aminocaproic acid in neurosurgery. A preliminary report. *Neurochirurgia* (Stuttgart), **10**, 81.

Nornes, H. (1973) The role of intracranial pressure and arrested hemorrhage in patients with ruptured intracranial aneurysms. *Journal of Neurosurgery*, **39**, 226.

Ogata, M., Marshall, B. M. & Lougheed, W. M. (1973) Observations on the effects of intrathecal papaverine in experimental vasospasm. *Journal of Neurosurgery*, **38**, 20.

Okawara, S.-H. (1973) Warning signs prior to rupture of intracranial aneurysm. *Journal of Neurosurgery*, **38**, 575.

Olivecrona, H. & Ladenheim, J. (1957) *Congenital Arteriovenous Aneurysms of the Carotid and Vertebral Arterial Systems*. Berlin, Göttingen, Heidelberg: Springer.

Olivecrona, H. & Riives, J. (1948) Arteriovenous aneurysms of the brain. *Archives of Neurological Psychiatry*, **59**, 567.

Overgaard, J. (1973) Personal communication.

Pakarinen, S. (1967) Incidence, aetiology and prognosis of primary subarachnoid haemorrhage. A study based on 589 cases diagnosed in a defined urban population during a defined period. *Acta Neurologica Scandinavica*, **43**, (Suppl. 29), 1.

Paterson, A. (1968) Direct surgery in the treatment of posterior communicating aneurysms. *Lancet*, ii, 808.

Paterson, J. H. & McKissock, W. (1956) Intracranial angiomas. A clinical survey of, with special reference to their mode of progression and surgical treatment. A report of 110 cases. *Brain*, **79**, 233.

Perret, G. & Nishioka, H. (1966) Arteriovenous malformations. An analysis of 545 cases of craniocerebral arteriovenous malformations and fistulae reported to the cooperative study. *Journal of Neurosurgery*, **25**, 467.

Peterson, E. W., Searle, R. W., Mandy, F. F. & Leblanc, R. (1973) The reversal of experimental vasospasm by Dibutryl-3',5' adenosine monophosphate. *Journal of Neurosurgery*, **39**, 730.

Pool, J. L. (1968) Excision of cerebral arteriovenous malformations. *Journal of Neurosurgery*, **29**, 312.

Pool, J. L. & Potts, D. G. (1965) *Aneurysms and Arteriovenous Anomalies of the Brain: Diagnosis and Treatment*. New York, Evanston, London: Harper and Row.

Ransohoff, J., Goodgold, A. & Vallo Benjamin, M. (1972) Pre-operative management of patients with ruptured intracranial aneurysms. *Journal of Neurosurgery*, **36**, 525.

Raynor, R. B., McMurty, J. G. & Pool, J. L. (1961) Cerebrovascular effects of topically applied serotonin in the cat. *Neurology* (Minneap.), **11**, 190.

Rice Edwards, J. M. (1973) Personal communication.

Sahs, A. L. (1966) Report on the cooperative study of intracranial aneurysms and subarachnoid hemorrhage. Section VII, Part 2: Hypotension and hypothermia in the treatment of intracranial aneurysms. *Journal of Neurosurgery*, **25**, 593.

Shellshear, J. L. (1920) The basal arteries of the forebrain and their functional significance. *Journal of Anatomy* (London), **55**, 27.

Shulman, K., Martin, B. F. Popoff, N. & Ransohoff, J. (1963) Recognition and treatment of hydrocephalus following spontaneous subarachnoid hemorrhage. *Journal of Neurosurgery*, **20**, 1040.

Simeone, R. A., Ryan, K. G. & Kotter, J. A. (1968) Prolonged experimental cerebral vasospasm. *Journal of Neurosurgery*, **29**, 357.

Slosberg, P. (1973) Treatment and prevention of stroke. 1: Subarachnoid hemorrhage due to ruptured intracranial aneurysms. *New York State Journal of Medicine*, **73**, 679.

Sonntag, V. K. H. & Stein, B. M. (1974) Arteriopathic complications during treatment of subarachnoid hemorrhage with Epsilon-aminocaproic acid. *Journal of Neurosurgery*, **40**, 480.

Symon, L. (1966) Vascular spasm in the cerebral circulation. In *Background to Migraine. First Migraine Symposium, Nov. 8–9, 1966, ed. Smith, R.London: Heinemann*.

Symon, L. (1967) An experimental study of traumatic cerebral vascular spasm. *Journal of Neurology, Neurosurgery & Psychiatry*, **30**, 497.

Symon, L. (1971) Vasospasm in aneurysm. In *Cerebral Vascular Diseases. Proceedings of the 7th Princeton Conference on Cerebrovascular Diseases*, 1970, ed. Moossy, J. & Janeway, R. New York: Grune & Stratton.

Symon, L., Ackerman, R. *et al.* (1972) The use of the Xenon clearance method in subarachnoid haemorrhage: post-operative studies with clinical and angiographic correlation. In *Cerebral Blood Flow and Intracranial Pressure. Proceedings of the 5th International Symposium, Roma-Siena, 1971, Part II, European Neurology*, ed. Fieschi, C. Basel: Karger.

Symon, L. & Dorsch, N. W. C. (1975) The use of long-term intracranial pressure measurement in the assessment of hydrocephalic patients prior to shunt preparation. *Journal of Neurosurgery* (in press).

Symon, L., Dorsch, N. W. C. & Stephens, R. J. (1972) Pressure waves in so-called low-pressure hydrocephalus.*Lancet*, ii, 1291.

Troupp, H. (1965) Arteriovenous malformations of the brain. Prognosis without operation. *Acta Neurologica Scandinavica*, **41**, 39.

Uttley, D. & Richardson, A. E. (1974) E-aminocaproic and subarachnoid haemorrhage.*Lancet*, ii, 1080.

Wegmann, H. D. (1970) Dass shicksal operierter patienten met arterial venosen aneurysma des gehirns. *Scheizer Archiv für Neurologie, Neurochirurgie und Psychiatrie*, **106**, 53.

Weir, B., Erasmo, R., Miller, J., MacIntyre, J., Secord, D. & Mielke, B. (1970) Vasospasm in response to repeated subarachnoid hemorrhages in the monkey. *Journal of Neurosurgery*, **33**, 395.

Wilkins, R. H. & Levitt, P. (1970) Intracranial arterial spasm in the dog. A chronic experimental model. *Journal of Neurosurgery*, **33**, 260.

Wilkins, R. H., Silver, D. & Odom, G. L. (1966) The role of circulating substances in intracranial arterial spasm. 1: Serotonin and histamine. *Neurology* (Minneap.), **16**, 482.

Wilkins, R. H., Wilkins, G. K., Gunnells, J. C. & Odom, G. L. (1967) Experimental studies of intracranial arterial spasm using aortic strip assays. *Journal of Neurosurgery*, **27**, 490.

Yamamoto, Y. L., Feindel, W., Wolfe, L. S., Katoh, H. & Hodge, C. P. (1972) Experimental vasoconstriction of cerebral arteries by prostaglandins. *Journal of Neurosurgery*, **37**, 385.

Yasargil, M. G. & Carter, L. P. (1974) Saccular aneurysms of the distal anterior cerebral artery. *Journal of Neurosurgery*, **40**, 218.

Yasargil, M. G., Yonekawa, Y., Zumstein, B. & Stahl, H.-J. (1973) Hydrocephalus following spontaneous subarachnoid hemorrhage. Clinical features and treatment. *Journal of Neurosurgery*, **39**, 474.

13. Stroke Rehabilitation

R. Langton Hewer

A stroke is a catastrophic event both for the patient and his relatives. A previously normal, intelligent person may be suddenly rendered aphasic, paralysed, and incontinent. The shock is total. All too often nothing can be done, medically or surgically, to improve the situation in the acute phase. The quality of the remainder of the patient's life will thereafter largely depend upon the degree of functional recovery which occurs. It is the aim of rehabilitation to help the patient make the best of his residual capabilities.

The incidence of stroke is approximately 2 per 1000 in the general population, and it is probable that approximately one-third will be left with some degree of neurological disability—usually a hemiparesis or a hemiplegia. Some of these patients will be left with severe handicap, and Harris (1971) found that stroke is the commonest cause of severe handicap in the community. She estimated that there are 130 000 impaired stroke survivors living in private households in Great Britain. It needs to be remembered, however, that stroke is only one cause of neurological disability. Others include head injury, multiple sclerosis, spinal injury, muscular dystrophy, spina bifida, cerebral palsy, and various 'system degenerations' such as Parkinsonism, motor neurone disease, and Friedreich's Ataxia. Important non-neurological causes of physical disability include rheumatoid arthritis, other diseases of the osteoarticular system, and emphysema. At least 56 per cent of patients aged between 15 and 59 who are receiving long-term care in hospital for chronic disabilities, other than those due to long term mental illness or subnormality, are disabled as a result of neurological disease (Circular London, Ministry of Health, 1968).

The term rehabilitation implies the restoration of patients to their fullest physical, mental, and social capability (Mair, 1972) and embraces the many physical, social, and organisational aspects of the after-care for patients who require more than acute short-term definitive care. The problem has been the subject of two recent reports (Department of Health and Social Security Welsh Office, 1972; Scottish Home and Health Department, 1972) and it is perhaps sad that there were no neurologists on either of the relevant subcommittees. Nichols (1974) has briefly reviewed the practice of rehabilitation and includes the following principles:

A clear definition of the clinical problem and likely outcome must be made and discussed with all concerned as early as possible (the patient included).

A realistic programme for hospital admission and returning home and to work should be agreed as soon as possible.

Appropriate industrial or domestic resettlement must be phased in with the continuing physical treatment as soon as possible.

There must be no gaps in treatment—even for a few days.

Skilled assessment of the environmental needs, the aids and appliances, and the social support needed for people with long-term disabilities.

It is obvious that if such a programme is to be implemented there must be close cooperation between a large number of people from various disciplines—including doctors, social workers, and physical therapists. They must work together assessing, planning, and implementing a management programme. The importance of stroke rehabilitation has been highlighted by the recent Report of the Geriatrics Committee of the Royal College of Physicians, London (1974).

A number of workers in the United Kingdom have reported on supervised programmes of rehabilitation for stroke patients (Adams, 1974; Isaacs and Marks, 1973; Millard, 1973, Somerville *et al.*, 1974; and Wilkinson, 1973). The reports originate either in departments of geriatrics or in special rehabilitation units. There are no reports of the results of stroke rehabilitation in district general hospitals.

Stroke is commonly thought of as being a hospital based problem. In the acute phase this may be so (although our own unpublished study in Bristol indicates that only 40 per cent of stroke patients are admitted to hospital). In the later recovery phase, however, the value of long-term hospitalisation is open to much doubt. Weddell (1973) summarises the problem neatly—'The rehabilitation of people after a stroke must be considered first as a problem involving people, and people at home, rather than in hospital. Rehabilitation to achieve the fullest possible life at home must always be the target. Whether hospital services have a significant part to play needs to be questioned. It may be that the most effective measures are those that increase people's capabilities in their own homes, for example the installation of aids and adaptations as soon as possible after the stroke, together with much improved coordination between medical services and the local authorities and voluntary agencies'.

A number of different techniques of physical treatment and of speech therapy have been proposed. So far there have been few attempts at validation. One of the principal problems is the normal process of restoration. Whilst obviously highly desirable, natural recovery makes it difficult 'to prove' that one method of therapy is better than another—or indeed even better than none at all. Present work in this and related fields is being concentrated on trying to predict outcome at an early stage, thus forming the basis for the proper evaluation of therapeutic techniques.

There are many problems in stroke rehabilitation. This chapter seeks to outline the size and scope of the problem and to discuss the assessment and management of the patient.

DEFINITION AND QUANTIFICATION IN STROKE REHABILITATION

One of the main difficulties in evaluating rehabilitation methods used in stroke rehabilita-

tion, is the lack of agreed criteria of assessment. If comparisons are to be made between treatment in hospital and at home, between one unit and another, or between the effects of different treatment regimes, it is necessary to know whether the patients were comparable and whether the criteria were the same. At present, there is no general agreement even about the definition of stroke, there is no standard method of reporting the nature, severity, cause, or duration of neurological deficit. Furthermore, there are no agreed methods for evaluating outcome, other than death or survival.

For rehabilitation purposes the definition of stroke may be accepted as 'an acute disturbance of cerebral function of presumed vascular origin, with disability lasting for more than 24 hours' (Report of the Geriatrics Committee, 1974).

No two stroke patients are precisely the same, and an infinite number of different types of stroke can occur. Most, however, have a hemiplegia. The Geriatrics Committee considered that in describing the deficit note should be taken of:

1. The side of the stroke.
2. Whether the neurological deficit resulted in motor loss only (or predominantly) or whether this was accompanied by major perceptual, cognitive, or language deficit.
3. Whether the patient was in good, or fairly good health apart from the stroke or whether he suffered from one or more complicating conditions known to affect prognosis adversely, for example, previous stroke, heart disease, or hypertension.

Isaacs and Marks (1973) suggested a simple classification using the first two items mentioned above. This classification was:

1. Right hemiplegia with communication disorder.
2. Right hemiplegia, no communication disorder.
3. Left hemiplegia, perceptual loss.
4. Left hemiplegia, no perceptual loss.

They divided the cases into two main groups— complex and simple. The complex cases had a major communication or perceptual disturbance, simple cases had not.

Various attempts have been made to quantify

the various perceptual and intellectual abnormalities in elderly patients (Adams, 1974; Denham and Jeffreys, 1972; Hodkinson, 1972, Isaacs and Marks, 1973; and Wilson and Brass, 1973). The functional results can be described in various ways. The most usual appears to be that of Rankin (1957). His scaling system is used by Marquardsen (1969):

Grade I	No significant disability. Able to carry out all usual activities.
Grade II	Slight disability. Unable to carry out some previous activities, but able to look after own affairs without assistance.
Grade III	Moderate disability. Able to walk without assistance but requiring some help with dressing.
Grade IV	Moderately severe disability. Incapable of walking alone and unable to attend to own bodily needs without assistance.
Grade V	Severe disability. Bed-fast or chair-fast. Usually incontinent, requiring constant nursing care and attention.

Adams (1974) uses a slightly different system:

Recovered Grade I	Fully independent. Intellect clear. Some use of hand. Confident gait.
Grade II	Handicapped. Mental clouding. Arm disabled. Walks unaided.
Long Stay	Confined to chair or bed. May be confused. May be incontinent.

The above mentioned systems may be made compatible (Report of the Geriatrics Committee, 1974): Adams's grades I and II would include all patients in Rankin's grades I, II, and III. The long stay patients of Adams were made equivalent to Rankin's categories IV and V. No system is perfect and a balance has to be struck in dealing with a problem which is superficially simple, but in actuality complex.

Degrees of independence can also be described in terms of ADL (activities of daily living). Katz *et al.* (1973) reported on an index of ADL which was developed to study the results of treatment and prognosis in the elderly and chronically sick. Grades of the index summarise performance in bathing, dressing, going to the toilet, transferring, continence, and feeding. There are thus six grades (A–F), A being independent in the six activities listed above and F being dependent in all six functions. This scale has been extensively used by many workers to measure the abilities of patients disabled by a variety of causes.

Another much used functional evaluation system was described by Mahoney and Barthel (1965) and is known as the Barthel Index. This has a ten point scale which includes feeding, transferring, personal toilet, getting on and off the toilet, bathing oneself, walking on a level surface, ascending and descending stairs, dressing, controlling bowels, and controlling bladder. Scheening and Iversen (1968) gave details of the Kenny self-care evaluation. This is a numerical rating system utilising a five point scale of the patient's abilities in six categories of self-care activities. Included in the six categories are 17 specific activities—thus 'locomotion' includes three subgroups, walking, stairs, and wheelchairs. This is a particularly detailed system and has been used for the construction of 'learning curves' for several groups of patients, including hemiplegics (Scheening and Iversen, 1968).

In summary, there are three main ADL scales in current use, reflecting in part the disagreement that exists over the number of activities that should be covered by these scales. This matter is fully discussed by Diller (1970).

MEDICAL ASSESSMENT

Whereas most stroke survivors have a hemiplegia this is not necessarily the most important result of a stroke. Adams and Hurwitz (1963) have reviewed a group of 45 bed-fast, hemiplegic patients in order to determine why they were unable to recover the ability to walk and look after themselves. Physical disabilities, such as dense paralysis complicated by severe sensory loss or limited exercise tolerance, were responsible in only half the patients. The others had cerebral deficits which the authors classified into four groups—impaired learning ability, disturbed awareness of self or space, disordered integrative action, and emotional disorders. Within these groups they identified a number of 'mental barriers to recovery from strokes':

1. Inability to learn (clouded consciousness, aphasia, memory defects, dementia).

2. Disturbed perception and attitude towards illness disordered by separation from reality (for example, neglect or denial of the hemiplegic limbs or disordered spatial orientation).

3. Disordered integrative action (impaired postural function, agnosia, apraxia, perseveration, and synkinesia).

4. Disturbance of emotional behaviour (emotional instability, apathy, loss of confidence, fear, unwillingness to try, catastrophic reactions, depression).

It was pointed out that the patient seldom has the insight to appreciate these barriers. Unless the physician is aware of these problems and plans his examination appropriately and systemically, it is likely that these all important deficits will be overlooked. Adams (1974) gives six general points which should be considered when assessing stroke survivors. What follows is based mainly on his account.

It is first necessary to know something about the patient's personality and morbid state of health. Such information usually needs to be acquired from a relative or friend.

1. EXERCISE TOLERANCE

It is particularly important to know about the presence of associated vascular symptoms such as angina, claudication, and possible postural hypotension, chronic bronchitis, emphysema, and osteoarthritis, which may alter the patient's mobility.

2. MOTIVATION

In assessing motivation it is important to know what the patient was like before the stroke. Information will be required about his interests, his energy and drive, and his psychological stability—particularly his reaction to previous stressfull situations. It is important to recognise that the patient's apparent unwillingness to help himself may in fact be due to associated disorders such as severe depression or defective memory. Such patients may be wrongly blamed for 'not trying'. Adams (1974) stresses the importance of reassurance: the patient should be told that he stands a good chance of eventually becoming independent and that the various humiliating features of the early weeks following the stroke will probably not persist.

3. SENSORY DEFICITS

Gross disturbances of memory, abnormalities of visuo-spatial orientation, and visual agnosia are examples of the type of sensory abnormality which may not be obvious at first glance but which profoundly affects the patient's ability to undertake everyday tasks. All too frequently such deficits go unnoticed, thus making the efforts of the rehabilitation team both illogical and frequently unsuccessful. In general, lesions of the left hemisphere produce verbal disorder, notably dysphasia, whereas lesions of the right hemisphere tend to produce defects of visual perception and spatial integration. Some of the main deficits are outlined in Table 13.1.

The method of assessment proposed by Adams is unconventional in that sensory function is tested before motor function. Adams makes out a good case for grouping together all sensory modalities, vision and hearing being included with disorders of proprioception and spatial integration.

4. MENTAL CAPACITY

Any method of assessment for brain damaged patients must include a test battery which will identify the important deficits mentioned in Table 13.2. The method should be comprehensive. It must also be simple to use, capable of being administered by a wide range of persons (not only psychologists), capable of being performed without complex apparatus, and unlikely to cause stress or embarrassment to the patient. It should also give a quantifiable estim-

Table 13.1   Table of principal 'sensory deficits'

	Deficit	Comment
Vision	Refractive errors	Ask the relatives to get the patient's glasses.
	Hemianopia	The patient may totally ignore people and objects placed in the blind field. The relatives and staff should stand, in the early stages at least, in the 'seeing field'. Bed lockers and food should be similarly placed. Some patients with a right hemisphere stroke may deny the existence of a left homonymous hemianopia. Such patients, if asked to draw, may leave out the left side of what they are drawing. They may also ignore food placed on the left side of the plate.
	Cortical blindness	This usually results from vascular or anoxic changes occurring bilaterally in the occipital cortex. Such patients are often unaware of blindness and are thought to be simply 'confused'.
	Visual agnosia (mind blindness)	The patient is not blind but is unable to recognise what he sees. He is unable to assess the size, shape, and position of objects, although he may be able to do so if he is able to use a non-visual modality such as taste or smell.
Hearing	Deafness	Removal of wax or the provision of a hearing aid are simple remedies which should not be forgotten. Social isolation and depression are fostered by deafness.
Disorders of body image and spatial orientation	Auditory agnosia Agnosia for the paralysed side	In this condition the patient can hear satisfactorily but cannot interpret what is said. In some patients there is loss of the normal awareness of the integrated representation of body segments. Some such patients may cease to be aware of the paralysed side of the body and may deny the existence of paralysis (anisognosia). Such patients are frequently unable to draw symmetrical objects such as a house, a person, or a clock — usually omitting, or poorly representing, objects on the affected side. A few patients experience complex delusions about the paralysed limbs, sometimes describing them as being longer or shorter than normal, covered with hair, or having a highly abnormal shape. Such delusions are frightening to the patient, who may be unwilling to acknowledge them.
	Impairment of space perception	Disturbances of the perception of the horizontal and vertical have been described in a series of papers, and it is likely that such disturbances are important barriers to recovery (Bruell, Peszczynski, & Volk, 1957) (Birch et al., 1961) (Birch et al., 1960)
Tactile and postural sensation in the limbs		Pin-prick sensation, touch localisation, and the ability to recognise objects placed in the hand are tested in the conventional way. Loss of proprioceptive sensation is usually easily detected by getting the blindfolded patient to put the index finger of the good hand on to that of the paralysed hand, which is held in different positions by the physician. The results of this test need to be interpreted with caution in patients who have disorders of body image.

ate of impairment and must be capable of validation.

It may be argued that it would be impossible to meet all these requirements. Therefore a number of test batteries have been devised in an attempt to meet them all. These include those of Adams (1974), Hodkinson (1972), Isaacs (1971), and Denham and Jeffreys (1972). Some of the tests involve the use of simple toys such as a post box or paper board. All involve a simple scoring system. It will be readily appreciated that any test will depend on a number of different factors. Thus, the ability to read and to paraphrase a sentence depends upon the intactness of vision, the ability to recognise the relevant letters and words, the ability to understand the concepts and subtleties of what is written, and the ability to remember what has been read. Even the simplest test will frequently depend upon several different modalities. The 'ultimate' test has yet to be devised but it is to be hoped that before long some degree of standardisation will become apparent so that the results of therapy in different centres can be compared.

5. MOTOR DEFICIT

Some of the observations required when assessing recovery from motor deficit in hemiplegia are itemised in Table 13.3. The subject is discussed more fully in a later section.

Table 13.2   Mental capacity

	Deficit	Comment
General assessment of appearance and mood	Dysphasia	The patient's ability to understand and to express himself must be tested initially, as much of what follows will depend on this. If dysphasia is present, detailed testing will need to be undertaken at a later stage.
	Perseveration	The patient persists in making the same response to different stimuli — for example, when asked to add two and two he will correctly say four, but if asked to add two and three he will still say four.
	Level of alertness	
	Comprehension and insight	Distractability and inattentiveness make rehabilitation difficult
	Ability to concentrate Reasoning ability	This is easily tested by setting the patient a simple problem or getting him to paraphrase proverbs.
	Arithmetic	Simple addition and subtraction
Speech		Detailed testing will be undertaken at this stage, if relevant.
Memory		Both registration and recall should be tested. Tests include digit retention, forwards and backwards, and the ability to repeat the salient features of a simple story or to remember an address correctly.
Behaviour and mood	Initiative Spontaneity	Does the patient spontaneously attempt to do things himself or does he wait to have everything done for him?
	Sense of humour	
	Continence	
	Emotional state	Depression is common and is a very important cause of lack of progress. Some patients show marked emotional lability.
Performance		The patient's capacity to undertake self-care and other activities would usually be assessed by the nursing staff and others

6. POSTURAL CONTROL

The control of posture is frequently defective following a stroke. The patient may not be able to sit straight and in this event will not be able to stand or to walk. This sort of posture is particularly common during the first days and weeks after onset. Sometimes the patient appears to be quite oblivious of the problem; some probably have disturbances of spatial orientation. When the problem persists it is sometimes due to spasticity of trunk muscles on the affected side.

The deficits which occur after a stroke are frequently complex. It is of great importance that the assessment should be carefully undertaken so that no important deficits are overlooked. Failure to do this will probably result in misdirection of the efforts of the rehabilitation team. A systematic approach to the problem such as that outlined by Adams (1974) is clearly essential.

PRACTICAL MANAGEMENT

The first medical person to be involved when a patient has a stroke is usually the general practitioner. He will have to decide whether or not to admit the patient to hospital. Factors influencing his decision include doubt about the diagnosis, the possibility of providing treatment in the acute phase, and nursing and social factors. Frequently, the patient's immobility is the reason for admission — i.e., the elderly spouse is unable to lift the patient in and out of bed.

If the patient is not admitted to hospital, the

Table 13.3 Motor deficit

Deficit	Comment
Trunk balance	The ability to sit up unsupported on the side of the bed or on a mat must be tested. Later trunk balance can be tested in standing and walking.
Voluntary movement in the limbs	The degree and distribution of returning voluntary movement in the limbs must be recorded. It must be noted whether or not this is occurring independently or, as frequently happens, as a mass movement. The patient's ability to stand and walk should be tested, if there has been sufficient recovery.
Contractures	These are particularly likely to occur at the elbows, hips, and knees. Pain and restriction of movement of the shoulder is particularly common.
Apraxia	Apraxia is the inability to perform a previously established pattern of movement, although muscle strength, sensation, and coordination appear to be normal. Various types of apraxia occur. Praxis may be tested by asking the patient to shut his eyes, wave good-bye, or to brush his hair. Apraxia involving the weak side of the body may be very difficult to detect.

family will require practical help and advice immediately. Advice needs to be given, amongst other things, about:

1. Lifting and transferring. They must be shown how to help the patient to get from one side of the bed to another and from the bed to the chair or commode and vice versa.

2. Management of incontinence.

3. Management of dysphasia. Some assessment of the patient's dysphasic difficulty must made and the relatives shown how to communicate with the patient.

It may be necessary to get the local authority to supply a commode and other relevant aids. If physiotherapy treatment is to be given the patient will usually have to attend hospital on a daily basis, but this may involve long ambulance journeys which are frequently poorly tolerated by the patient. It must be conceded that in practice it is currently difficult to achieve efficient

management of the severely disabled stroke patient in a *purely* home environment. In most areas of the United Kingdom domiciliary care is still at a very early stage of development.

If the patient is admitted to hospital even for a short while, it should be possible to plan the rehabilitation programme. This programme involves a number of distinct but interrelated stages. These are assessment, definition of objectives, planning and implementation of a treatment programme, and long-term follow up. When carrying out this programme it is important that the various members of the team should work closely together.

Assessment. Assessment involves finding out as much about the patient as possible, so that realistic objectives can be defined. This includes information about his previous employment, his interests, his personality, how he has reacted to previous stress, and about his family. Because recovery is often a lengthy process it may be necessary to carry out several assessments over a period of months.

Objectives. The first objective is usually independence—the ability to wash, dress, feed, and manage his own toilet together with some degree of independent mobility. Sometimes the objectives are less ambitious. They may be limited to being able to feed, transfer from bed to a chair, and regain some degree of continence. Other patients who may be more ambitious may eventually return to work. Objectives need to be reviewed from time to time as recovery occurs.

Planning and implementation of treatment programme. All too often the stroke patient is given only a few minutes of physiotherapy, occupational therapy, and speech therapy per day, usually at irregular intervals. He spends much of his time in the ward or at home doing nothing. Such a haphazard approach is demoralizing for all concerned. A planned and integrated management programme needs to be worked out for each patient. The patient should be consulted and told what is planned for him. He should be given a weekly written timetable, so that he and his family know what to expect.

The various members of the rehabilitation team need to work closely together and ideally there should be shared responsibilities between the hospital and the community. It is particularly important to involve the community services at an early stage, so that the transfer of the patient from hospital to home is smooth. Home adaptations must be organised and 'aids' ordered at an early stage.

Long-term follow-up. Recovery from brain damage is frequently slow and may continue for many months or even years; rehabilitation does not always stop three to four months after the stroke. Some form of intermittent treatment may need to be continued for a while. For those patients who are left with a substantial disability it may be necessary to provide some type of long-term support, for instance, at a Day Centre.

At each stage it is important constantly to bear in mind the objectives of rehabilitation. There is, for example, no point in continuing to give physiotherapy or speech therapy to a patient who has long since ceased to benefit.

Composition of the rehabilitation team

A large number of people are involved in attempting to get the stroke patient to make the best of his residual capabilities. The patient's own family, notably the husband or wife and the children, are amongst the most important. They are easily forgotten in spite of the fact that it is they who will probably eventually have to shoulder a large part of the burden. Similarly, the family doctor is in a unique position because of his knowledge of the patient and his background.

Members of the rehabilitation team will each have their own defined areas of responsibility, but inevitably there will be a considerable amount of overlap. Thus, the nursing staff, the physiotherapist, and the occupational therapist will all be involved in helping the patient to stand and walk. The hospital rehabilitation team will usually include:

1. The *consultant* and his junior supporting staff. They will be responsible for making a medical assessment and for coordination of the activities of the team.

2. *Nursing staff* (see below).

3. *Social worker*. The social worker's main functions include home assessment, coordination of the various 'helping agencies' in the community (both statutory and voluntary), and follow-up visits, as necessary. The social worker is well placed to assess the various stresses and problems faced by the patient and his family. In addition he or she will need to be aware of legislation relevant to the care of the handicapped.

4. *Physiotherapist*. The physiotherapist will be responsible for helping the patient to regain control over the paralysed limbs and to achieve some degree of independent mobility. The question of which techniques of physical therapy should be used are discussed in the next section. It is essential that the various members of the team should use the same methods of treatment. Different, and possibly contradictory, treatment methods will only confuse.

5. *Occupational therapist* (see below).

6. *Speech therapist* (see below).

7. *Neuropsychologist*. Unfortunately, there are very few neuropsychologists. There is little doubt that such a person is a very valuable member of the team, both in identifying cognitive and other disorders and also in developing treatment methods for those conditions which are not always obvious but very important. In practice, the doctor, with the help of other members of the team, will usually undertake the psychological assessments.

8. *Psychiatrist*. Depression is a particularly important complication of stroke. The psychiatrist may be able to give valuable advice on the management of this and other psychiatric complications.

9. *Employment officer*. The employment officer must be involved at an early stage, particularly if the patient was employed immediately before the stroke. The patient's job may need to be safeguarded and the employer must be kept informed.

10. *Orthotist*. The provision of orthotic devices, e.g. foot drop support, is a specialised task, and the orthotist, if one is available, should be consulted.

11. *Orthopaedic surgeon*. The place of surgery in the management of hemiplegic patients is briefly discussed below. Surgery may be indicated for the correction of contractures and the alleviation of spasticity.

Nursing

The patient in hospital, and his family, are more likely to confide in the nurse than anyone else; certainly, they see a great deal of her. The nurse will be partly responsible for helping the patient to regain independence and for teaching him, for instance, to feed and wash. Similarly, the district nurse will be closely involved with the patient's home management. Some general points relevant to the nursing of stroke patients may be mentioned.

1. *Correct positioning in bed*

The patient should not remain in bed during the day without a very good reason. It is usually possible to get the patient sitting up within a few days of the acute event.

The bed itself should be neither too high nor too low; ideally it should be of variable height. The height of the bed is particularly important when the patient is being nursed at home—a bed that is at the wrong height may make it impossible for the patient to be got in and out of bed (see Fig. 13.1). The mattress should be firm and should not sag in the middle. There should be a backrest.

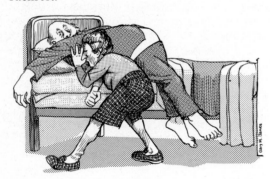

Fig. 13.1

The patient should be nursed in such a way as to minimise the likelihood of deformities. Failure to do so may result in deformities of the type shown in Figure 13.2. In particular, the arms should be maintained on a pillow in a partially abducted position, with the elbow slightly flexed. The leg should be kept in an extended position with a cradle over the foot, to eliminate

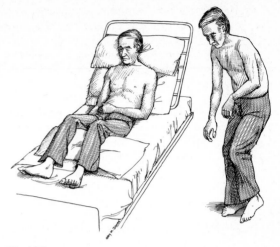

Fig. 13.2

pressure by the bedclothes (Fig. 13.3A and 13.3B).

If a hemianopia is present relatives should be instructed to sit on the normal side. Similarly, bed lockers and food should be placed within the 'seeing' field.

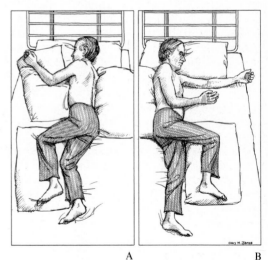

A   B

Fig. 13.3

2. *Correct positioning in chair*

The height of the chair and the depth of the seat should be correct. Many chairs are much too low and involve the dangers of flexion contractures of hips and knees. The back of the chair should have a variable rake so that the patient can, if necessary, fall asleep without being awakened by his head falling forwards or sideways due to lack of support. The arm should be supported on a pillow or specially designed armrest, with the shoulder partially abducted and the elbow partially flexed (Fig. 13.4).

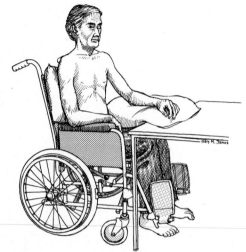

Fig. 13.4

3. Lifting and transferring

The nursing staff and physiotherapist must adopt a standardised approach to lifting and transferring (see Figs. 13.5 and 13.6).

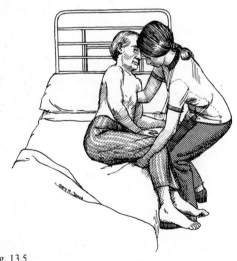

Fig. 13.5

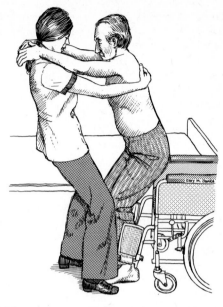

Fig. 13.6

4. Feeding

Initially, the patient will need to use his *good* arm for feeding. The nursing staff must be particularly alerted if there is a hemianopia and if there is anisognosia. Such patients may ignore food placed on the affected side.

5. Sphincters

Bladder training is a vital nursing function. Walking is very difficult when there is a catheter, or Paul's tube and the urinary bag, *in situ*. Training is likely to involve regular attempts at micturition—hourly in some cases. Bowel training is not usually a major problem. Faecal incontinence may be due to a faecal impaction.

6. Avoidance of pressure sores

Pressure sores delay rehabilitation and can usually be avoided. Frequent turning of the patient by day and night is essential. Sores are particularly liable to occur on the heels and over the malleoli as well as in the lumbo-sacral area and over the greater trochanters. Heel sores may be prevented by using a specially shaped calf pad and by enclosing the heel in tube gauze.

7. Dressing

Pyjamas or a nightdress are probably the least suitable clothing for patients undergoing active rehabilitation. Frequently the donning of ordinary day clothes affects a remarkable psychological change in previously depressed patients. For a man trousers and shirt are usually satisfactory. Alternatively, a track suit could be worn—this fosters the idea that something active is expected. Proper lace-up shoes should be provided when the patient first starts to walk. Bedroom slippers are quite unsuitable.

Occupational therapy

The occupational therapist must cooperate closely with the physiotherapist, nursing staff, and speech therapist. Much of her work will be undertaken in the patient's home. Her duties will include:

1. *ADL activities.* The occupational therapist will need to be particularly familiar with the ADL scale mentioned previously. Regular monitoring of the patient's progress is probably best done by the use of such scales. She will also be concerned with the re-training of various practical activities such as feeding and dressing.

2. *Assessment in the patient's home.* The occupational therapist will need to look at such practical points as the presence or absence of a hand rail on the stairs, the height of the cooker, whether the doors are wide enough to take a wheelchair, and whether there are steps in the house which make mobility difficult. Having made her assessment, she would need to liase with the local authority in arranging to get the necessary alterations undertaken as quickly as possible, so that the patient's discharge from hospital is not delayed.

3. *Aids and appliances.* Examples of practical aids which may help the disabled stroke patient include 'Velcro' instead of buttons, elastic shoe laces instead of the conventional type which need to be tied, one handed potato peelers, and non-slip mats to be used under plates. The occupational therapist must be in a position to select such aids and to teach the patient and his relatives in their use. It should, however, be noted that many patients dislike 'gadgets' feeling that they emphasise the fact of disability. The number of aids should be kept to a minimum.

4. Providing the patient with something *inter-esting* to do. Inevitably, the range of activities available to the severely disabled patient is limited. It requires considerable imagination to find things that he can do and enjoy. It is all too easy to sit the patient down in front of the television screen. An activity enjoyed by many disabled people is gardening.

5. *Hand exercises.* The occupational therapist is usually responsible for teaching hand exercises to hemiplegic patients. Regretfully, however, many patients never reach the stage of being able to use the affected hand usefully. This is an obvious area for future research.

TREATMENT OF HEMIPLEGIA BY PHYSICAL METHODS

Despite the evident importance of physical therapy in the management of hemiplegia, there is considerable disagreement about which methods are best. A number of techniques are advocated (See Bobath, 1970; Knott, 1967; Rood, 1969; Brunnstrom, 1970). To date, however, little attempt has been made at validation. Amongst the factors which have influenced the development of techniques of physical therapy are the following:

The importance of sensory input to movement.

The presence of abnormal patterns of movement.

Spasticity.

The phenomena of inhibition and facilitation of movement.

SENSORY INPUT AND MOVEMENT

Mott and Sherrington (1895) studied a series of monkeys with complete sensory denervation of a limb produced by section of the posterior nerve roots. The limb was rendered useless. This devastating effect, however, only occurred when denervation was complete—if one root was spared the motor deficit was much less. Twitchell (1951) repeated and extended these experiments and noted, in particular, the loss of the ability to use the hand when denervation was complete. However, when one sensory root supplying a portion of the hand was spared, the animal was able to use the limb in a nearly normal manner, for walking, climbing, feeding, and grooming.

Twitchell emphasised the importance of both exteroceptive and proprioceptive impulses in motor function.

Brodal (1973), in describing his own stroke, noted the value of passive movement in training. Initially, he was unable to make a voluntary movement at a joint. However, when the movement had been made passively several times by the therapist, he was able to perform the movement, albeit with minimal force.

Practically all physiotherapists use passive movement and emphasise its importance. The fact remains that for at least 23 hours out of 24 the totally paralysed hemiplegic limb is lying perfectly still. It is possible that recovery might be hastened if passive movement, providing some degree of sensory feed-back, could be given for several hours daily.

THE PRESENCE OF ABNORMAL PATTERNS OF MOVEMENT: THE EXISTENCE OF 'LIMB SYNERGIES'

The flaccidity that follows the stroke is, within a matter of weeks, usually replaced by spasticity. During this phase the hemiplegic 'synergies' make their appearance. These synergies are stereotyped movements consisting either of a gross flexion movement or a gross extensor movement. The muscles activated in each synergy cannot, in the early stages, be recruited for different movement patterns. There is a 'loss of selective movement patterns' (Bobath, 1970). The sequence of recovery in the hemiplegic limb was described in Twitchell's classic paper (1951), which has greatly influenced the development of various physiotherapy techniques.

It has been argued (Bobath, 1970) that pathological reflex responses of the type mentioned above should not be employed in training for fear that they will prevent the return of normal movement. According to this view, the patient should not be allowed to use the basic limb synergies of flexion and extension, but rather attempts should be made, from the beginning, to develop normal motor responses. Any movement, according to this view, in the direction of the abnormal response should be prevented, and the patient's limbs, at rest, should be placed in a 'reflex-inhibiting posture'—usually the opposite position of the dominant synergy.

Brunnstrom (1970) after a review of the evidence comes to the opposite conclusion and considers that the patient should be encouraged to gain control of basic limb synergies. She considers that once the syngeries can be performed it should be possible to train the patient to modify the pattern of movement. She notes that the synergies appear to constitute a necessary intermediate stage of further recovery and cites the work of Twitchell (1951) in support of the view that the gross movement synergies of flexion and extension always precede the restoration of advanced motor function following hemiplegia in man. Brunnstrom makes use of 'associated reactions' in training. Thus, for example, a strong voluntary effort involving the normal arm may produce an involuntary movement on the paralysed side. Unfortunately, the studies of Twitchell have never been repeated and extended; it is clear that much basic work needs to be done in order to establish the stages through which the weak limbs pass during recovery.

SPASTICITY

Spasticity, when severe, can obscure residual movement; all major physiotherapy techniques involve some method of trying to reduce spasticity. Bobath (1970) considers that the physiotherapist should not allow an active movement until she has made sure that it will not be resisted by spastic muscle groups. She describes various manoeuvres for inhibiting spasticity.

INHIBITION AND FACILITATION OF MOVEMENT

Voluntary movement can be inhibited by many factors, some of them 'psychological'. For example, a long and tedious ambulance journey, or contact with a bad-tempered member of staff, may make the patient tense, unable to relax, and thus not able to benefit from treatment.

It is known that certain stimuli can be used to produce excitation and inhibition of different muscle groups. Thus, for example, Hagbarth (1960) studied the effects, electro-myographically, of the stimulation of the skin of the lower limb in terms of excitation and inhibition of flexor and extensor motoneurones. Skin stimulation in certain specific areas causes excitation of extensor motoneurones and inhibition of flexor motoneurones. Skin stimulation may be used therapeutically, for instance, by brushing the skin of the relevant segment (Rood, 1969).

Another example of facilitation is given by Twitchell (1951). He showed that the relaxation phase of a finger jerk could be much prolonged by the willed effort of the patient, despite the absence of voluntary movement. In some patients the attempt to pull against the fingers of the examiner whilst intermittent finger jerks were being delivered produced flexion of the wrist, elbow, and shoulder. These and other responses he called proprioceptive facilitation. A series of clinical therapeutic techniques involving PNF (proprioceptive neuromuscular facilitation) have been described (Knott 1967).

Thus there are several approaches to the treatment of spastic hemiplegia. These are summarised by Manning (1974). The patient can be trained to use the unaffected side for all tasks previously undertaken by both together—the affected side being neglected and the leg being used purely as a prop. Alternatively, an attempt can be made to retrain the affected side—as much as the patterns of spasticity will allow.

The Bobath techniques are widely used, partly because they deal specifically and effectively with the problems of spasticity. They aim to suppress abnormal movement patterns produced as a result of spasticity before allowing normal movement to occur. The techniques of PNF are also employed in combination with those of Bobath. The techniques of Brunnstrom, however, are not so much used in the U.K.

EVALUATION OF THERAPEUTIC TECHNIQUES

A number of attempts have been made to ascertain the usefulness, or otherwise, of different methods of physical rehabilitation.

In 1961 Feldman et al. reported on a controlled study of the rehabilitation of an unselected group of 82 stroke patients admitted to Bellvue Hospital with a hemiplegia or hemiparesis. The control group of 40 patients was given functionally orientated medical care including training in sitting, standing, balancing, walking, and self-care activities. The other 42 comprising the rehabilitation group were given a programme which was 'prescribed individually' and was varied according to the patient's needs and progress. Forty-two and a half per cent of the controls and 45 per cent of the rehabilitation group achieved a level of function at which they were able to perform the activities of daily living independently in a satisfactory manner. Fifty-five per cent of the control group were discharged home compared with 66 per cent of the rehabilitation group. The authors conclude that 'the results suggest that the great majority of hemiparetic stroke victims can be rehabilitated adequately on medical and neurological wards, without formal rehabilitation services, if proper attention is given to ambulation and self-care activities'.

Marquardsen (1969) after reviewing the literature and his own large series, concludes that 'it would seem, therefore, that few stroke patients would benefit from long continued and extensive treatment in rehabilitation institutions'.

Stern et al. (1970) reported on the effects of facilitation exercise techniques in stroke rehabilitation. Sixty-two patients with hemiplegia were divided randomly into two groups. The control group received no specialised therapy. The 'exercise group' was given a special exercise programme which included proprioceptive neuromuscular facilitation. The motility index test of knee-flexion and extension strength and the Kenny Rehabilitation Institute Self-Care Evaluation were the measurements used to determine improvements. The authors concluded that no significant difference existed in improvement between the control and the 'exercise group'. The results have been questioned (Inaba et al. 1973) on various grounds including the nature of the evaluation methods used which, with the exception of the assessment of activities of daily living, are poor measures of improvement in patients with hemiplegia.

Peacock et al. (1972) reported on an epidemiological study undertaken in Birmingham, Alabama. Fifty-two patients were included in this study on rehabilitation. They were first assessed by a multidisciplinary team on their personal care and occupational status and potential.

Then they were randomised into a control group of 23, who were given standardised hospital care, and an experimental group of 29, who were given intensive rehabilitation. Reevaluation at the time of maximum improvement showed little or no advantage for the group receiving intensive rehabilitation.

Inaba *et al.* (1973) studied 77 hemiplegic patients. The patients were divided into three treatment groups. Group I patients served as a control group and received functional training only and 'selective stretching'. Group II patients received active exercises in addition to functional training and 'selective stretching'. Group III patients received progressive resistive exercises, as well as functionally orientated training and 'selective training'. The results indicated that a one month programme of progressive resistive exercises and training in ADL is more effective than a programme of ADL alone, or when this is combined with simple active exercises. However, following two months of treatment no difference was evident between the groups in levels of achievement in activities of daily living. The results were claimed to demonstrate that the same level of function can be achieved in half the time providing the most effective treatment procedures are utilised.

The above studies do not give clear answers about the usefulness or otherwise of rehabilitation procedures. Further controlled studies are required, and these must include sensitive and relevant assessment techniques and a clear idea of what procedures are being evaluated. It has not yet been established that any one physical technique is better than another, or indeed that any particular treatment method is better than simple functionally orientated therapy. It is perhaps surprising that there have been no attempts to validate the very widely used Bobath techniques. In assessing the usefulness or otherwise of therapeutic techniques, it must be remembered that rehabilitation inevitably involves a 'package deal'. A large number of different factors are involved—making the control of each one difficult.

For many years there has been interest in the problem of exciting peripheral nerves electrically for the purpose of producing a functional muscle contraction. In particular, several devices have been developed to stimulate the common peroneal nerve by superficial surface stimulation in order to correct the 'foot-drop' occurring in hemiplegic patients. This and other aspects of the problem were reviewed in 1972 (Functional Neuromuscular Stimulation, 1972). The use of proportionally controlled functional electrical stimulation at the hand has been reported (Rebersek & Vodovnik, 1973). Programmed electrical stimulation of areas of the brain in order to produce skilled movements have been investigated in monkeys (Pinneo *et al.*, 1972). The applicability of this technique to man is still uncertain.

The possibility of using bio-feedback techniques in training have been investigated by a number of workers. This subject is reviewed generally by Blanchard, Young, and Jackson (1974) and specifically in relation to disorders of voluntary movement by Brunday *et al.* (1974). Most workers have used EMG signals obtained from limb muscles, which are then appropriately amplified, rectified, integrated, and displaced in a visual or auditory manner.

It is clear that there is potential for the very close collaboration of a number of different people coming from different disciplines. These would include physical therapists and neurologists, in addition to neurophysiologists, neuropsychologists, and engineers.

COMMUNICATION DISORDERS AND APHASIA

Inability to communicate is one of the most serious results of a stroke for many patients and their families. This section briefly discusses the incidence of aphasia, diagnostic tests, and practical management.

Marquardsen observed aphasia or dysphasia in 33 per cent of the three week survivors of an acute stroke. Thygeson *et al.* (1964) found aphasia in 35 per cent of his stroke series and noted that at least 75 per cent of patients with a lesion in the dominant hemisphere had some degree of dysphasia. Ellams (1964) surveyed 748 hemiplegic patients who had survived their acute stroke by at least three months and were aged between 16 and 65 years. Of those with a right hemiplegia 72.6 per cent were found to have some degree of dysphasia or dysarthria. Only 1.2 per cent of patients with a left hemiplegia showed a language deficit.

The above mentioned studies have been undertaken on patients seen either in hospital or in a rehabilitation centre. There are no published studies of the incidence or prevalence of dysphasia in the community. This latter figure would, in any event, need to take account of non-vascular causes — notably head injury. Our own, unpublished, observations indicate that there might be between 40 and 50 new cases of dysphasia due to stroke each year in the notional population of 200000 serviced by one district general hospital.

INCIDENCE AND NATURAL HISTORY

The natural history of aphasia is still the subject of considerable debate. Contributions to the subject include those of Vignolo (1964), Culton (1969), Kevin and Swisher (1972) and Mohr and Sidman (1973). Many attempts have been made to assess the effectiveness of speech therapy, but for a number of reasons, including difficulty with prediction of natural history, the results are still inconclusive. Important papers on this subject include those of Butfield and Zangwill (1946), Vignolo (1964), Leannenberg (1967) and Hagen (1973).

DIAGNOSIS

The subject matter is complex and theories of language function abound. It is therefore hardly surprising that many tests of communication ability have been devised. Furthermore, it must always be remembered that when an aphasia test is administered the errors the patient makes may not necessarily be aphasic errors (Darley, 1970). The nature of the errors, the existence of non-language dysfunctions, and the affective behaviour of the patient must all be considered before drawing conclusions about the nature of the patient's communication problem. The ideal test of aphasia would have the following characteristics:

1. Easy to use. A test that cannot easily be learned by therapists engaged in routine clinical practice is unlikely to be of widespread value.

2. Relatively short. Many aphasic patients tire rapidly and testing cannot be undertaken for more than 15 to 20 minutes at a time.

3. Comprehensive. The test must assess all the important speech modalities.

4. Relevance. It should have functional, and thus therapeutic, relevance.

5. Encompass a wide range. The test must be able to be used for patients with very mild defects on the one hand and major ones on the other.

6. Accuracy. It must give consistent results and be capable of validation.

At least eight tests are in use at present. These include those of Schuell (1974) and Porsch (1971). A new British test has recently been described by Whurr (1974).

Space does not permit a detailed analysis of each test. Some are too long and some insufficiently comprehensive; others lack the necessary range to test widely differing abilities. No test is perfect and it is usually necessary to choose the test most suitable for particular situations.

PRACTICAL MANAGEMENT

It has been said that strokes happen to families and not to individuals. The family can indeed be invaluable, if guided correctly, in stimulating the patient to make the most of his residual abilities. The speech therapist, the family, and the whole of the rehabilitation team should collaborate so that the patient is not confused by a number of uncoordinated attempts to help him.

The type of treatment to be given will depend upon the results of the initial assessment. *Treatment and guidance should start without delay.* The material presented by the therapist should be meaningful to the patient in his immediate environment (Ellams, 1974) and will depend upon his previous interests and educational attainments. There is no point in trying to discuss gardening with someone whose sole, lifelong preoccupation has been horse racing. Planning of such individual programmes necessitates the gathering together of a large amount of biographical material on many subjects.

The methods of treatment used are highly individual and there are no standardised procedures (Darley, 1970). Treatment methods are of two kinds. The first may be called the stimulation approach—therapy being based not upon formal re-education but upon goal-directed stimulation derived from the patient's needs, drives, and motivation. The second is programmed instruction. This latter approach views language rehabilitation as an educative process and concentrates upon the basic structural patterns of language. In practice, each therapist develops her own combination of techniques. Table 13.4 gives some general points which may be helpful when dealing with dysphasic patients.

The use of machines in language rehabilitation has been described by a number of authors (Wepman and Moreney, 1973; Gordon, 1969; Hatfield, 1971). Holland (1969) devised programmes of progressive levels of difficulty for use in an auditory teaching machine.

The place of machine-based, or machine-assisted, therapy has yet to be fully explored. It seems, however, that such an approach does offer an opportunity for the structuring of therapy, for increasing the amount of therapy given, and for controlling the degree of personal intervention. In this way it might, hopefully, be possible to undertake a realistic evaluation of the usefulness of different therapeutic techniques.

COMPLICATIONS

Complications are those events which occur at some point after the onset of the stroke. Those that affect rehabilitation can conveniently be divided into those that are primarily cerebral and those that involve the limbs. These subjects have been thoroughly reviewed by Moskowitz (1969). Some of the more important complications are listed below.

DEPRESSION

Depression is very easily overlooked or misdiagnosed as 'poor motivation', particularly in patients with a significant communication disorder. Indeed, it seems likely that most patients with a severe stroke do become depressed at some point. An attempt must be made to understand the patient's problems, which may be highly complex. Problems include worries about finance, employment, the possibility of permanent disablement, and marital relations. One member of the stroke team must be responsible

Table 13.4 Practical advice on helping the aphasic patient to communicate

Never hurry the patient. Remember that he may take much longer than normal to understand what is said, and to formulate his reply.	Find out what interests the patient has and centre discussion around these. The patient will probably perform best when talking about things that are familiar to him.
Any attempt at communication by the patient should be encouraged—if only with a 'thumbs-up' sign.	If the patient uses a one word sentence, e.g. 'toilet', encourage him to expand the sentence by saying 'I want to go to the toilet'.
Do not 'talk over' the patient when he is able to answer questions himself. Avoid 'Does he take sugar in his tea'. Speak *to* the patient. Do not leave him out, for example, he should not be left out on a ward round.	Remember that fatigue and emotional disturbance adversely affect both comprehension and expression. Make sure that the patient is relaxed. He may perform best if there is nobody else in the room.
Any attempt on the part of the patient should be accepted and encouraged. Remember that many patients feel embarrassed, humiliated, and frustrated.	Aphasic patients are highly distractable. Avoid background noise.

Practical advice on helping patients who have a problem with comprehension
Remember that most patients have, at the least, a mild receptive disability.

Never under-estimate the patient's comprehension.

Avoid long, rambling conversations—the patient will not understand.

Speak a little slower than normal. Do *not* shout!

Stand in front of the patient so that he can *see* your facial movements and expression.

for establishing rapport with the patient and must be prepared to spend time helping sort out the patient's problems. Antidepressive drugs may be used in some cases but cannot be regarded as a panacea.

EPILEPSY

The incidence of epilepsy was noted to be 6 per cent in Marquardsen's series (1969) and 7.7 per cent in that of Louis and McDowell (1967). Moskowitz (1969) quotes an incidence of over 15 per cent in a long-term follow-up of older patients.

VENOUS THROMBOSIS IN THE HEMIPLEGIC LEG

Cope, Reyes, and Skversky (1973) undertook a phlebographic study of patients who had survived the acute stroke and found a 33 per cent incidence of acute venous thrombosis in the hemiplegic leg. In about one-third the thrombosis was undiagnosable by clinical examination. The practical importance of this complication has not yet been fully explored.

PAINFUL STIFF SHOULDER

Pain and stiffness in the shoulder of a hemiplegic arm is very common. It is frequently the result of faulty lifting technique and poor positioning of the limb in the early flaccid stage. Any attempt to assist the patient into a sitting or standing position must avoid load-bearing on the affected joint. In addition, the weight of the arm itself tends to distract the shoulder capsule, and for this reason it may be helpful to put the arm into a sling when the patient is walking. Pain and stiffness can sometimes be alleviated by local injections of hydrocortisone. Other causes of a painful shoulder are:
—Fracture of the neck of the humerus.
—Dislocation of the shoulder joint (particularly liable to occur in the flaccid stage).
—Contracture due to the later development of spasticity. In some cases this may necessitate surgical division of the major muscles which cause internal rotation and adduction of the shoulder (Braun et al., 1971).
—Shoulder/hand syndrome. This complication has been also named 'post-hemiplegic reflex sympathetic dystrophy' (Moskowitz, Bishop, and Shibutani 1958). This problem occurs in

about 5 per cent of stroke patients. In severe cases there is de-mineralisation of the head and neck of the humerus. Oral steroids and vigorous passive exercises are usually effective.
—Inflammation in soft tissues around the shoulder joint. Inflammation may occur in a number of different sites including the acromioclavicular and glenohumeral joints, the biceps tendon, and in the subdeltoid bursa (Braun et al., 1971).
—Ectopic calcification in the periarticular structures. This is a rare complication and the diagnosis can only be made by X-ray.

GROSS SPASTICITY

Mild degrees of spasticity are the rule in the latter stages of hemiplegia and there are various physiotherapeutic techniques available for its reduction (Bobath, 1970). Sometimes, however, the spasticity cannot be controlled by simple positioning and relaxing techniques and other measures may need to be adopted. These include:
—Cooling. A temporary reduction in the severity of spasticity can often be achieved by applying ice-bags or by immersing the spastic limb in cold water (Hedenberg, 1970; Lee and Warren, 1974).
—Drugs. A large number of drugs have been used to reduce spasticity. The use of diazepam was evaluated in various neurological conditions by Nathan (1970). The practical experience of most workers is that drugs are of very limited value in the management of spasticity occurring in the hemiplegic patient.
—Intraneural, intramuscular, and intrathecal phenol injections. A temporary reduction in spasticity lasting for about six months can sometimes be achieved by selective injections of phenol into the nerve sheaths of peripheral nerves (Braun et al., 1973). Phenol injections can be a valuable supplementary form of treatment when combined with tendon transplant or vigorous physical therapy. Similar results have been reported with intramuscular motor point injections (Halpern and Meelhuysen, 1966; Awad, 1972). When spasticity in the leg is very severe, rendering nursing impossible, it may occasionally be necessary to resort to intrathecal phenol

injections (Roper, 1975). Such procedures are usually reserved for incontinent patients.

— Destructive surgery. Occasionally spasticity can only be overcome by destructive surgery involving division of muscles, tendons, or nerves. For example, where there is severe finger flexion there can be odoriferous maceration in the palm of the hand. Division of the flexor tendons at the wrist will relieve this (Roper, 1975).

CONTRACTURES AND DEFORMITIES

Contractures are liable to follow prolonged unrelieved severe spasticity — the result of irreversible changes in the soft tissues around the joints. Contractures may occur at all the main limb joints. Sometimes there is a combination of spasticity and contracture. Two examples may be given:

1. Equinovarus deformity. In moderate cases this can be controlled with a short leg brace which must not incorporate a spring as this will accentuate the stretch reflex. In other cases the deformity can be corrected by elongation of the Achilles tendon and transfer of half of the tibialis anterior to the outer border of the foot (Roper, 1975).

2. Pronation-flexion deformity of the forearm and hand. This can sometimes be partially corrected, in carefully selected cases, by surgical release of the flexor origins of the relevant muscles (Braun, Mooney, and Nickel 1970).

The potential for surgery of hemiplegic deformities has been pioneered at Rancho Los Amigos Hospital, Downey, California (Nickel, 1969; Roper, 1975).

Splinting and calipers

Light-weight splints are sometimes used in order to maintain the flaccid paralysed limb in a satisfactory position. Splints alone are useless when there is marked spasticity. One of the most used devices is a below-knee brace, sometimes combined with a T strap. The usefulness of this brace is debated, and many physiotherapists claim that there is rarely a need for any type of foot drop support. The author's experience however is that a brace can sometimes be very useful, particularly in the early stages before marked spasticity has developed.

FRACTURE OF LONG BONES

Fractures of the neck of the femur are particularly likely to occur in patients with an equinovarus deformity of the ankle because of the obvious tendency for the foot to catch on the ground (Treanor, 1969).

PERIPHERAL NERVE PALSIES

A variety of root and nerve compression lesions can occur, particularly if the paralysed limbs are allowed to rest in an incorrect position (Moskowitz, 1969). Nerve palsies readily go undiagnosed when they occur in an already partially paralysed limb. Lesions of the C_{5-6} root, the long thoracic nerve, and the radial nerve all occur if the unsupported arm is allowed to hang out of bed. In the case of the radial nerve the back of the upper arm may rest against the hard edge of the bed. Ulnar nerve lesions can occur if the inner side of the elbow is allowed to rest on the unpadded rail of a wheelchair. Common peroneal and sciatic nerve lesions can both occur with faulty positioning.

The future

It is clear that much requires to be done in the field of stroke rehabilitation. The problems range from the organisation of care services, including a definition of the inter-related roles of the hospital and of the community, to the physiology of motor control. Here, indeed, is a field in which useful collaboration between people with widely differing skills should be possible.

Rehabilitation of the neurologically disabled is one of the most exciting fields in neurobiology today. It is at once worthwhile and offers the opportunity for helping some of those who need help most.

LONG-TERM MEDICAL TREATMENT

R. W. Ross Russell

Anticoagulant treatment

While there is general agreement that anticoagulant drugs have a part to play in the treatment of transient ischaemic attacks, there is still no consensus of opinion on their role in patients with established stroke. It became apparent soon after the introduction of anticoagulants, firstly, that they did not offer a complete protection against recurrence of stroke and, secondly, that they carried a serious risk of haemorrhage. The balance for and against their use could be assessed only by a controlled clinical trial. The variable natural history of stroke, the difficulty of making an accurate diagnosis, and the vagaries of anticoagulant control made this a formidable undertaking.

A number of trials have been conducted and it is possible to find fault with most of them. The large multi-centre projects have contributed impressive numbers of patients but at the expense of variation in selection, treatment of patients, accuracy of prothrombin control, and completeness of follow-up. In most trials except that of Hill, Marshall, and Shaw (1962) treatment has begun at a variable interval after the stroke. In many trials the treated and control groups are not comparable with respect to important variables such as blood pressure, cardiac status, associated disease, and severity of stroke.

The criteria of assessment in all trials have been death, recurrent stroke, and haemorrhagic complications. Unless the patient is under constant surveillance and unless an autopsy is permitted in cases of death it may be impossible to decide whether a recurrent or fatal stroke is occlusive or haemorrhagic, and whether an episode of sudden death is due to cardiac or cerebral causes.

It is thus not surprising that most of the larger trials have given results which are inconclusive (Baker *et al.*, 1962; Hill *et al.*, 1962). In these two trials the recurrence rate of infarction, approximately 30 to 40 per cent in two years, was actually higher in the treated group, and severe haemorrhagic complications varied from 4 to 11 per cent.

Millikan (1971) has recently summarised the findings of these studies (Table 13.5) concluding that anticoagulants cannot be recommended for the overall category of occlusive stroke. He stresses the risk of haemorrhage especially in hypertensive patients, stating that in this category anticoagulants are contraindicated.

Against these negative conclusions must be considered the beneficial effects obtained in a stresses the frequency of haemorrhage especially in hypertensive patients, stating that in this category of patients anticoagulants are contraindicated.

Against these negative conclusions must be considered the beneficial effect obtained in a few centres. These have usually included smaller numbers of patients, but selection and conditions of patient care and control have been more standard and in general the laboratory supervision superior. In the careful study of Enger and Boysen (1965) 100 institutionalised patients randomly allocated to treatment and placebo were treated for two years and followed for a further six months. Recurrent events were 11 in placebo as against five in the treatment group; one death occurred in the treatment group as against three in the placebo. The authors suggested a moderate protective effect on recurrence rate, but there was an unavoidable risk of haemorrhage. A similar protective effect on recurrent stroke was shown by McDowell and McDevitt (1965) and by Howell, Tatlow, and Feldman (1964) during the period when their patients were receiving anticoagulants. However, after stopping treatment many patients developed a stroke and there was no difference in the numbers alive after six years.

From this large amount of work it is possible to draw some tentative conclusions (Groch, 1961) Long-term anticoagulants seem to have only a marginal beneficial effect on secondary prevention of stroke and are suitable only for a proportion of patients. Patients with hypertension or mental impairment and those who cannot be given regular and expert haematological supervision should be excluded. The prothrombin time should not be excessively prolonged. The maximum benefit is obtained in the early stages after stroke, and treatment should probably not be continued longer than two years. Finally there is little benefit in treating patients with a very severe permanent disability who have little prospect of an independent existence.

The value of anticoagulants in the primary prevention of venous thrombo-embolism has

Table 13.5 Results of controlled clinical trials of anticoagulant treatment in patients with completed stroke (*from* Millikan, 1971).

		Number of Patients	Months of follow-up	Cerebral infarct	Died Cerebral infarct	Severe haemorrhage
Baker *et al.* (1962)	Controls	60	16	16 (27%)	5 (8%)	0
	Treated	72	10	30 (42%)	6 (8%)	7 (10%)
Hill *et al.* (1962)	Controls	65	31	19 (29%)	1 (2%)	0
	Treated	66	28	22 (33%)	5 (8%)	7 (11%)
McDowell & McDevitt	Controls	99	33.5	22 (22%)	7 (7%)	2 (2%)
	Treated	92	42.2	1 (1%)	1 (1%)	7 (8%)
Enger & Boyesen (1965)	Controls	49	39.2	8 (16%)	3 (6%)	0
	Treated	51	22.8	4 (8%)	1 (2%)	3 (6%)
Howell *et al.* (1964)	Controls	92	36	28 (3%)		0
	Treated	103	16	7 (7%)		4 (4%)

been established, and if it is decided to use anti-coagulants in an individual patient there is much to be said for starting treatment early, within a few days of the ictus while the patient may be confined to bed or chair and at a time when venous thrombo-embolism is most likely to occur. Caution is often advised over the early use of anticoagulants in case an ischaemic infarct becomes haemorrhagic, but this theoretical danger does not appear to have been confirmed in practice.

Long-term treatment of blood pressure

The relationship between raised blood pressure and stroke has been emphasised in Chapters 1 and 2. The conclusions may be summarised as follows:

1. Pathological examination shows that atheroma is more severe and extensive in patients having raised blood pressure during life and that a specific pathological change (lipohyalinosis) occurs in small intracerebral arteries.

2. Prospective epidemiological studies have established hypertension as the dominant risk factor predisposing to stroke.

3. Approximately half the patients with stroke have elevated blood pressure, and this group has a worse immediate prognosis, a greater number of recurrences, and greater long-term mortality than normotensive patients. These last two features are proven only for males (Marshall and Kaeser, 1961; Acheson and Hutchinson, 1971).

When the association between hypertension and cerebrovascular disease first became clear the question arose whether antihypertensive treatment would prevent the occurrence of stroke in hypertensive patients (primary prevention) or would reduce the incidence of recurrence in patients who had already suffered a stroke (secondary prevention). It was also considered at that time that reduction in blood pressure in a patient with cerebrovascular disease might be positively harmful and might provoke further cerebral thrombosis or ischaemia. While this may occur in a few patients it is usually easily recognised and prevented, and the theoretical dangers of hypotension have not been borne out in practice.

Breckenridge, Dollery, and Parry (1970) who compared two seven-year periods before and after 1960 were able to show an improved five-year survival for severely hypertensive patients treated during the latter period due principally to a reduction in deaths from renal failure and from cerebrovascular accidents. The incidence of myocardial infarction was not reduced.

There are also a number of reports dealing with secondary prevention notably from Carter (1970), who compared the prognosis of treated and untreated hypertensive patients with stroke over a four year period. A total of 99 patients were studied. The mortality rate was 46 per cent in the untreated and 26 per cent in the treated group. Recurrent strokes numbered 21 in the untreated (10 deaths) compared with 10 in the treated group (three deaths).

Beevers *et al.* (1973) also treating hypertensive patients with established cerebrovascular disease showed that the recurrence rate of cerebral episodes was related to the effectiveness of control of blood pressure varying from 5 per cent in two years in those patients who are well controlled to 28 per cent within two years in those with poor control.

An even more striking effect was obtained in the Veterans Administration Cooperative Study Group from the U.S. (1967), which included 143 hypertensive patients with established stroke followed for a mean period of 18 months, and divided into treated and untreated groups. There were 27 further cerebral events and two deaths in the untreated group compared with two events (no deaths) in the treated group.

These results no longer allow any doubt on the overall value of antihypertensive agents in cerebrovascular disease. The probable mode of action is to retard the progress of arterial lipohyalinosis, the lesion which underlies both cerebral haemorrhage and lacunar infarction. The failure of antihypertensive drugs to influence myocardial infarction recurrence rates suggests they have no preventative action on the processes of atheromatous degeneration and thrombosis in larger arteries.

It is, however, still necessary to exercise care in prescribing hypertensive drugs to individual patients, especially those with extracranial arterial occlusion. Although autoregulation is preserved in hypertension the range of effective homeostasis is altered to a higher level with the result that patients are less efficient in tolerating a reduction in blood pressure without a fall in cerebral perfusion. It is advisable to avoid excessive reduction in systemic blood pressure such as may be produced by ganglion blocking agents with a powerful postural effect. Methyldopa or propranolol in association with a thiazide diuretic give adequate control in the great majority of patients.

Cerebral vasodilators

In health the blood supply to cerebral tissues is adjusted to metabolic requirements and it is known that any increase in metabolic activity either local or general will be matched by an increase in blood supply to the relevant region, this being brought about by alteration in the biochemical environment of small blood vessels. Vasodilator therapy is based on the doubtful premise that the regulatory mechanisms are disturbed, that because of vascular disease the brain receives insufficient blood for its metabolic requirements, and that cerebral perfusion and function will both improve if the arteries are dilated.

Dilator therapy is applied in two situations, firstly, in the short term to increase the amount of blood available by collateral channels immediately after a stroke, secondly, as a long-term treatment for chronic occlusive arterial disease.

Short-term vasodilatation has been considered in Chapter 9. Its value is doubtful because of the many variables involved. Regional CBF measurements shortly after an acute stroke may show regions of high as well as low flow and the action of a vasodilator agent in this situation is complex. There may be an increase in flow to the ischaemic region but at other times the flow may be reduced. Whether this is the result of diversion of blood (intracerebral steal) or because of increase in cerebral oedema or venous or CSF pressure produced by the drug is debatable.

In chronic cerebral arteriosclerosis the situation is different; many patients with primary cerebral degeneration such as Huntington's chorea who have a reduction in the weight and volume of brain have a normal total and regional cerebral blood flow in terms of perfusion rate per weight of brain tissue. On the other hand patients with clinical evidence of arteriopathic dementia often show focal or generalised reduction in perfusion rate. This may be due either to a reduced metabolism in surviving areas of brain with a corresponding reduction in requirement for blood or to primary occlusive process in blood vessels limiting the amount of blood available. If the blood vessels are primarily at fault and blood supply can be restored to normal by causing dilatation of diseased vessels or of collaterals then there are theoretical reasons for vasodilator therapy.

The requirements for an ideal vasodilator are:

1. It should increase blood flow to the whole brain including the underperfused regions.

2. Its action on cerebral vascular resistance must not be accompanied by corresponding reduction in blood pressure.

3. It must be easily administered, its action must be sustained and unaccompanied by dangerous side effects.

4. It must be shown to produce clinical benefits in terms of improved performance or prognosis.

There are certainly drugs which increase cerebral blood flow but few are suitable for long-term use. Papaverine has been shown to increase mean hemisphere blood flow and to improve significantly flow to regions of low flow (McHenry, Jaffe, and Kawamura, 1970). However, it requires intravenous injection and its effects are short term. A short-term increase in flow has also been noted after intravenous administration of hexobendine and the carbonic anhydrase inhibitor acetazolamide (McHenry, 1972).

Cyclandelate, the mandelic acid ester of trimethylcyclohexanol, has been the subject of a number of studies. This is given orally in a dose of 1600 mg per day in divided doses and there are no serious side effects. Some workers have shown a slight short-term increase in cerebral perfusion (O'Brien and Veal, 1966). There have also been several clinical trials showing mental and neurological improvement in demented patients thought to be suffering from cerebral arteriosclerosis, but clinical improvement shows a poor correlation with increased blood flow. In a recent randomised cross-over trial in patients with arteriopathic dementia Young, Hall, and Blakemore (1974) showed that some aspects of mental function including memory and ability to converse declined less during treatment with cyclandelate than with placebo. No changes were found in neurological signs.

Hydergine, a combination of the mesylates of dihydroergocornine and dihydroergokryptine, has not been convincingly shown to improve cerebral perfusion (McHenry, 1972), but clinical trials in elderly patients believed to be suffering from cerebrovascular insufficiency have again shown some improvement in terms of mental function. The absence of any definite effect on blood flow suggests that this improvement may be due to a nonspecific alerting or antidepressant action.

REFERENCES

Acheson, J. & Hutchinson, E. C. (1971) The natural history of focal cerebral vascular disease. *Quarterly Journal of Medicine*, **40**, 15.

Adams, G. F. & Hurwitz, L. J. (1963) Mental barriers to recovery from strokes.*Lancet*, ii, 533.

Adams, G. F. (1974) *Cerebrovascular Disability and the Ageing Brain*. Edinburgh and London: Churchill Livingstone.

Awad, E. A. (1972) Intramuscular neurolysis for stroke. *Minnesota Medicine*, **55**, 711.

Baker, R. N., Broward, J. A., Fang, H. C., Fisher, C. M., Groch, S. N., Heyman, A., Karp, H. R., McDevitt, E., Sheinberg, P., Schwartz, D. & Toole, J. F. (1962) Anticoagulant therapy in cerebral infarction: report on a co-operative study. *Neurology*, **12**, 823.

Beevers, D. G., Hamilton, M., Fairman, M. J. & Harpur, J. E. (1973) Antihypertensive treatment and the course of established cerebrovascular disease.*Lancet*, i, 1407.

Benton, A. L. (Ed.) (1970) *Behavioural Change in Cerebrovascular Disease*. New York: Harper & Row.

Birch, H. G., Belmont, I., Reilly, T. & Belmont, L. (1961) Visual verticality in hemiplegia. *Archives of Neurology*, **5**, 444.

Birch, H. G., Proctor, F., Bortner, M. & Lowenthal, M. (1960) Perception in hemiplegia: 1. Judgement of vertical and horizontal by hemiplegic patients. *Archives of Physical Medicine and Rehabilitation*, **41**, 19.

Blanchard, E. B., Young, L. D. & Jackson, M. (1974) Clinical applications of biofeedback training. *Archives of General Psychiatry*, **30**, 573.

Bobath, B. (1970) *Adult Hemiplegia: Evaluation and Treatment*. London: Heinemann.

Braun, R. M., Hoffer, M. M., Mooney, V., McKeever, J. & Roper, B. (1973) Phenol nerve block in the treatment of acquired spastic hemiplegia in the upper limb. *Journal of Bone and Joint Surgery*, **55-A**, 580.

Braun, R. M., West, F., Mooney, V., Nickel, V. L., Roper, B. & Caldwell, C. (1971) Surgical treatment of the painful shoulder contracture in the stroke patient. *Journal of Bone and Joint Surgery*, **53-A**, 1307.

Braun, R. M., Mooney, V. & Nickel, V. L. (1970) Flexor-origin release for pronation-flexion deformity of the forearm and hand in the stroke patient. An evaluation of the early results in 18 patients. *Journal of Bone and Joint Surgery*, **52-A**, 907.

Breckenridge, A., Dollery, C. T. & Parry, E. H. O. (1970) Prognosis of treated hypertension. *Quarterly Journal of Medicine*, **39**, 411.

Brunday, J., Korein, J., Levidow, L., Grynbaum, B. B., Lieberman, A. & Friedmann, L. W. (1974) Sensory feedback therapy as a modality of treatment in central nervous system disorders of voluntary movement. *Neurology* (Minneapolis), **24**, 925.

Brodal, A. (1973) Self-observations and neuro-anatomical considerations after a stroke. *Brain*, **96**, 675.

Bruell, J. H., Peszczynski, M. & Volk, D. (1957) Disturbance of perception of verticality in patients with hemiplegia: second report. *Archives of Physical Medicine and Rehabilitation*, **38**, 776.

Brunnstrom, S. (1970) *Movement Therapy in Hemiplegia. A Neurophysiological Approach.* New York: Harper and Row.

Butfield, E. & Zangwill, O. L. (1946) Re-education in aphasia: a review of 70 cases. *Journal of Neurology, Neurosurgery & Psychiatry*, **9**, 75.

Carter, A. B. (1968) *All about Strokes.* London: Nelson.

Carter, A. B. (1970) Hypotensive therapy in stroke survivors. *Lancet*, i, 485.

Circular London, Ministry of Health (1968) *Care of Younger Chronic Sick Patients in Hospitals.* London: H.M.S.O. (68) 41.

Cope, C. Reyes, T. M. & Skversky, N. J. (1973) Phlebographic analysis of the incidence of thrombosis in hemiplegia. *Radiology*, **109**, 581.

Culton, G. L. (1969) Spontaneous recovery from aphasia. *Journal of Speech and Hearing Research*, **12**, 825.

Darley, F. L. (1970) Article in *Behavioural Change in Cerebrovascular Disease*, Benton, A. L. New York and London: Harper & Row.

Denham, M. J. & Jeffreys, P. M. (1972) Routine mental testing in the elderly. *Modern Geriatrics*, **2**, 275.

Department of Health and Social Security Welsh Office (1972) *Rehabilitation. Report of a Sub-Committee of the Standing Medical Advisory Committee (Tunbridge Report).*

Diller, L. (1970) Article in *Behavioural Change in Cerebrovascular Disease*, ed. Benton, A. L. New York and London: Harper & Row.

Ellams, J. (1974) Speech therapy for the hemiplegic patients. *Nursing Mirror*, August 9, 1974, 66.

Enger, E. & Boyesen, S. (1965) Long term anticoagulant therapy in patients with cerebral infarction: a controlled clinical study. *Acta Medica Scandinavica* (Suppl.) **438**, 1.

Feldman, D. J., Lee, P. R., Unterecker, J., Lloyd, K., Rusk, H. A. & Toole, A. (1961) A comparison of functionally orientated medical care and formal rehabilitation in the management of patients with hemiplegia due to cerebrovascular disease. *Journal of Chronic Diseases*, **15**, 297.

Gordon, M. T. (1969) An experiment in audio and audio-visual group therapy. *British Journal of Disorders of Communication*, 83.

Groch, S. N. (1971) Discussion on anticoagulant therapy. *Neurology* (Minneapolis), **11**, 141.

Hagbarth, K. E. (1960) Spinal withdrawal reflexes in human lower limb. *Journal of Neurology, Neurosurgery and Psychiatry*, **23**, 222.

Hagen, C. (1973) Communication abilities in hemiplegia. effect of speech therapy. *Archives of Physical Medicine and Rehabilitation*, **54**, 454.

Halpern, D. & Meelhuysen, F. E. (1966) Phenol motor point block in the management of muscular hypertonia. *Archives of Physical Medicine and Rehabilitation*, **47**, 659.

Harris, A. I. (1971) *Handicapped and impaired in Great Britain. Part 1.* London: H.M.S.O.

Hatfield, F. M. (1971) Some uses of video-tape recording in language rehabilitation after brain damage. *Medical and biological Illustration*, **21**, 166.

Hedenberg, L. (1970) Functional improvement of the spastic hemiplegic arm after cooling. *Scandinavian Journal of Rehabilitation Medicine*, **2**, 154.

Hill, A. B., Marshall, J. & Shaw, D. A. (1962) Cerebrovascular disease: trial of long term anticoagulant therapy. *British Medical Journal*, ii, 1003.

Hodkinson, H. M. (1972) Evaluation of a mental test score for assessment of mental impairment in the elderly. *Age and Ageing*, **1**, 233.

Holland, A. L. (1969) Some current trends in aphasia rehabilitation. *Asha: Journal of the American Speech and Hearing Association* (Washington), **11**, 3.

Howell, D. A., Tatlow, W. E. T., Feldman, S. (1964) Observations on anticoagulant therapy in thromboembolic disease of the brain. *Journal of Canadian Medical Association*, **90**, 611.

Inaba, M., Edberg, E., Montgomery, J. & Gillis, M. K. (1973) Effectiveness of functional training, active exercises, and resistive exercise for patients with hemiplegia. *Physical Therapy*, **53**, 28.

Isaacs, B. (1971) Identification of disability in the stroke patient. *Modern Geriatrics*, **1**, 390.

Isaacs, B. & Marks, R. (1973) Determinants of outcome of stroke rehabilitation. *Age and Ageing*, **2**, 139.

Katz, S., Ford, A. B., Moskowitz, R. W., Jackson, B. A. & Jaffe, M. W. (1963) Studies of illness in the aged. *Journal of the American Medical Association*, **185**, 914.

Kenin, M. & Swisher, L. (1972) A study of patterns of recovery of aphasia. *Cortex*, **8**, 56.

Knott, M. (1967) Introduction to and philosophy of neuro-muscular facilitation. *Physiotherapy*, **53**, 1.

Lee, J. M. & Warren, M. P. (1974) Ice, relaxation and exercise in reduction of muscle spasticity. *Physiotherapy*, **60**, 296.

Lennenberg, E. H. (1967) *Biological Foundations of Language*. New York: John Wiley.

Louis, S. & McDowell, F. (1967) Epileptic seizures in nonembolic cerebral infarction. *Archives of Neurology*, **17**, 414.

Luria, A. R. (1973) *The Working Brain. An Introduction to Neuropsychology*, ed. Foss, B. M. London: Allen Lane Penguin Press.

Mahoney, F. I. & Barthel, D. W. (1965) Functional evaluation: the Barthel index. *Maryland State Medical Journal*, **14**, 61.

Manning, J. (1974) Article in *Hemiplegia in Neurology for Physiotherapists*, ed. Cash, J. London: Faber and Faber.

Marquardsen, J. (1969) *The Natural History of Acute Cerebrovascular Disease*. Copenhagen: Munksgaard.

Marshall, J. & Kaeser, A. C. (1961) Survival after nonhaemorrhagic cerebrovascular accidents. *British Medical Journal*, ii, 73.

Millard, J. B. (1973) Medical rehabilitation and hemiplegia. *Proceedings of the Royal Society of Medicine*, 66, 1003.

Millikan, C. H. (1971) Reassessment of anticoagulant therapy in various types of occlusive cerebrovascular disease. *Stroke*, **2**, 201.

McDowell, F. & McDevitt, E. (1965) Treatment of the completed stroke with long term anticoagulants. In *Cerebral Vascular Disease 4th Princeton Conference*, ed. Siekert, R. G. & Whisnant, J. New York: Grune & Stratton.

McHenry, L. C., Jaffe, M. E., Kawamura, J. (1970) Effect of papaverine on regional blood flow in focal vascular disease of the brain. *New England Journal of Medicine*, **282**, 1167.

McHenry, L. (1972) Cerebral vasodilator therapy in stroke. *Stroke*, **3**, 686.

Mohr, J. P., Sidman, M., Stoddard, L. T., Leicester, J. & Rosenberger, P. B. (1973) Evolution of the defect in total aphasia. *Neurology* (Minneapolis), **23**, 1302.

Moskowitz, E. (1969) Complications in the rehabilitation of hemiplegic patients. *Medical Clinics of North America*, **53**, 541.

Moskowitz, E., Bishop, H. F. & Shibutani, K. (1958) Posthemiplegic reflex sympathetic dystrophy. *Journal of the American Medical Association*, **167**, 836.

Mott, F. W. & Sherrington, C. S. (1895) Experiments upon the influence of sensory nerves upon movement and nutrition of the limbs. *Proceedings of the Royal Society of Medicine*, **57**, 481.

Nathan, P. W. (1970) The action of diazepam in neurological disorders with excessive motor activity. *Journal of the Neurological Sciences*, **10**, 33.

Nichols, P. J. R. (1971) *Rehabilitation of the Severely Disabled. 2. Management*. London: Butterworth.

Nichols, P. J. R. (1974) Rehabilitation in the reorganised national health service. A King's Fund Centre talk. *Occupational Therapy*, July 1974, 113.

Nickel, V. L. (Ed.) (1969) *Symposium on the Orthopaedic Management of Stroke*. Reprinted from Clinical Orthopaedics No. 63. Philadelphia: J. B. Lippincott.

O'Brien, M. D. & Veall, N. (1966) Effect of cyclandelate on cerebral cortex perfusion rate in cerebrovascular disease. *Lancet*, ii, 729.

Peacock, P. B., Riley, C. P., Lampton, T. D., Raffel, S. S. & Walker, J. S. (1972) The Birmingham stroke, epidemiology and rehabilitation study. In *Trends in Epidemiology*, ed. Stewart, G. T. Springfield, Illinois: Charles C. Thomas.

Pinneo, L. R., Kaplan, J. N., Elpel, E. A., Reynolds, P. L. & Glick, J. H. (1972) Experimental brain prosthesis for stroke. *Stroke*, **3**, 16.

Porsch, B. E. (1971) Multi-dimensional scoring in aphasia testing. *Journal of Speech and Hearing Research*, **14**, 776.

Rankin, J. (1957) Cerebral vascular accidents in patients over the age of 60. II. Prognosis. *Scottish Medical Journal*, ii, 200.

Rebersek, S. & Vodovnik, L. (1973) Proportionally controlled functional electrical stimulation of the hand. *Archives of Physical Medicine and Rehabilitation*, **54**, 378.

Report of the Geriatrics committee Working Group on Strokes. (1974) London: Royal College of Physicians.

Ritchie, D. (1974) *Stroke. A Diary of Recovery*. London: Faber and Faber.

Rood, M. (1969) Unpublished observations.

Roper, B. A. (1975) Surgical aspects of stroke rehabilitation. *Modern Geriatrics*, **5**, 4.

Rudinger, E. (Ed.) (1974) *Coping with Disablement*. London: Consumers' Association.

Rusk, H. A. (1971) *Rehabilitation Medicine*. 3rd edn. Saint Louis: Mosby.

Scheening, H. A. & Iversen, I. A. (1968) Numerical scoring in self-care status: a study of the Kenny self-care evaluation *Archives of Physical Medicine and Rehabilitation*, **49**, 221.

Schuell, H. (1974) *Aphasia Theory and Therapy*. New York: MacMillan.

Scottish Home and Health Department (1972) *Medical Rehabilitation: The Pattern for the Future* (*Mair report*). Edinburgh: H.M.S.O.

Somerville, J. G., Wilkinson, M., Canning, M., D'Alton, A., Langridge, J. C., Keane, W., Wycherley, J. & Draper, J. (1974) A symposium on the rehabilitation of the stroke patient. *Nursing Mirror*, August 9, 1974, 57.

Stern, P. H., McDowell, F., Miller, J. M. & Robinson, M. (1970) Effects of facilitation exercise techniques in stroke rehabilitation. *Archives of Physical Medicine and Rehabilitation*, **51**, 526.

Thygesen, P., Christensen, E., Dyrbye, M., Eiken, M., Frantzen, E., Gormsen, J., Lademann, A., Lennox-Buchthal, M., Ronnov-Jessen, V. & Therkelsen, J. (1964) Cerebral apoplexy. *Danish Medical Bulletin*, **11**, 233.

Treanor, W. J. (1969) The role of physical medicine treatment in stroke rehabilitation. Clinical Orthopaedics, **63**, 14.

Twitchell, T. E. (1951) The restoration of motor function following hemiplegia in man. *Brain*, **47**, 443.

Veterans Administration Cooperative Study Group. (1967) Antihypertensive agents. *Journal of American Medical Association*, **202**, 1028.

Vignolo, L. A. (1964) Evolution of aphasia and language rehabilitation: A retrospective exploratory study. *Cortex*, **1**, 345.

Weddell, J. M. (1973) Rehabilitation after stroke—a medico-social problem. In *The Skandia International Symposia: Rehabilitation after Central Nervous System Trauma*, ed. Bostrom, H., Larsson, T. & Ljungstedt, N. Stockholm: Nordiska Bokhandelns Forlag.

Wepman, J. M. & Morency, A. (1973) Filmstrips as an adjunct to language therapy for aphasia. *Journal of Speech andLearning Disorders*, **28**, 191.

Wilson, L. A. & Brass, W. (1973) Brief assessment of the mental state in geriatric domiciliary practice. *Age & Ageing*, **2**, 92.

Whurr, R. (1974) Personal communication.

Wilkinson, M. (1973) Rehabilitation after stroke. *British Journal of Hospital Medicine*, **10**, 278.

Young, J., Hall, P. & Blakemore, C. (1974) Treatment of the cerebral manifestations of arteriosclerosis with cyclandelate. *British Journal of Psychiatry*, **124**, 177.

14. Less Common Varieties of Cerebral Arterial Disease

R. W. Ross Russell

CONGENITAL ABNORMALITIES

Absence of one or both internal carotid arteries is a rare congenital defect; only about 25 cases have been recorded (Turnbull, 1962; Hills and Sament, 1968). The condition may be discovered by chance in infants dying from other malformations. In later life patients may present with haemorrhage from dilated collateral arteries or from a co-existent berry aneurysm, or with multiple lower cranial nerve palsies caused by pressure from a greatly enlarged basilar artery. Absence of the carotid canals may be detected radiologically.

Hypoplasia of the internal carotid arteries on one or both sides is also a rarity. It affects the whole length of the artery except for the proximal two centimetres. It also is associated with malformation of the Circle of Willis, berry aneurysm, or abnormal collateral channels, and the condition usually comes to light during investigation of intracerebral or subarachnoid haemorrhage (Lhermitte, Gautier, and Poirier, 1968; Smith, Nelson, and Dooley, 1968).

Congenital looping and kinking

Looping and tortuosity of the internal carotid artery may be found at any age. In children the condition has a prevalence of 15 per cent and is undoubtedly congenital since the fetal carotid artery is normally tortuous at the point where it is crossed by the glossopharyngeal nerve. In adults tortuosity and coiling becomes exaggerated as a result of degenerative arterial disease and the prevalence rises to 25 per cent (Weibel and Fields, 1965). Kinking or angulation of the artery is usually regarded as an acquired condition affecting a previously tortuous artery.

Any relationship between these extracranial abnormalities and cerebral ischaemia is uncertain, but a number of possible mechanisms have been suggested. Tortuous arteries may become kinked or occluded during movements of the neck (Bauer, Sheehan, and Meyer, 1961). The endothelium of the kinked segment may become damaged and act as a source of embolism; during kinking the carotid sinus may be distended and cause reflex hypotension and bradycardia (Sarkavi, Holmes, and Bickerstaff, 1970).

It is difficult to assess the clinical relevance of tortuosity in individual patients. In one report, for instance (Metz, *et al.* 1961), there were slightly more ischaemic episodes in patients with tortuosity of the carotid artery than in normal patients. In another (Bauer *et al.*, 1961) the frequency of carotid and vertebral tortuosity in patients with clinical cerebral vascular disease was 25 per cent, the same frequency as in a random sample. It is probable that tortuosity is only rarely a primary cause of symptoms in adults, but a group of children has been described with seizures, transient hemiparesis, hemianopia, and dysphasia in association with looping of the internal carotid artery on the appropriate side usually just below the base of the skull (Sarkavi *et al.*, 1970).

Fibromuscular dysplasia

Fibromuscular dysplasia, a condition first recognised in the renal arteries, refers to alternating segments of stenosis and ectasia, the narrowed segments having a constant and sharply localised 'string of beads' appearance. The proximal portion of the internal carotid artery is not involved. Patients are usually females over the age of 50, and occasionally there may be occlusion of an intracerebral artery (Frens *et al.*, 1974). Twenty-five per cent of cases have an intracranial berry aneurysm (Houser and Baker, 1968). Narrowing of the lumen is a constant feature but complete obstruction is most unusual; in 75 per cent of cases the condition is bilateral (Fig. 14.1).

Histological studies show alternating zones of fibrous medial thickening and thinning. The thinned areas show a loss of elastic tissue (mural aneurysm) and the muscle coat may be entirely absent.

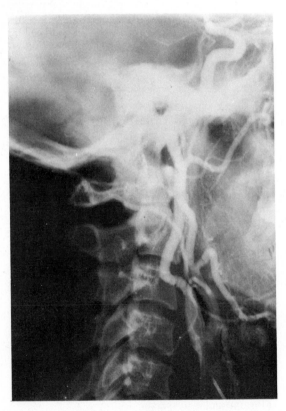

Fig. 14.1   Fibromuscular dysplasia affecting the proximal segment of the internal carotid artery.

Fibromuscular dysplasia must be distinguished from two other conditions; the first is a localised band-like or tubular stenosis of the internal carotid artery not usually associated with vascular disease or with significant obstruction to blood flow. The second is the stationary arterial wave, often an incidental angiographic appearance but sometimes found with retarded blood flow in the carotid artery. It differs from fibromuscular hyperplasia in the absence of dilated segments. Some authors interpret stationary arterial waves as artefacts of contrast injection and state that they may disappear on a second injection (New, 1966).

ACQUIRED ARTERIAL DISEASE

Aneurysms of the carotid artery

Dissecting aneurysm of the cervical portion of the internal carotid artery is an unusual cause of occlusion in youth and middle age. It may be related to cystic medial necrosis where there is deposition of mucoid metachromatic material in the arterial wall (Thapedi, Ashenhurst, and Rozdilsky, 1970). Dissection usually occurs between the medial and the adventitial coats and the split begins near the origin of the internal carotid artery extending up to the base of the skull (Brice and Crompton, 1964).

Clinical symptoms consist of severe unilateral headache and facial pain sometimes with partial oculosympathetic palsy. Transient retinal or cerebral ischaemia may occur as a prelude to a dense hemiplegia. The carotid artery on arteriography may show irregular narrowing throughout its length (string sign) or may show a tapering occlusion (Anderson and Schechter, 1959; Ojemann, Fisher, and Rich, 1972). The origin of the dissection may be visible as the contrast medium tracks into the wall of the artery. On rare occasions the condition has been treated by arterial excision and grafting (Barnes and Jacoby, 1962) (Fig. 14.2).

Very occasionally dissecting aneurysms have been reported in intracerebral arteries due to trauma, atheroma, or syphilitic arteritis, and causing either occlusion or subarachnoid haemorrhage (Wolman, 1959). Saccular atheromatous aneurysm of the carotid sinus is rare, but has been described as a cause of transient cerebral ischaemia progressing to carotid occlusion. Embolism of mural thrombus is suggested as the cause of transient symptoms (Schwartz, Mitchell, and Hughes, 1962).

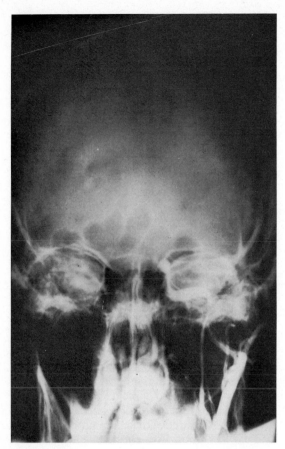

Fig. 14.2 Dissecting aneurysm of the internal carotid artery in the neck. The artery is markedly narrowed up to the base of skull (string sign).

Infraclinoid aneurysm

The cavernous portion of the carotid artery is a frequent site for aneurysm. At this point the artery is extradural and although the aneurysm may rupture into the cavernous sinus, massive subarachnoid haemorrhage is exceptional. The aneurysm may arise at the origin of a small hypophyseal branch vessel and although originally saccular it slowly expands to distend the sinus taking up the original artery wall as it does so and stretching the nerves on the lateral wall of the sinus (Barr, Blackwood, and Meadows, 1971). The aneurysm may eventually occupy much of the floor of the middle fossa.

Patients are almost always elderly women and present as a painful unilateral cavernous sinus syndrome. The pain may be severe, has a constant boring quality, and is felt behind the eye, in the forehead, and root of the nose. Pain is followed by the development over a few days of ophthalmoplegia involving first the sixth then third and fourth cranial nerves (Meadows, 1951). The pupil is usually smaller on the affected side due to damage to the sympathetic fibres around the carotid artery; its reactions to light and near are reduced or absent. Some disturbance of facial sensation over the first two divisions of the trigeminal nerve is often present and the corneal reflex is reduced, though not lost. Proptosis is slight and vision normal. Plain X-rays of the skull may be normal or may show erosion of the anterior clinoid process and sella turcica. The wall of the aneurysm itself may be calcified and may erode the superior orbital fissure and middle fossa. Orbital venograms show obstruction of the cavernous sinus; carotid angiography is diagnostic.

If untreated the aneurysm slowly enlarges although pain and ophthalmoplegia usually improve after some weeks. For intractable pain the carotid artery may be ligated in the neck but there is a considerable risk of hemiplegia in elderly patients.

Caroticocavernous fistula

This complication may affect small aneurysms which have not filled the sinus, or may follow basal skull fracture. A large proportion of the carotid blood flow may be re-routed directly into the sinus and the hemisphere becomes dependent for its blood supply on the contra-lateral carotid artery. The cavernous sinus and its tributaries become distended with arterial blood. The patient presents with pulsating tinnitus, proptosis, chemosis, and venous engorgement and rapidly develops a cavernous sinus syndrome with complete external and internal ophthalmoplegia. One or both eyes may be affected. The sixth nerve is the most vulnerable and the last to recover. Vision is usually normal but may deteriorate from ischaemic retinopathy. The retina shows many haemorrhages, microaneurysms, dilated veins, and macular oedema.

The fistula may close spontaneously or after angiography. Carotid ligation in the neck is useless and may be dangerous. For progressive proptosis or visual failure the fistula may be isolated by a surgical trapping procedure, or blocked by a muscle embolus or balloon introduced up the carotid artery.

Basilar aneurysm

Although less frequent than on the anterior part of the Circle of Willis, berry aneurysms may occur on the posterior cerebral arteries, at the bifurcation of the basilar artery, or on any of its branches in the posterior fossa. The presenting symptom is subarachnoid haemorrhage and is discussed in Chapter 12. The basilar artery is also the site of an unusual type of vascular ectasia, the fusiform aneurysm, often though not invariably found in association with extensive atheroma and hypertension (Alajouanine, Le Beau, and Houdart, 1948). The basilar artery is extensively dilated and lengthened, becoming serpiginous and extending laterally into one cerebello-pontine angle to involve the lower cranial nerves. Thrombosis occurs in successive layers on the luminal surface and may finally occlude the artery. The carotid arteries may be affected by a similar process.

The clinical presentation is diverse; many patients present with symptoms of transient vertebrobasilar ischaemia including brain stem and posterior cerebral territories. Headache and neck pain is prominent and may be made worse by head movements. A special diagnostic feature is the involvement of cranial nerves mainly the seventh and eighth and including attacks of hemifacial spasm (Denny-Brown and Foley, 1952).

Large aneurysms act additionally as mass lesions and simulate posterior fossa tumours usually in the cerebellopontine angle or foramen magnum regions. There may be progressive ataxia, spastic quadriplegia, and pseudobulbar palsy from progressive compression of the brain stem by the aneurysm. Any of the cranial nerves from third to twelfth may also be involved (Yaskin and Alpers, 1944). Raised intracranial pressure and organic dementia are also reported

(Michael, 1974). Cerebrospinal fluid examination normally shows a raised protein content with or without xanthochromia. Vertebral angiography is diagnostic but may underestimate the size of the aneurysm because of thrombus within the lumen.

Prognosis is poor, death occurring from basilar occlusion or haemorrhage within two years of diagnosis in the great majority of patients.

Aortic arch syndrome

Occlusion of the origins of the major brachiocephalic-arteries gives rise to a distinctive symptomatology related to long-term reduction in blood flow to external and internal carotid territories. As arterial narrowing develops in a major extracranial artery it reaches a point at which there is restriction of blood flow; under usual circumstances this is minimised by an increased blood flow via the remaining arteries and Circle of Willis so that total cerebral blood supply is little affected. If, however, the remaining arteries are also diseased other homeostatic mechanisms come into operation notably a generalised vasodilatation in intracerebral resistance vessels, the development of collateral channels bypassing the occlusion and a compensatory hypertension from baroceptor reflexes in the carotid sinus. The effectiveness of homeostasis is illustrated by the reports of symptomless patients with occlusion of three or even four of the main extracranial arteries (Vitek, Halsey, and McDowell, 1972).

A temporary insufficiency can arise either as a consequence of increased metabolic tissue demand (e.g. in the muscles supplied by the external carotid artery) or by minor reductions in systemic blood pressure, caused for example by oversensitivity of the carotid sinus baroceptors to mechanical distension. The compensatory decrease in cerebral vascular resistance which would normally accompany a fall in blood pressure cannot take place since the cerebral resistance vessels are already maximally dilated; consequently cerebral blood flow falls and in the long term ischaemic changes in both intracranial and extracranial tissues may result. Although the aetiology of the aortic arch syndrome is diverse, the symptomatology is uniform and varies only in degree and duration (Ross and McKusick, 1953). The symptoms may be transient or permanent. Episodes of vertigo, confusion, or lightheadedness are the commonest complaints and are present in over half the patients; there may be actual loss of consciousness or true seizures. Some patients experience episodic hemiparesis, dysarthria, deafness, tinnitus, or rarely, an unusual type of drop attack without change in consciousness but with incontinence of urine (Currier, De Jong, and Bole, 1954). Intense occipital headache and claudicating pain in the jaw on eating are commonly reported. Visual symptoms are often present and may affect one or both eyes. These may be provoked by sudden standing or by exercise. When the defect is uniocular the cause must be a reduction in blood flow to one eye but in bilateral or altitudinal field loss the mechanism may be ischaemia of the occipital cortex (Russell, 1973). Ischaemic pain in the arms on exercise is an unusual symptom, although pallor and coldness may be noted on examination. Chronic ischaemia in the external carotid territory may lead to facial atrophy, ulceration of the scalp, palate, or nasal septum. In the brain there may be memory loss, progressive intellectual impairment and dementia, with focal signs suggesting bilateral parieto-occipital lesions (Russell, 1973).

Chronic ocular ischaemia may present as progressive visual impairment with low pressure retinopathy, scattered retinal and vitreous haemorrhages, slowing of blood flow in small veins, optic atrophy, peripheral microaneurysms, and arterial attenuation (Knox, 1965). The peripapillary anastomosis described by Takayasu (1908) is seen only in severe cases.

The principal findings on examination are reduced or absent arterial pulsations in the head, neck, and arms (Fig. 14.3). The ophthalmic and brachial pressures are reduced or unrecordable. Vascular bruits around the neck or scapula may be detected. In spite of occlusion of the subclavian arteries blood flow to the arms may be normal at rest but fails to increase on exercise (Held, Jipp, and Schreier, 1972). There may also be evidence of aortic regurgitation, aortic dilatation, renal artery stenosis, and ischaemic

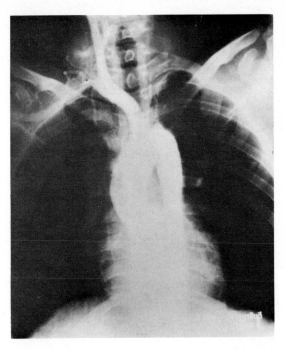

Fig. 14.3   Takayasu's arteritis: occlusion or severe narrowing affects both subclavian arteries and the left common carotid artery.

changes in the legs. Angiography shows segmental dilatation and stenosis of the aorta with occlusion at the origin of the great vessels (Strachan, 1966).

Various types of arterial pathology may be responsible. Many of the early cases occurred in young Oriental women and showed histological evidence of low grade arteritis of unknown cause. The artery wall is thickened due to fibrous proliferation and there is mononuclear infiltration and occasional giant cells. Fibrinoid change or eosinophils are absent (Danaraj, Wong, and Thomas, 1963). Some patients show predominant involvement of the descending aorta and in some there is concurrent tuberculous infection. A fibrous, hyperplastic type of atheroma accounts for most of the less florid examples of pulseless disease seen in India or in Europe (Dalal, 1973). Syphilitic aortitis with or without aneurysm formation is now rarely encountered.

In the younger age group, including some patients reported from the Orient, there is evidence of a systemic disorder which may precede arterial occlusion by some years. The features are fever, anaemia, pleurisy, haemoptysis, arthralgia, Raynaud's syndrome, and erythema nodosum. The sedimentation rate is markedly raised (Strachan, 1966). It is suggested that this variety is due to a hypersensitivity angiitis to vascular elastic tissue. Corticosteroid treatment is recommended for these patients. Atheromatous and non-inflammatory types of aortic arch syndrome may be amenable to reconstructive surgical procedures.

Moya-moya disease

This unusual variety of cerebral vascular disease occurs chiefly in female infants and young adults and is characterised by narrowing or occlusion of the terminal portions of both internal carotid arteries and the Circle of Willis and by the development of a fine vascular anastomotic network involving both the perforating and pial arteries. In the later stages other anastomotic networks are formed including the orbital and ethmoidal branches of the external carotid, leptomeningeal, and transdural anastomoses. The cervical part of the internal carotid artery is also narrowed (Fig. 14.4). The disease was first thought to be confined to Japanese (Kudo, 1968) but has now been described in many parts of the world. The cause is unknown but most writers favour a form of acquired arteritis related to nasopharyngeal infection or trauma rather than a congenital malformation or persistence of an embryonic vascular pattern (Levesque et al., 1974). To date few convincing autopsy reports have been published. There is hypoplasia of the media with subintimal proliferation but no inflammatory lesions (Picard et al., 1974). The symptoms vary according to age. Infantile forms account for 70 per cent of cases in the literature. In children the disease presents with repeated episodes of cerebral ischaemia, hemiparesis, dysphasia, headache, or mental retardation. Occasionally there are seizures or involuntary movements (Susuk and Takaku, 1969). With increasing age the episodes become fewer but mental retardation may persist. A fatal outcome is exceptional. In adults the presentation

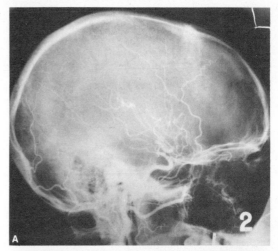

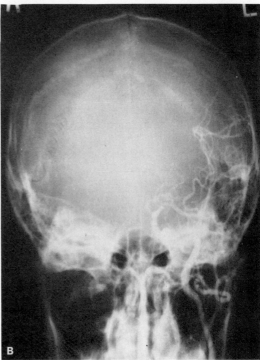

Figs. 14.4A and 14.4B   Moya-moya disease: narrowing of the terminal portion of the internal carotid artery with dilatation of the striate branches of the middle cerebral artery.

is with subarachnoid or sometimes cerebral haemorrhage (Higashi, Hateno, and Maza, 1974). Basal anastomoses are less prominent but ethmoidal and meningeal anastomoses may be extensive. Carotid stenosis rarely extends below the level of the third cervical vertebra (Picard et al., 1974).

In Western Europe and America a similar angiographic pattern of collateral vessels may be seen in children with acute hemiplegia or in older patients with occlusive atheromatous or thromboembolic disease involving the terminal carotid artery (Solomon et al., 1970). This particular type of collateral enlargement occurs only if the posterior communicating arteries are hypoplasic or diseased. Neurofibromatosis or a history of cranial X-ray therapy may be associated (Taveras, 1969).

Traumatic thrombosis of the carotid and vertebral arteries

Direct trauma to the neck by laceration, missile injury, or skull fracture near the carotid canal may cause the artery to thrombose. Propagation of thrombus intracranially to involve the ophthalmic artery, the Circle of Willis, and its main branches is found in fatal cases (Caldwell and Hadden, 1948). The carotid artery may also be injured during tonsillectomy or by penetrating injuries to the tonsillar fossa or soft palate in children (Fairburn, 1957). A more difficult diagnostic problem is posed by those cases resulting from indirect trauma, which need not be severe. As a result of sudden stretching during violent turning or extension of the head the internal carotid artery may develop a transverse intimal tear 2 to 3 cm above its origin. Extravasation of blood into the arterial wall and carotid sheath occurs and the intimal injury acts as a nidus for mural intravascular thrombosis which may propagate upwards and downwards. Propagation does not normally extend beyond the carotid siphon and for that reason it may be asymptomatic. However, there may be extension of the thrombus into the middle or anterior cerebral arteries or embolism of portions of thrombus before all blood flow through the artery is arrested (Cairns, 1942).

Traumatic thrombosis of the internal carotid artery should be suspected when signs of cerebral or retinal ischaemia suddenly develop some hours after indirect hyperextension injury to the neck. Patients are usually young men and may exhibit facial abrasion, bruising of the neck, fracture of the jaw, clavicle, or first rib. In the 16 cases reviewed by Hockaday (1959) motor involvement of the arm and leg was equally severe in 10, in four the arm was the more severely affected and in two the leg. Immediate angiography is indicated to confirm the condition and to exclude other intracranial lesions. If occlusion is complete there is little to be gained by exploring the artery but if flow is continuing and if the thrombus is visible within the lumen the artery should be ligated to prevent cerebral embolism. Immediate anticoagulant treatment using heparin intravenously is advisable.

In patients with **cervical rib** or congenital fibrous band the subclavian artery may be stretched and angulated as it crosses the first rib. During movements of the arm the artery may be compressed between the first rib and clavicle and continued trauma may result in a local area of fibrosis and internal damage sometimes with the formation of an aneurysm. Mural thrombosis in this segment of artery gives rise to distal embolism with occlusion of digital and palmar arteries and attacks of pain due to ischaemia of arm muscles. On rare occasions the thrombus may propagate in a retrograde direction to involve the origin of the vertebral arteries and on the right side the brachiocephalic trunk. Cerebral embolism may then occur in the territory of the vertebral or right carotid arteries (Gunning et al., 1964).

The vertebral arteries may be damaged in acute or chronic trauma to the cervical spine (Schneider and Schemm, 1961). There are three vulnerable points: (1) at the intervertebral foramina, (2) at the atlantoaxial joint when there is subluxation leading to stretching and angulation of the artery, (3) at the occipitoatlantal joint where the condyle slides forward over the groove in the lamina of the atlas. Thrombosis with distal embolism to basilar and posterior cerebral arteries has followed manipulation of the neck (Ford and Clark, 1956) but more often the condition presents as intermittent vertebrobasilar insufficiency, the artery being obstructed as a result of extension or rotation of the neck or by atlantoaxial subluxation or fracture dislocation (Ford, 1952). Spontaneous atlantoaxial subluxation is frequent in severe rheumatoid arthritis of the cervical spine (Schneider and Crosby, 1959; Kao et al., 1974) and death from vertebral artery thrombosis has been reported in this condition (Webb, Hickman, and Brew, 1968).

Acute carotid arteritis

Local inflammation of the retropharyngeal tissues and regional lymph nodes may spread to the walls of the carotid artery in the neck. A number of such cases were reported in children in the pre-antibiotic era but are now rare (Litchfield, 1938). Thrombosis of the artery may be indicated by the occurrence of a transient or permanent hemiplegia often with headache and convulsions; the symptoms are due to distal propagation or embolisation of thrombus. At an earlier stage angiography may show an irregularity of the lumen in relation to the infected region or narrowing of the whole internal carotid and its branches (Bickerstaff, 1964). A few instances of acute hemiplegia in apparently healthy infants (usually male) or in children with congenital heart disease have been shown to be caused by idiopathic internal carotid artery thrombosis without an obvious source of infection (Bickerstaff, 1964).

In septic cavernous sinus thrombosis there may be occlusion or narrowing of the intracavernous portion of the carotid artery with distal occlusion of anterior or middle cerebral arteries (Mathew et al., 1971). In pneumococcal or meningococcal meningitis the intracerebral branches of the carotid or vertebral arteries in the subarachnoid space and on the pial surface of the brain are surrounded by inflammatory exudates. Histological evidence of arteritis is described in fatal cases in the form of fibrin deposition in the lumen, foci of pan-arteritis, and phlebitis and local cerebral necrosis (Cairns and Russell, 1946). Cerebral ischaemia is rarely recognised clinically in the acute stage since the clinical state of the patient is dominated by the features of acute meningitis. When antibiotic treatment has been used the acute inflammatory reaction in the artery wall may progress to fibrinoid necrosis and at a later stage to a proliferative fibrous endarteritis. Progressive narrowing of the vascular lumen may then lead to ischaemia in the territory of one of the carotid branches, usually the middle cerebral artery.

MALARIA

The cerebral vascular complications of malaria occur almost exclusively in infections due to *Plasmodium falciparum*. Cerebral malaria is a diffuse encephalopathy due to disseminated small vessel occlusion by pigment clumps of infected erythrocytes and fibrin. There is often endothelial oedema and proliferation as well as multiple petechial haemorrhages. Multiple small areas of softening are responsible for the neuropsychiatric symptoms of intense headache, confusion, depressed consciousness, toxic delirium, and seizures which make up the clinical picture. Focal neurological signs due to major vessel occlusion occur much less frequently (Musoke, 1966).

Chronic arteritis

Chronic inflammation and fibrosis of the meninges at the base of the brain frequently involves the Circle of Willis and its major branches as well as the adjacent cranial nerves. In **tuberculous meningitis** miliary tuberculous nodules may be detected histologically within the walls of both arteries and veins, the outer coats being most severely affected (Blackwood, 1958). **Syphilitic arteritis** affects large and medium-sized meningeal vessels causing inflammatory infiltration of the middle and outer coats with a secondary fibrosis. The medial coat is thin and a fusiform aneurysm may form although rupture is rare; the elastic lamina is intact. The intima shows fibroplastic and later collagenous thickening (endarteritis obliterans) with eccentric narrowing of the lumen and sometimes thrombosis (Blackwood, 1958).

Mucor mycosis is a rare fungus infection which may cause a localised meningitis by spread from the nasal sinuses. Most patients are severe diabetics or have an immunological abnormality. Inflammatory cells may invade the cerebral cortex and the walls of the arteries leading to thrombosis and to extensive infarction

(Kurrein, 1954). The angiographic changes in the various forms of chronic meningitis are similar and have been especially well studied in tuberculous meningitis in the Far East where the disease is still prevalent (Fig. 14.5). Narrowing or occlusion of the distal internal carotid and the proximal segment of anterior and middle cerebral arteries are described. Smaller branches may also be affected. Various patterns of collateral circulation may be seen according to the site of occlusion; the collateral vessels may be the striate arteries (moya-moya type), transdural internal-external carotid anastomoses, and pial anastamoses (Mathew, Abraham, and Chandy, 1970).

The diagnosis of chronic infective arteritis of the cerebral vessels rests on the recognition of its two major components, meningitic and vascular, together with detection of any source of infection in the sinuses or chest. The disease usually affects young patients at an age when degenerative arterial disease is uncommon. The occurrence of headache, fever, personality change, seizures, cranial nerve palsies, or signs of raised intracranial pressure in the days or weeks before the onset of hemiplegia is an indication of preceding basal meningitis, and the diagnosis is confirmed by the finding of inflammatory cellular reaction and positive serological tests in the cerebrospinal fluid. The causative organism may be visible on a stained smear of CSF.

The ischaemic cerebral symptoms, being caused by thrombosis of the inflamed vessel, are usually abrupt in onset and vary in severity according to size of the infarcted zone. Any of the main carotid or basilar branches may be occluded. Provided that appropriate treatment is given for the primary infection the degree of recovery is often greater than would be expected in ischaemic stroke secondary to arterial disease.

A non-specific **granulomatous periarteritis** confined to the cavernous segment of the internal carotid artery was first described by Tolosa (1954). The carotid artery may show a localised stenosis and the adventitial coat is thickened. The condition presents in adult patients as a painful cavernous sinus syndrome involving the third to sixth cranial nerves and responds rapidly to steroids. Ischaemic cerebral symptoms do not occur.

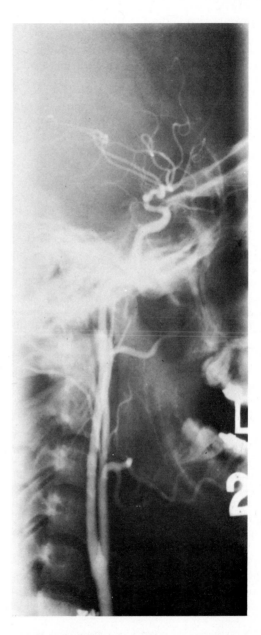

Fig. 14.5 Carotid arteritis: narrowing of the supraclinoid portion of the internal carotid artery in a patient with chronic basal meningitis.

COLLAGEN DISEASES

Polyarteritis nodosa

Polyarteritis nodosa is a widespread destructive inflammatory disorder of small arteries and arterioles sometimes also involving larger vessels. It tends to heal by granulation and fibrosis with occasional aneurysm formation. The cause is thought to be a hypersensitivity reaction to a variety of antigenic stimuli (Miller and Daley, 1946).

The disease principally affects visceral, renal, and pulmonary arteries but those of the brain and spinal cord may also be involved (Rose and Spencer, 1957). Estimates of the frequency of cerebral involvement vary widely from 8 to 60 per cent. Both intracerebral and pial branches and occasionally major cerebral arteries may be affected and may have a beaded appearance due to multiple aneurysms (Facon, Mestes, and Georgesco, 1960; Ford and Siekert, 1965). Pathologically there are foci of cortical necrosis surrounded by an acute inflammatory reaction with eosinophilia and sometimes by chronic inflammatory cells. Affected arteries show fibrinoid change in the media sometimes with giant cells. Areas of haemorrhage are frequently found.

About one-third of patients show clinical symptoms of central nervous system involvement throughout the course of the illness (Parker and Kernohan, 1949). The symptoms are extremely variable; sometimes multiple small vascular occlusions and sometimes haemorrhage. The symptom most commonly recorded is sudden hemiparesis or hemianopia (15 to 20 per cent) sometimes with an organic confusional state or with headache and seizures. At other times the clinical picture may suggest a slowly evolving cerebral abscess or glioma (Roger, Poursines, and Roger, 1955). Diabetes insipidus and choreic involuntary movements are also recorded. Rupture of aneurysms is not common but subarachnoid haemorrhage is the presenting feature in 5 per cent of cases (Ford and Siekert, 1965).

A further third of patients show neurological features only in the terminal illness. These are usually related to severe hypertension and consist of seizures, hypertensive encephalopathy, brain stem signs, and subarachnoid haemorrhage (Roger et al., 1955). At autopsy multiple haemorrhages in the hemispheres and brain stem may be found (Haft et al., 1957).

Treatment consists of corticosteroids in a dose sufficient to control the symptoms and reduce the sedimentation rate to normal. Large amounts may be required and side effects are common. In some patients it may be possible to control the disease by administration of corticosteroids on alternate days.

Systemic lupus erythematosus

Involvement of the blood vessels of the central nervous system is common in systemic lupus erythematosis. Pathological cerebral changes were found in 72 per cent of fatal cases in the series of Johnson and Richardson (1968). Cerebral involvement may occur at any time but is most often encountered in the late stages of the disease. Presenting features are seizures (52 per cent), cranial nerve signs (42 per cent), and mental changes (37 per cent) ranging from a mild affective disorder to a florid psychosis. Less commonly there may be hemiparesis, paraparesis, cranial nerve palsies, involuntary movements (chiefly choreic), hypothalamic involvement, or subarachnoid haemorrhage. The majority of these symptoms can be attributed to small ischaemic lesions in the brain stem, basal ganglia, and hemispheres. The pathological basis is a necrotic and proliferative change in arterioles and capillaries. Fibrin is found outside the blood vessels suggesting increased permeability (Gold and Yahr, 1960). Small and medium-sized haemorrhages may be present (Glaser, 1952), the cerebrospinal fluid may show an increased protein or cell content; more often it is normal. Cerebrospinal fluid complement levels may be increased. Arteriography occasionally shows occlusion of a major cerebral vessel but is usually normal. The level of DNA antibody, which relates well to the activity of the disease in other organs, is of little help in those with cerebral involvement. The pathological changes are distinct from those found in polyarteritis nodosa but are similar to those in acute rheumatic fever, hypertensive encephalopathy, and thrombotic thrombocytopenia. They are probably not due to embolism from a verrucose endocarditis.

Giant cell arteritis

In this type of arteritis there is a granulomatous reaction involving arteries of many different sizes from the aorta down to small branch vessels (Armsworth and Gresham, 1961; Crompton, 1959). Cranial arteries derived from external carotid and vertebral are the most commonly affected (Wilkinson and Russell, 1972). The disease is almost unknown under the age of 60 and runs a chronic course of 1 to 10 years.

Pathologically there is subintimal cellular proliferation and a chronic inflammatory reaction with giant cells, centered on the elastic tissue which is largely destroyed. The arterial lumen is greatly narrowed and thrombosis may occur. Arteritis of scalp vessels and of maxillary and facial branches accounts for the principal symptoms of headache, scalp tenderness, trismus, pains in the jaw, tongue, and throat. The scalp arteries are often irregular, thickened and tender to palpation; angiography shows irregular narrowing of the lumen. Ischaemic neuropathy of the optic nerve and of the oculomotor nerves is due to arteritis affecting the ciliary arteries and other branches of the ophthalmic artery within the orbit (Crompton, 1959).

Although cervical portions of the internal carotid and vertebral arteries are frequently involved, features of cerebral ischaemia occur only rarely (Fisher, 1959). Intracranial portions of the carotid arteries are practically free from inflammation, possibly because they contain smaller amounts of elastic tissue (Wilkinson, 1972).

Microscopic granulomas have occasionally been found in middle cerebral artery branches (Greenfield, 1951) but in the other reported cases of hemisphere ischaemia in giant cell arteritis there has been either complete occlusion of the internal carotid usually with thrombosis (Macmillan, 1950) or evidence of cerebral embolism from carotid thrombosis. The intracerebral arteries themselves have not been inflamed.

Similarly in the posterior cerebral circulation there have been a small number of reports of ischaemic episodes in brain stem (most often the lateral medullary syndrome) or in both occipital lobes due to embolism from a source of thrombus in the vertebral arteries (Wilkinson and Russell, 1972).

The symptomatology of cerebral involvement is not distinctive and consists of one or more sudden episodes of ischaemia often accompanied by an organic confusional state in a senile patient. A history of preceding headache and scalp pain, muscle pains, ischaemic optic neuritis, tenderness of scalp arteries or of the carotid artery in the neck may provide a diagnostic clue (Hamilton, Shelley, and Tumulty, 1971). The sedimentation rate and serum alkaline phosphatase (liver fraction) are constantly elevated, and these examinations should be a routine test in all elderly patients with ischaemic stroke.

Treatment consists of corticosteroids, initially in high dosage, which are then slowly reduced after a few days to a level sufficient to keep the sedimentation rate within normal limits. Treatment should be started as soon as the diagnosis is suspected because of the risk of permanent visual loss. It may be necessary to continue treatment for some years (Russell, 1959).

GRANULOMATOUS ANGIITIS

A pathological entity distinct from giant cell arteritis is the rare condition of giant cell granulomatous angiitis of the central nervous system. This disease, the cause of which is unknown, occurs at any age and in either sex and runs a progressive course to a fatal outcome in a few weeks or months (Nurick, Blackwood, and Mair, 1972). The symptoms of headache, memory loss, seizures, and impaired consciousness are those of an organic psychosis due to diffuse ischaemia affecting chiefly grey matter of both hemispheres. Some patients show disturbances of eye movement, pupillary abnormalities, facial sensory loss, or blurred vision. The cerebrospinal fluid, which is under raised pressure, usually contains an excess of mononuclear cells and protein. The electroencephalogram is diffusely abnormal and angiography shows no abnormality. Corticosteroids may lead to temporary improvement. Pathologically the lesion may be confined to intracerebral blood vessels; unsuspected visceral arteritis may be found in a minority of cases. There is necrosis of the walls of small leptomeningeal and intracerebral arteries and veins which are infiltrated with chronic inflammatory cells. The brain shows foci of ischaemic necrosis with or without haemorrhage (Hughes and Brownell, 1966).

RHEUMATIC FEVER

There are many reports in the older literature of cerebral complications in acute rheumatic fever (Winkelman and Eckel, 1932). In fatal cases the brain is swollen and shows numerous perivascular haemorrhages and focal areas of cell loss. The arterioles and capillaries show endarteritis with proliferative, hyaline, and fibrotic changes in the walls. These changes are non-specific and are found in other varieties of severe infection. The primary damage may be widespread hypersensitivity angiitis with abnormal permeability of the vessel wall (Costero, 1949). Early symptoms consist of abnormal restlessness and delirium with meningism and sometimes chorea. This may lead on to impairment of consciousness and finally death in coma. Hyperpyrexia is usual but not invariable.

Although fibrin-platelet vegetations are frequently found on the heart valves and although occasional patients with embolic obstruction of the retinal arteries have been described in chorea (Hearn and Roper-Hall, 1961), there is general agreement that the vascular changes found in fatal cases of rheumatic fever are unlikely to be due to embolism alone.

SCLERODERMA

In contrast to other forms of collagen disease, involvement of the cerebral arteries in scleroderma is exceptionally rare. Occasional case reports have appeared of cerebral infarction secondary to stenosis and occlusion of the terminal carotid artery with thrombosis of the major branches (Lee and Haynes, 1967). The carotid artery shows marked medial fibrosis and thickening due to proliferation of normal collagen fibres. Smaller arteries show medial and intimal hyperplasia with fibrinoid necrosis and some cellular infiltration.

BLOOD DISEASES

Polycythaemia

In polycythaemia, either the primary disorder or when secondary to cardiac or pulmonary disease, there is excessive production of red blood cells leading to an increased red cell mass and blood volume. The abnormal proportion of cells to plasma is reflected in a raised haematocrit (PVC) over 52 per cent. In many patients with polycythaemia vera there is also an increase in plasma volume so that the haematocrit is not an exact estimate of red cell overproduction. In polycythaemia vera, leucocytes and platelets are also increased.

The red cells are the major factor influencing the viscosity of blood in the circulation although there are other components notably the plasma protein fibrinogen. In general, viscosity is greatest under conditions where blood is flowing slowly in the capillary bed (i.e. at low shear rates). As PVC rises there is a logarithmic increase in viscosity. A relatively small increase in PVC thus produces a much larger increase in viscosity and so in peripheral resistance. This effect may be buffered to some extent by peripheral vasodilation and by an increase in blood pressure, but cerebral blood flow measurement in patients with polycythaemia indicates that these compensatory mechanisms are insufficient to offset the increased viscosity. Very low values of cerebral perfusion rate have been recorded at normal levels of $P_a\text{CO}_2$ (Kety, 1950).

Peripheral vasodilatation and slowed cutaneous blood flow are responsible for the dusky plethoric appearance of polycythaemic patients and for the conjunctival injection. The retina shows engorged cyanosed veins with evidence of retarded blood flow and hypoxic changes such as haemorrhages and microaneurysms. These haemodynamic changes are also present in patients with secondary polycythaemia and in the group of benign erythrocytosis where red cell mass is increased without change in leucocytes and platelets (Modan, 1971).

It is not surprising in a disease characterised by increased viscosity, slowed blood flow, and often by thrombocytosis that vascular symptoms are prominent. In the large series of Chievitz and Thiede (1962) 63 per cent of patients suffered some form of thrombosis of which cerebral thrombosis comprised more than half. In 15 per cent of patients cerebral thrombosis was the cause of death and cerebral haemorrhage accounted for a further 4 per cent.

The Mayo Clinic group (Millikan, Siekert, and Whisnant, 1960) first drew attention to the minor symptoms of cerebral vascular insufficiency which may precede a stroke. Twenty-two polycythaemic patients were described having transient symptoms in either the vertebrobasilar or carotid territory (including retina) and with no evidence of other provoking features such as hypotension or arterial degeneration. The attacks were relieved by control of the polycythaemia. In the large review of Silverstein, Gilbert, and Wasserman (1962) transient symptoms of this kind occurred in one-tenth of polycythaemic patients in the following order of frequency: headaches (41 per cent), vertigo (30 per cent), paraesthesiae (15 per cent), visual symptoms (11 per cent).

It is equally common, however, for patients to present with a completed stroke due to cerebral thrombosis or a progressive stroke due to intracerebral or subdural haematoma. A fluctuating dementia, confusional state, or a choreic syndrome due to multiple small vessel occlusions in the cortex and basal ganglia are also recorded.

The life expectancy and the occurrence of further cerebral vascular episodes is favourably influenced by treatment, either by repeated venesection or by radioactive phosphorus (Harman and Leslie, 1967; Lawrence, Berlin, and Huff, 1953).

Sickle cell disease

A recent study of the cerebral vascular complications in sickle cell disease (haemoglobin type SS) (Portnoy and Herion, 1972) showed that 25 per cent of patients experienced one or more strokes during a five year period. This compared with an incidence of 5 per cent in sickle haemoglobin C disease and 1.7 per cent in sickle cell trait. Many of the affected patients were young, over half under the age of 15 years, and the youngest being aged 2 years. The underlying pathology was occlusion of cerebral arteries by sickled erythrocytes. The vessels showed some endothelial hyperplasia and frequent perivascular haemorrhages but no thrombi were seen. There were ischaemic infarcts of various sizes and numerous small areas of cortical necrosis.

The commonest clinical syndrome was hemiparesis, but seizures, transient uniocular blindness, subarachnoid haemorrhage, acute psychosis, and ocular motor palsy were also recorded. One-third of the hemiplegic patients made a complete recovery, one-third improved but were left with a residual deficit, one-third showed no improvement or died. Anaesthesia and angiography carry an added risk in patients with sickle cell disease. Abnormal carotid angiograms have been reported in the form of partial or complete occlusion of the internal carotid artery or its major branches (Stockman et al., 1972). Repeated studies may show progressive narrowing of the supraclinoid carotid artery with the development of an extensive collateral circulation of moya-moya type.

Thrombotic thrombocytopenia purpura

Thrombotic thrombocytopenia purpura is a rare disease occurring at any age, in which many systemic arteries and capillaries are occluded by homogeneous eosinophilic material, possibly fibrin. Platelet deposition occurs on damaged endothelium. The clinical features are haemolytic anaemia, thrombocytopenia, fever, and renal involvement. Symptoms relating to the central nervous system are present in 90 per cent of patients and form the principal complaint in 47 to 60 per cent (Silverstein, 1968). The onset is usually acute and the course rapid and progressive, but fluctuating or remittent cases may occur.

Pathologically there are numerous small cerebral infarcts and petechial haemorrhages. Less commonly there may be larger areas of haemorrhage and occlusion of major cerebral vessels, or cerebral embolism from endocardial vegetation (Jones and Sim, 1961). The neurological features may be generalised (such as coma, confusional state, or seizures) or focal (such as hemiparesis, dysphasia, hemisensory loss, visual field defect). The cerebrospinal fluid may be normal or show increased protein content; electroencephalography is diffusely abnormal.

Improvement has been claimed following intensive corticosteroid treatment with or without splenectomy. Exchange transfusion with fresh blood combined with high dose heparin treatment has also been advocated (Rubenstein, 1959).

Macroglobulinaemia

Waldenstrom's macroglobulinaemia is a rare chronic disease of late adult life, characterised by anaemia, a haemorrhagic tendency, lymphadenopathy, and hepatosplenomegaly. There is a relative lymphocytosis and thrombocytopenia in the peripheral blood and the bone marrow is infiltrated with plasma cells. Marked elevation of serum globulin and erythrocyte sedimentation rate is present. Abnormal protein may be detected in the blood before overt signs of disease appear (Matzke, Clausen, and Guttier, 1964). The relatively slow progression, the absence of osteolytic bone lesions, and the rarity of urinary Bence-Jones protein distinguish the condition from myelomatosis. Life expectancy is 2 to 10 years from diagnosis (Logothetis, Silverstein, and Coe, 1960).

About one-quarter of patients have evidence of central nervous system vascular complications at any time from a few months to two years after the onset. The symptoms usually suggest intermittent ischaemia of vertebrobasilar type with fluctuating vertigo, gait ataxia, leg weakness, dysarthria, and hemiparesis. Other patients present an encephalitic syndrome with seizures, headache, organic psychosis, and clouding of consciousness without localising signs (Nutter and Kramer, 1965). A third type presents earlier in the course of the disease with subarachnoid or intracerebral haemorrhage (Cohen, Bohannon,

and Wallerstein, 1966).

Intermittent blurring of vision is noticed by one-third of patients and is caused by reduced retinal perfusion. Marked retinal venous dilatation and scattered haemorrhages are a constant finding (McCollister et al., 1967).

Many of these features can be explained by overall reduction in cerebral blood flow with its maximum effect in the vertebrobasilar territory. Cerebrovascular resistance is markedly increased due to an increased blood viscosity and exceeds the regulatory reserves of cerebral vasodilatation. This explanation is supported by the rapid improvement in symptoms and retinal appearances which follows plasmophoresis. Pathological vessel changes are inconspicuous but there may be some perivascular infiltration in brain and meninges and multiple intracerebral zones of haemorrhage (Logothetis et al., 1960). Treatment with chlorambucil is beneficial in the majority of patients (McCollister et al., 1967).

Other blood diseases

When **severe anaemia** is combined with cerebral arterial disease the oxygen carrying capacity of the blood may occasionally be reduced to a degree which may provoke episodes of transient ischaemia, affecting carotid or more commonly vertebrobasilar territories. Restoration of haemoglobin levels to normal may abolish the attacks. This simple and remediable cause of cerebral ischaemia is often overlooked (Siekert, Whisnant, and Millikan, 1960).

Cerebrovascular complications in the form of large and small intracerebral haemorrhages are found in 50 per cent of children dying from **acute leukaemia** and in many they are the cause of death. Leukaemic intracerebral infiltration is rare and in most cases the haemorrhage is due to thrombocytopenia (Groch, Sayre, and Heck, 1960).

In **primary thrombocytosis**, a rare disease of childhood, there is widespread vascular thrombosis and infarction including myocardium and brain. An onset with hemiparesis, cortical blindness, and confusion is recorded (Spach, Howell, and Harris, 1963).

CARDIAC EMBOLISM

The occurrence of stroke in a patient unlikely to have disease of the cerebral arteries should always direct attention to the heart as a possible source of embolism. Pathological studies show that 20 per cent of systemic arterial emboli derived from the heart are carried to the cerebral circulation (Darling, Austen and Linton, 1967). A large embolus may lodge at the carotid bifurcation or the terminal internal carotid. Most smaller emboli enter the middle cerebral artery occluding the main trunk or one of its branches (Lhermitte, Gautier, and Poirier, 1968). Emboli composed of thrombus may be displaced distally down the arterial tree and may disappear entirely as a result of lysis or organisation (Dalal, Shali, and Aiyer, 1965). Pathologically no occlusion may be found in the regional artery, but fragments of thrombus may be visible in small vessels within the infarct, which tends to be haemorrhagic in type (Adams, 1950).

There are certain clinical features which point to cardiac embolism as a cause of stroke, although in many cases the distinction from cerebral thrombosis cannot be made with certainty. Of first importance is the finding of heart disease (Table 14.1) and the detection of signs of major or minor embolism in other organs such as the retina, fingernails, spleen, kidney, or skin. Of lesser importance are the features of the stroke itself. The majority occur during waking hours and have an onset which is more abrupt than in other varieties of stroke reaching a maximum disability within a few seconds or minutes. A focal or generalised seizure (12 per cent) or loss of consciousness (28 per cent) occurring at the onset is also a pointer towards embolism (Wells, 1959).

Premonitory symptoms in the days or hours before the stroke are experienced by 16 per cent of patients either in the form of minor ischaemic attacks or localised headache. The latter may be due to an embolus lodged at the carotid bifurcation (Wells, 1961). Recurrent episodes are also a characteristic of most types of embolism and various arterial territories may be involved at different times.

Table 14.1 A comparison of the cardiovascular features of thrombotic versus embolic cerebral vascular occlusions[a].

	Thrombotic group (42%)	Embolic group (37%)
Cardiac failure	13.5%	33.3%
Myocardial infarction	24.3	42.4
Valvular disease	21.6	30.3
Atrial fibrillation	32.3	82.1
Other severe arrhythmias	16.1	7.1
Lone atrial fibrillation	6.4	25.0
Endocardial thrombi	0	45.5
Systemic arterial occlusion	18.9	36.4
Extensive atherosclerosis	78.4	57.6

[a]Seventy-nine patients from unselected autopsy series of Jorgensen and Torvik (1966).

Rheumatic heart disease

The small fibrin platelet vegetations which form on the valves during acute rheumatic carditis rarely cause clinical symptoms; occasional patients develop occlusion of the central retinal artery (Hearn and Roper-Hall, 1961). However, in chronic rheumatic endocarditis many patients notice transient uniocular attacks of visual loss probably as a result of retinal embolism with fibrin platelet clumps dislodged from scarred heart valves (Swash and Earl, 1970). Transient ischaemic attacks affecting the brain, in either the carotid or vertebrobasilar territories, are present in 14 per cent of patients (Hutchinson and Stock, 1963). Micro-embolism again probably accounts for the majority of these.

Intracardiac thrombus in chronic rheumatic heart disease secondary to involvement of the mitral valve is responsible for a large proportion of fatal cerebral emboli although the frequency may be declining (Darling, Austen, and Linton, 1967). In a recent large series of cardiac emboli the proportion due to this cause was 30 per cent (Torvik and Jörgensen, 1966). In 97 per cent of the rheumatic group there was a mitral valve lesion, usually stenotic, and in 90 per cent atrial fibrillation was present. All patients had one or other of these two features.

Although some patients are in cardiac failure at the time of embolism, a greater number are in good health and many are symptomless. When atrial fibrillation is present it is usually of long-standing and in only a few cases is there any relationship to changing cardiac rhythm (Daley *et al.*, 1951). Approximately half the episodes of systemic embolism which are detected clinically involve the cerebral circulation but many visceral and limb emboli may escape notice. As in other forms of embolism, recurrent episodes are the rule; 60 per cent of patients experience further episodes, mostly during the first six months. After two years the risk of recurrence appears to decline. Anticoagulant treatment significantly reduces the risk of recurrence and may also improve the prognosis in recovery from the initial stroke (Carter, 1965).

Endocarditis

Bacterial endocarditis appears to be changing its clinical characteristics; the acute form of the disease with large vegetations capable of blocking major cerebral arteries is now rarely seen. Subacute bacterial endocarditis in its turn has been influenced by antibiotics and by improved dental hygiene, and streptococcus viridans is giving way to enterococcus and to other less common organisms such as yeast, fungi, histoplasma, and rickettsiae. Endocarditis is also becoming commoner in elderly patients (Anderson and Staffurth, 1955).

Cerebrovascular complications of various types are the presenting feature in 20 to 40 per cent of patients. A meningoencephalitic illness, with drowsiness, headache, impaired concentration, vertigo, and irritability and with nuchal rigidity is common. The cerebrospinal fluid may be normal or meningitic and culture is sterile. Various cranial nerve palsies, central retinal artery occlusion, dyskinesias with tremor, rigidity, or chorea are also recorded. Micro-emboli causing multiple occlusions of small intracerebral arteries combined with low grade infection are responsible (Ziment, 1969).

Acute stroke is an uncommon presentation but a frequent complication of the established disease. The infected embolus may be large enough to occlude a major cerebral artery causing an ischaemic infarction. The stroke is often preceded by TIA and is easily mistaken for the effect of degenerative arterial disease (Siekert and Jones, 1970). Less commonly a mycotic aneurysm may rupture causing subarachnoid, intracerebral, or ventricular haemorrhage. Mycotic aneurysms may be suspected from the angiographic appearances since they are often multiple and situated on peripheral parts of the arteries (Roach and Drake, 1965).

As acute endocarditis declines, abacterial or **marantic endocarditis** increases in frequency. Friable thrombotic vegetations form on the cardiac valves, most commonly the mitral (60 per cent), the aortic (12 per cent), or both, and when detached they may be carried to the brain to occlude a small, or rarely a major, cerebral artery (Rosen and Armstrong, 1973). Cardiac murmurs are inconspicuous and may be absent.

The condition is usually a terminal event in advanced malignant or wasting diseases and thrombosis may also involve the venous side of the circulation. Pancreatic and gastric carcinomas and bronchial carcinomas are particularly prone to this condition and the mechanism is thought to be a hypercoagulable state. It is proposed that mucus or some other product of tumour cells is released into the circulation where it acts as a tissue thromboplastin initiating intravascular coagulation.

Ischaemic heart disease

Ischaemic heart disease is an increasingly common cause of systemic embolism. Myocardial infarction was found in 22 per cent of a large series of systemic emboli (Darling, Austen, and Linton, 1967) and in 42 per cent of a series of cerebral emboli (Torvik and Jörgensen, 1966) (Table 14.1).

Embolism is strongly correlated with the presence of intracardiac thrombus which forms on the endocardium of the left ventricle over a region of recent infarction. Pathological studies show that one-third of patients who show intracardiac thrombus at autopsy also have evidence of systemic embolism. Clinically the great majority of embolic episodes occur 4 to 12 days following myocardial infarction although recurrence of embolism may continue for up to six months. One-third of patients have atrial fibrillation. The recurrence rate is significantly reduced by anticoagulants (Carter, 1965).

The fact that cerebral arterial occlusion also occurs frequently in patients with healed myocardial infarction is probably a reflection of widespread atheromatous disease rather than due to continuing embolism.

Other types of heart disease

Systemic embolism may be encountered in other types of heart disease and in such patients a cerebral embolus is often the terminal event. Isolated atrial fibrillation without valvular disease or myocardial infarction has been found in as many as 25 per cent of patients dying of systemic embolism (Table 14.1). Widespread atherosclerosis and cardiac failure are contributary factors in many cases. It is notable that atrial fibrillation occurring with thyrotoxic heart disease rarely causes embolism.

Primary myocardial disease comprises a group of disorders of diverse aetiology but with common clinical characteristics consisting of cardiac failure with cardiomegaly, various arrhythmias, cardiac and other chest pain, and recurrent systemor or pulmonary embolism. Specific types may be caused by infections (e.g. viral or protozoan) toxic (e.g. emitine), infiltrative (e.g. amyloid disease), avitaminosis (e.g. thiamine deficiency) and alcoholic cardiomyopathy. Neuromuscular disorders such as progressive muscular dystrophy, including Duchenne and myotonic types or Friedreich's ataxia, are also recorded (Holt and Lambert, 1964). Finally there is a large idiopathic group including endomyocardial fibrosis and African cardiomyopathy.

In all these conditions mural thrombus may form either on the right or left side of the heart and result in pulmonary or systemic embolism. The prevalence of embolism in the idiopathic group (8 per cent) is greater than in the specific group (4 per cent) (Segal, Harvey, and Gurel, 1965).

Cardiac myxoma deserves special attention because of the possibility of radical cure. It is a rare condition usually affecting young women and presents as refractory cardiac failure, constitutional disturbance, or embolism. The cardiac failure is due to the obstructive tumour in the left atrium causing fluctuating cardiac murmurs, rhythm changes, and pulmonary oedema. Constitutional effects include fever, anaemia, raised sedimentation rate, and hyperglobulinaemia. Emboli occur in 50 per cent of patients and are due to blockage of small arteries with myxomatous tissue or thrombus (Goodwin, 1963). Local invasion of the artery wall may produce pseudoaneurysms and fatal haemorrhage (Price et al., 1970). Echocardiography is useful as a diagnostic screening test.

Postoperative systemic embolism is a major hazard after **cardiac valve replacement**, emboli to the cerebral and coronary arteries being the commonest in terms of death and disability. With earlier types of valve prosthesis the frequency was 25 to 30 per cent, but this has progressively declined, partly as a result of effective anticoagulant treatment but more significantly as a result of changes in valve design. Of these, covering of the metal parts of the valve with Dacron or Teflon is the most important. In earlier reports it was claimed that consistent prolongation of prothrombin time resulted in better control of embolism (Friedli et al., 1971). There was no agreement as to whether patients in atrial fibrillation were more at risk. The incidence of emboli decreased in the third and fourth year after operation. Some workers found the addition of an antiplatelet agent such as dipyridamole to the standard anticoagulant regime gave improved results (Sullivan, Harken, and Gorlin, 1968).

More recent experience shows that the incidence of embolism with a cloth-covered aortic valve is so low that the hazard of long-term anticoagulants exceeds the benefit. In aortic valve replacement only a few weeks of anticoagulant treatment are now recommended and aspirin or dipyridamole are used thereafter. In the case of the mitral valve long-term anticoagulants still seem to be of value (Isom et al., 1973).

METABOLIC DISORDERS

Diabetes mellitus

The effect of diabetes on the occurrence of ischaemic vascular symptoms during life and on arterial pathology after death has long been a matter for debate; for many years it was held that degenerative vascular disease was no different in diabetics and non-diabetics. More recently it has been conclusively shown in a population study that ischaemic symptoms occur at a significantly younger age in diabetics than in a matched control group, and that the probability of ischaemic symptoms is related to the blood sugar level (Keen *et al.*, 1965). It is also established that the mortality from occlusive vascular disease is twice as high in diabetics as non-diabetics (Entmacher, Root, and Marks, 1964) and that the prevalence at autopsy of cerebral infarction and lacunar infarction (focal encephalomalacia) is significantly greater in the brains of diabetics than in others (Alex *et al.*, 1962). On the other hand cerebral haemorrhage does not show any increased prevalence at autopsy and hypertension occurs with significantly greater frequency only in diabetics over the age of 70 (Freedman, Moulton, and Spencer, 1958).

The occlusive vascular changes fall into two groups, those affecting large arteries and those affecting small arterioles and capillaries; it is the second group which accounts for the increased incidence of vascular disease (Alex *et al.*, 1962). The large vessel changes are those of atheroma and are non-specific; the small arterioles throughout the body and including the brain show patchy hyalinization with accumulation of PAS-positive material in the subintimal zone and with variable amount of fibrous and cellular proliferation. Capillaries show thickening of the basement membrane (Warren, Le Compte, and Legg, 1966).

Large vessel atheroma and thrombosis lead to regions of cerebral infarction in the territories of the major arteries, usually the internal carotid and middle cerebral arteries. Microangiopathy affecting the small intracerebral arteries of the striate system and cortical penetrating arteries produce small deep areas of infarction and encephalomalacia (lacunes) similar to those found in hypertensive and senile brains.

The symptomatology of these lesions is described elsewhere (see Chapter 10). Microangiopathy also affects the vasa nervorum of the cranial nerves and is responsible for the occurrence of oculomotor or abducens palsy in diabetic subjects (Asbury *et al.*, 1970). There is focal demyelination of a segment of the oculomotor nerve in the region of the cavernous sinus, and hyalinization (which need not block the vessel completely) of the vasa nervorum arising from the internal carotid and other large arteries. The palsy characteristically spares the pupil and recovers completely in a few weeks without faulty regeneration.

The management of established cerebral vascular disease in diabetic patients consists of optimal control of hyperglycaemia and body weight in an attempt to retard the progress of vascular degeneration. In obese diabetics with hyperlipaemia fat is restricted as well as carbohydrate and saturated fats are replaced by unsaturated. If the lipid abnormality persists in spite of weight and diabetic control the type of hyperlipidaemia is determined and specific therapy given. Hypertension and extracranial arterial stenotic lesions are treated as in the non-diabetic patient.

HOMOCYSTINAEMIA

Homocystinaemia is a rare inborn error of metabolism due to a deficiency of the enzyme cystathionine synthase. Homocystine accumulates in plasma and tissues and may be detected in the urine. The main features are ectopia of the lens, a moderate degree of mental defect, and skeletal deformities. There is a strong tendency to progressive cardiovascular disease and a high incidence of thromboembolism which may occur within the first year of life. One-third of patients die before the age of 30 (Carson, Dent, and Field, 1965).

Pathological changes affect arteries of all sizes and include medial degeneration, intimal fibrosis, and hyperplasia. Thrombosis is frequent and may occlude the carotid artery (Schimke *et al.*, 1965).

Experimental homocystinaemia in animals causes loss of vascular endothelium, a rise in platelet consumption, and thrombosis, and it is suggested that arterial thrombi are secondary to endothelial injury. It has been shown that a reduction in plasma homocystin by pyridoxin stops the excessive consumption of platelets. Dipyridamole has the same effect (Harker *et al.*, 1974).

Hyperlipaemia

Although there is strong evidence from prospective studies that subjects with elevated serum cholesterol are at increased risk from myocardial infarction, the association between lipid levels and stroke is less definite. The Framingham prospective study showed that an elevated serum cholesterol carried a slightly increased risk of brain infarction only in men under the age of 50 (see Chapter 1). When combined with other risk factors, cholesterol levels may become more significant.

Many reports of lipid levels in patients with established cerebrovascular disease have been published although most can be criticised on the grounds of varying diagnostic criteria, lack of homogeneity, imperfectly matched control groups, and arbitrary limits of lipid normality. Most workers have found no difference in cholesterol levels between patients with any type of cerebrovascular disease and controls (Meyer *et al.*, 1959; Cumings *et al.*, 1967; Ballantyne *et al.*, 1974). On the other hand Heyman, Nefzger, and Estes (1961), who studied a stroke group including patients with hypertension, heart disease, and diabetes, found a significant elevation of serum cholesterol compared with a healthy control group. The mean cholesterol level for all patients was 227 mg per 100 ml and for controls 205 mg per 100 ml.

In recent years lipid abnormalities other than cholesterol have also been included. Jakobsen (1967) found no difference between 52 patients and controls with respect to cholesterol or triglycerides although lipid levels in the controls were unusually high.

Fogelholm & Aho (1973) studied 213 patients under 50 with cerebral infarction most of whom had angiography. They showed a significant rise in triglycerides in men between 40 and 50 and in women between 30 and 50. The group contained an excess of young women some taking the contraceptive pill, a factor known to increase triglyceride levels.

Definite conclusions must await the results of further studies, but the present consensus is that of the two main types, pre-beta lipoproteinaemia, having markedly elevated triglycerides and a modest increase in cholesterol, shows the stronger link with premature peripheral vascular disease including stroke. Patients in this group also have an increasing incidence of heart disease but not as great as in beta lipoproteinaemia (hypercholesterolaemia). There is no explanation for the lesser correlation between hypercholesterolaemia and stroke except that coronary artery disease develops at a younger age, and that in cerebral arterial disease hypertension predominates as a risk factor. It should be noted that a patient with hypercholesterolaemia may either be at the upper end of a normal distribution curve or may be a heterozygote for familial hypercholesterolaemia, two conditions which may carry a different prognosis.

There are a number of dietary or drug regimes which can reduce elevated blood lipids and it is customary to advise treatment for patients with established disease. At present there is little evidence that reducing blood lipids will reduce existing arterial lesions or symptoms (Acheson and Hutchinson, 1972) although skin xanthomata and hard retinal exudates may become smaller.

For pre-beta lipoproteinaemia reductions of lipid level ranging from 10 to 50 per cent may be achieved by diet and clofibrate, which decreases hepatic synthesis and increases faecal excretion of cholesterol.

For beta lipoproteinaemia, cholestyramine, which increases the faecal excretion of bile acids, is used with or without restriction of dietary saturated fat and cholesterol. Younger relatives should be screened for lipid abnormality since in them preventative treatment is more likely to be effective.

INHERITED DISORDERS
OF CONNECTIVE TISSUE

In **pseudoxanthoma elasticum**, characteristic skin lesions are found in association with amblyopia, gastrointestinal haemorrhage, coronary, peripheral, and cerebral vascular disorders. Patches of loose wrinkled skin are found on the neck or flexural folds. The retina shows dark angioid streaks radiating from the disc, and pigmentary and haemorrhagic lesions at the macula lead to progressive visual loss. The retinal appearances are caused by degeneration in Bruch's membrane and similar change affects the media and internal elastic laminae of muscular arteries throughout the body (Robertson and Schroder, 1959). Patients with pseudoxanthoma may have hypertension, widening of the aorta, aneurysm formation, or medial calcification. They may present as cerebral or subarachnoid haemorrhage (Dixon, 1951).

Ehlers Danlos syndrome is an uncommon disorder of connective tissue possibly due to a defect in collagen fibres. The main features are fragile and hyperextensible skin and subcutaneous tissue, abnormal mobility of joints, and bleeding disorders. Inheritance is usually of autosomal dominant type. Affected subjects are liable to dissection of the aorta, rupture of arteries, and gastrointestinal haemorrhage (Beighton, 1970).

The cerebral arteries may be involved and patients are reported with multiple intracranial aneurysm and subarachnoid haemorrhage (Rubenstein and Cohen, 1964). There is also a tendency to spontaneous caroticocavernous fistula presenting as pulsating exophthalmos (Graf, 1965). Because of fragility of the arterial walls carotid angiography carries an increased risk in this condition.

The **Marfan syndrome** is a related disorder of mesenchymal development having its main expression in the cardiovascular and musculoskeletal systems. The commonest mode of inheritance is autosomal dominant. Affected arteries show fragmentation of the elastic elements with distortion and degeneration of muscle fibres, replacement fibrosis, and accumulation of pools of mucoid metachromatic material within the wall.

Skeletal features include arachnodactyly, funnel deformity of the chest, high-arched palate and increased joint mobility (Parish, 1960). Cardiovascular abnormalities are present in 25 per cent of cases and are very varied, the commonest being aortic dilatation, dissecting aneurysm, aortic reflux, dilatation of the pulmonary artery, atrial septal defect, cardiac dysrhythmias, and dextroversion (Sinclair, Kitchin, and Turner, 1960). Coarctation of the aorta is also an associated feature and these patients may present with subarachnoid haemorrhage from an aneurysm of the Circle of Willis.

The chief importance of the syndrome is as a cause of aneurysmal enlargement or dissection of the extracranial carotid arteries affecting external, common, or internal segments (McKusick, 1966). Such cases have been treated surgically (Hardin, 1962).

Angiokeratoma corporis diffusum (Fabry's disease) is a rare familial disorder characterised by vascular cutaneous lesions, progressive renal disease, and paroxysmal attacks of severe pain in the extremities (Wise *et al.*, 1962). Cerebral vessels are also affected and show deposits of glycolipid in the media of small arteries in the leptomeninges. Larger arteries are dilated. There are scattered small areas of infarction in hemisphere and brain stem (Kahn, 1973). Cerebral vascular symptoms and renal failure occur in the third to fifth decade.

Neurocutaneous syndromes

Under this heading are included a group of inherited developmental anomalies of brain, skin, and retina, some associated with mental retardation. In **neurofibromatosis** (von Recklinghausen's disease) symptoms due to vascular disease are exceptionally rare, but carotid angiography may show vascular dysplasia with alternating segments of stenosis and dilatation (Hilal, 1974). Occlusion may affect the internal carotid artery.

In **Sturge Weber syndrome** (encephalotrigeminal angiomatosis) a port wine naevus over the face is associated with failure of development of the underlying brain. Although earlier reports showed no intracerebral vascular abnormality modern angiography can detect an abnormality in small arteries, capillaries, and veins in about 50 per cent of patients. The most frequent finding is capillary-venous telangiectasia with increased density of the capillary bed but no abnormality of larger vessels. Occlusion or dysplasia of branches of the peripheral leptomeningeal arteries may also occur. Large arteriovenous angiomas are excessively rare (Poser and Taveras, 1957). Occasionally the facial naevus may fill from the internal carotid artery. Cerebral calcification occurs in 60 per cent of patients.

Patients with **tuberose sclerosis** may also show excessive tortuosity affecting intracranial arteries with segments of stenosis and ectasia (Hilal, 1974).

IATROGENIC ARTERIAL DISEASE

Oral contraceptives

An association between oral contraceptive agents and the development of cerebral infarction has been suspected since 1965 (Illis et al., 1965), when an increase was noted in the number of strokes occurring in young women. Bickerstaff and Holmes (1967) found a five-fold increase in the incidence of stroke in this group of patients in their practice after 1964 when the use of contraceptives became widespread. Further retrospective studies established a definite statistical link between venous thromboembolism and oral contraceptives (Inman and Vessey, 1968), and the collaborative group for the study of stroke in young women (1973) has recently issued its findings in a group of 598 women aged 15 to 44 with cerebral vascular disease compared with age-matched pairs. Women on oral contraceptives were found to have a nine-fold increased risk of cerebral thromboembolism and a slightly increased risk of cerebral haemorrhage. Cigarette smoking was also much more prevalent in the stroke group. It appears that the thrombotic tendency is related to the oestrogen content of the preparation (Inman et al., 1970).

The pathogenesis is not yet clear; a number of coagulation changes have been shown to follow oestrogen ingestion including a rise in plasma antiplasmin, plasmogen, and fibrinogen and a decrease in serum antithrombin activity (Howie et al., 1970). Platelet adhesiveness also increases (Caspary and Peberdy, 1965).

There are no specific clinical features which distinguish this type of stroke (Heyman et al., 1969). Angiography may show occlusion of the internal carotid artery or a major cerebral branch and the appearances often suggest embolism rather than thrombosis in situ (Enzell and Lindemalm, 1973). The arteries do not appear unduly atheromatous and it is suggested that emboli may originate in the pulmonary veins. The increased incidence of haemorrhagic as distinct from thrombotic cerebrovascular disease may possibly be related to the effect of oral contraceptives in raising blood pressure (Weir et al., 1971).

DRUG ADDICTION

A link between chronic drug abuse and cerebral angiitis has been proposed. Citron and colleagues (1970) published 14 fatal cases showing widespread fibrinoid vascular necrosis with thrombosis in many cerebral arteries. Intracerebral arteries are the most affected and show irregular constriction and dilatation (Lognelli and Buchhert, 1971). It is not clear which of many drugs are responsible.

EFFECT OF IRRADIATION

There are a number of reports of damage to blood vessels following the therapeutic use of X-rays and such changes have also been produced experimentally.

The immediate changes of exposure of cerebral tissue to X-rays are an acute inflammatory vasculitis and meningitis with neuronal damage. After a latent period of 7 to 12 months further proliferative changes become evident in vascular tissues and in astrocytes. The small arteries appear to show the greatest change, notably a marked fibrinoid infiltration of the subintima and various degrees of cellular infiltration with lipid containing histiocytes. Fragmentation of elastic tissue, fibrosis, mural thrombosis, and recanalisation are also evident. Large arteries including carotid and aorta also show inflammatory changes or fibrosis. Some of the cerebral changes are undoubtedly a result of multiple vascular occlusions, but these are thought unlikely to account for all the damage, which shows a predilection for subcortical white matter in brain stem and spinal cord in a pattern not seen in vascular disease (Fig. 14.6).

The clinical presentation results from the combined effects of irradiation necrosis of the brain and blood vessels; affected patients have usually been irradiated for pituitary tumour (Peck and McGovern, 1966) or lymphoma (Zeman, 1968). A specifically vascular presentation is unusual. A recent report describes a patient who developed, six months after cobalt treatment for Hodgkin's disease, transient ischaemic attacks followed by a stroke. Foam cell arteritis and multiple ischaemic areas were found at autopsy and the terminal carotid and its main branches showed irregular narrowing (Kagan, Bruce, and Di Chiro, 1971).

OTHER VARIETIES OF CEREBRAL VASCULAR DISEASE

Migraine

This is not the place to consider in detail the pathogenesis of migraine. However, there is ample clinical evidence to show that the pain arises in arteries, mainly those of the external carotid system. During the headache, when the patient is frequently pale, the superficial temporal artery may be seen to be engorged and tender, and pressure on the artery or over the carotid artery in the neck relieves the pain for a short time. Later in the attack the artery and surrounding tissue feel thickened and oedematous.

The prodromal visual symptoms of classical migraine, which consist of coloured shimmering jagged crescents starting near the fixation point and slowly expanding into one half-field, probably arise in the occipital cortex and are rarely encountered in other forms of arterial disease.

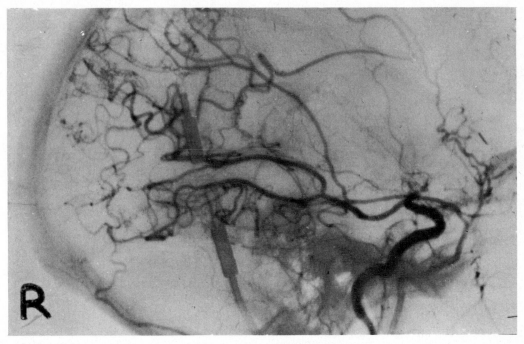

Fig. 14.6   Irradiation arteritis: extensive occlusion of branches of the middle cerebral artery following irradiation of a craniopharyngioma of the third ventricle. Extensive collateral circulation linking posterior and middle cerebral artery territories.

It has now been confirmed that arterial narrowing and a regional reduction in blood flow occurs during the migrainous aura (Skinhøj and Paulson, 1969).

These changes are often ascribed to vascular spasm, but a transient oedema of the arterial wall affecting both internal and external carotid systems is an alternative explanation. At the onset of an attack there is an increase in plasma serotonin which falls rapidly as the headache develops (Anthony, Hinterberger, and Lance, 1968). In a susceptible subject an injection of reserpine, which reduces plasma serotonin, will provoke an attack and this can be relieved by a further injection of intravenous serotonin (Kemball, Friedman, and Vallejo, 1960).

Various complications of migraine may be encountered and require to be distinguished from more serious forms of vascular disease. In hemiplegic migraine the headache is succeeded by an episode of hemiparesis with or without dysphasia which clears slowly and completely over 4 to 10 days. The diagnosis can be made with confidence only when there is a history of a previous attack affecting one or other side and in such a case arteriography is best avoided. There is usually a strong family history of the disorder (Whitty, 1953).

In ophthalmoplegic migraine the headache is succeeded by a third or sixth nerve palsy clearing over some weeks, sometimes leaving a residual cycloplegia. As in hemiplegic migraine, the patient is usually a child or young adult with a past and family history of similar headaches. The cause of the ophthalmoplegia is thought to be oedema of the cavernous portion of the carotid artery and a narrowed segment may be seen angiographically (Walsh and O'Doherty, 1960). In rare instances complete vascular occlusion may occur during a migraine attack leaving a permanent residual deficit. This has been recorded in the retina (Graveson, 1949), in the optic nerve (McDonald and Sanders, 1971), and in the middle cerebral artery (Fisher, 1971), but

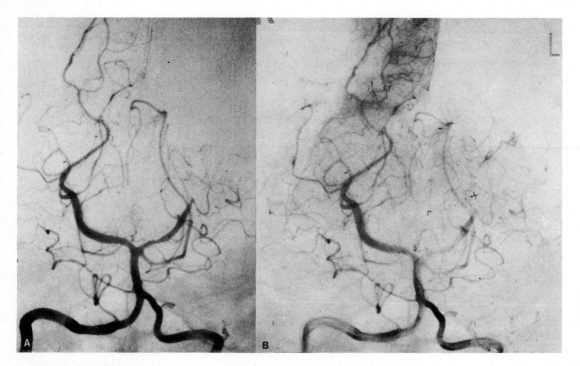

Fig. 14.7A   Occlusion of the left posterior cerebral artery after a severe migraine attack.
Fig. 14.7B   Delayed capillary filling in the posterior cerebral territory.

is commonest in the posterior cerebral artery where the main trunk or one of its branches such as the calcarine artery may be occluded (Fig. 14.7A and 14.7B). Sometimes no occlusion is visible but there is reduced capillary perfusion in a localised area (Kaul *et al.*, 1974). The defect in the visual field is a homonymous paracentral scotoma extending close to the fixation point. Central visual acuity is usually spared (Poliak, 1957). By contrast no angiographic occlusion has been found in those patients who developed a permanent hemiplegia during an attack of migraine (Fisher, 1971). Other instances of permanent hemisphere or brain stem infarction occurring in migrainous patients are recorded by Connor (1962).

Stroke related to pregnancy or the puerperium; occult thromboembolism

The development of an acute hemiplegia in the last four weeks of pregnancy or in the puerperium is well recorded but until recently was regarded as invariably due to cerebral venous thrombosis. Recent studies show that the majority of such cases are arterial in origin.

Cross, Castro, and Jennett (1968) described 31 such patients of whom 16 were pregnant (mostly in the third trimester) and the remainder puerperal (most from 1 to 16 days post partum). All had a hemiplegia and six had seizures. More than half the patients had occlusion of a major cerebral artery, internal carotid, or middle cerebral, shown at angiography or autopsy. Three fatal cases showed no significant arterial disease, source of embolism, or venous occlusion (Adams and Graham, 1967).

A further 21 patients were recorded by Fisher (1971). Some patients had clinical evidence of migraine or thrombophlebitis. One third of puerperal patients showed an arterial occlusion or stenosis. All angiograms on pregnant patients were normal.

The aetiology of this type of cerebral occlusive disease is unknown. It does not seem to be due to premature atherosclerosis, hyperlipaemia, or inflammatory arterial disease but to an abnormal tendency to thrombosis. By analogy with the thrombogenic effect of contraceptive medication it is suggested that increased levels of oestrogen may be responsible, but if this were true it is curious that no marked increase in cerebrovascular disease has been noted in male patients receiving oestrogen therapy for prostatic carcinoma.

It must not be forgotten that quite apart from the special risks of pregnancy and contraceptive medication a small group of premenopausal women present with occlusive cerebrovascular disease often involving the internal carotid artery or its middle cerebral branch (Illis *et al.*, 1965). They do not show coronary artery disease but may develop venous thrombi or thrombi in peripheral systemic arteries. Some may be examples of **paradoxical embolism** which is probably commoner than generally realised since 28 per cent of hearts have a potential route of right to left shunt via an unclosed foramen ovale (Johnson, 1951). Any condition such as pulmonary embolism which may raise the pressure in the right atrium to a level where the interatrial pressure gradient is reversed may cause shunting, and venous thrombi from the iliac or femoral veins may pass into the systemic arterial circulation. Septal defects of this kind can be closed surgically.

Occult embolism from a source of thrombosis in the heart or in the aorta (Fisher, 1971) also accounts for some puzzling cases of cerebral vascular occlusion in whom a diagnosis may only be reached after angiocardiography and arch aortography.

Patients with repeated minor episodes in whom no underlying abnormality, either cardiovascular, haematological, or hormonal, can be discovered are often treated with anticoagulants with cessation of attacks in some instances (Fisher, 1971). A history of heavy cigarette smoking is often present, and in the present state of knowledge it is advisable to proscribe the cigarette habit entirely in patients of either sex with occult cerebrovascular disease.

REFERENCES

Acheson, J. & Hutchinson, E. C. (1972) Controlled trial of clofibrate in cerebral vascular disease. *Atherosclerosis*, **15**, 177.

Adams, J. H. & Graham, D. I. (1967) Twelve cases of fatal cerebral infarction due to arterial occlusion in the absence of atheromatous stenosis or embolism. *Journal of Neurology, Neurosurgery and Psychiatry*, **30**, 479.

Adams, R. D. (1950) Observations on brain embolism with special reference to the mechanism of haemorrhagic infarction. *Journal of Clinical Investigation*, **29**, 795.

Alajouanine, T., Le Beau, J. & Houdart, R. (1948) La symptomologie tumorale des volumineux aneurysmes des arteres vertebrales et basilaires. *Revue Neurologique*, **80**, 321.

Alex, M., Baron, E. K., Goldenberg, S. & Blumenthal, H. T. (1962) An autopsy study of cerebrovascular accidents in diabetes mellitus. *Circulation*, **25**, 663.

Anderson, H. J. & Staffurth, J. S. (1955) Subacute bacterial endocarditis in the elderly. *Lancet*, ii, 1055.

Anderson, R. & Schechter, M. (1959) A case of spontaneous dissecting aneurysm of the internal carotid artery. *Journal of Neurology, Neurosurgery and Psychiatry*, **22**, 195.

Anthony, M., Hinterberger, H. & Lance, J. W. (1968) The possible relationship of serotonin to the migraine syndrome. In *Research and Clinical Studies in Headache*, ed. Friedman, A. P. Basel and New York: Karger.

Armsworth, R. W. & Gresham, G. H. (1961) Giant cell arteritis with rupture of aorta. *Journal of Pathology and Bacteriology*, **82**, 203.

Asbury, A. K., Aldredge, H., Hershberg, R. & Fisher, C. M. (1970) Oculomotor palsy in diabetes mellitus: a clinico-pathological study. *Brain*, **93**, 555.

Ballantyne, D., Groshart, K. W. G., Ballantyne, J. P., Young, A. & Lawrie, T. D. B. (1974) Relationship of plasma lipids and lipoproteins to cerebral atherosclerosis and ECG findings. In *Third International Symposium of Atherosclerosis, West Berlin*. Berlin and New York: Springer-Verlag.

Barnes, W. T. & Jacoby, G. F. (1962) Aneurysm of the common carotid artery due to cystic medial necrosis treated by excision or graft. *Annals of Surgery*, **155**, 82.

Barr, H. W. K., Blackwood, W. & Meadows, S. P. (1971) Intracavernous carotid aneurysms—a clinical pathological report. *Brain*, **94**, 607.

Bauer, R., Sheehan, S. & Meyer, J. S. (1961) Arteriographic study of cerebrovascular disease. *Archives of Neurology*, **4**, 119.

Beighton, P. (1970) *The Ehlers Danlos Syndrome*. London: Heinemann.

Bickerstaff, E. R. (1964) Aetiology of acute hemiplegia in childhood. *British Medical Journal*, ii, 82.

Bickerstaff, E. R. & Holmes, J. M. (1967) Cerebral arterial insufficiency and oral contraceptives. *British Medical Journal*, i, 726.

Blackwood, W. (1958) Vascular disease of the central nervous system. In *Neuropathology*, Greenfield, J. G., Meyer, A., Norman, R. M., McMenemey, W. H. & Blackwood, W. London: Arnold.

Brice, J. G. & Crompton, M. R. (1964) Spontaneous dissecting aneurysms of the cervical internal carotid artery. *British Medical Journal*, ii, 790.

Bryan, C. S. (1969) Non bacterial thrombotic endocarditis with malignant tumours. *American Journal of Medicine*, **46**, 787.

Cairns, S. H. (1942) *Lisboa Medica*, **19**, 375.

Cairns, H. & Russell, D. S. (1946) Cerebral arteritis and phlebitis in pneumococcal meningitis. *Journal of Pathology and Bacteriology*, **58**, 649.

Caldwell, H. W. & Hadden, F. C. (1948) Carotid artery thrombosis; report of 8 cases due to trauma. *Annals of Internal Medicine*, **28**, 1132.

Carson, N. A. J., Dent, C. E. & Field, C. M. B. (1965) Homocystinuria: a clinical and pathological review of 10 cases. *Journal of Paediatrics*, **66**, 565.

Carter, A. B. (1965) Prognosis of cerebral embolism. *Lancet*, ii, 514.

Caspary, E. A. & Peberdy, M. (1965) Oral contraception and blood platelet adhesiveness. *Lancet*, i, 1142.

Chievitz, E. & Thiede, T. (1962) Complications and causes of death in polycythaemia vera. *Acta Medica Scandinavica*, **172**, 513.

Citron, B. P., Halpern, M., McCarron, M., Lundberg, G. D., McCormick, R., Pincus, T. J., Tatter, D. & Halverback, B. J. (1970) Necrotising angiitis associated with drug abuse. *New England Journal of Medicine*, **283**, 1003.

Cohen, R. J., Bohannon, R. A. & Wallerstein, R. O. (1966) Waldenstrome's macroglobulinaemia. *American Journal of Medicine*, **41**, 274.

Collaborative Group for the Study of Stroke in Young Women (1973) Oral contraception and increased risk of cerebral ischemia or thrombosis. *New England Journal of Medicine*, **288**, 871.

Connor, R. C. R. (1962) Complicated migraine. *Lancet*, ii, 1072.

Costero, I. (1949) Cerebral lesions responsible for death of patients with active rheumatic fever. *Archives of Neurology and Psychiatry*, **62**, 48.

Crompton, M. R. (1959) Visual changes in temporal arteritis. *Brain*, **82**, 377.

Cross, J. N., Castro, P. O. & Jennett, W. B. (1968) Cerebral strokes associated with pregnancy and the puerperium. *British Medical Journal*, iii, 214.

Cumings, J. N., Grundt, I. K., Holland, J. T. & Marshall, J. (1967) Serum lipids and cerebrovascular disease. *Lancet*, ii, 194.

Currier, R. D., De Jong, R. N. & Bole, G. C. (1954) Pulseless disease: central nervous system manifestations. *Neurology* (Minneapolis), **4**, 818.

Dalal, P. M. (1973) Aortic arch syndrome. In *Tropical Neurology*, ed. Spillane, J. D. Oxford University Press.

Dalal, P. M., Shah, P. M. & Aiyer, R. R. (1965) Arteriographic study of cerebral embolism. *Lancet*, ii, 358.

Daley, R., Mattingly, T. W., Holt, C. L., Bland, E. F. & White, P. D. (1951) Systemic arterial embolism in rheumatic heart disease. *American Heart Journal*, **42**, 566.

Danarj, T. J., Wong, H. O. & Thomas, M. A. (1963) Primary arteritis of the aorta causing renal artery stenosis and hypertension. *British Heart Journal*, **25**, 153.

Darling, R. L., Austen, W. G. & Linton, R. R. (1967) Arterial embolism. *Surgery, Gynecology and Obstetrics*, **124**, 106.

Denny-Brown, D. & Foley, J. M. (1952) The syndrome of basilar aneurysm. *Transactions of the American Neurological Association*, **77**, 30.

Dixon, J. M. (1951) Angioid streaks and pseudoxanthoma elasticum with aneurysm of the internal carotid artery. *American Journal of Ophthalmology*, **34**, 1322.

Entmacher, P. S., Root, H. F. & Marks, H. H. (1964) Longevity of diabetic patients in recent years. *Diabetes*, **13**, 373.

Enzell, K. & Lindemalm, G. (1973) Cryptogenic cerebral embolism in women taking oral contraceptives. *British Medical Journal*, iv, 507.

Facon, E., Mestes, E. & Georgesco, T. (1960) Polyarteritis nodosa with lesions particularly in large cerebral arteries. *Revue Neurologique*, **103**, 147.

Fairburn, B. (1957) Thrombosis of internal carotid artery after soft palate injury. *British Medical Journal*, ii, 750.

Fisher, C. M. (1959) Ocular palsy in temporal arteritis. *Minnesota Medicine*, **42**, 1258.

Fisher, C. M. (1971) Cerebral ischaemia — less familiar types. *Clinical Neurosurgery*, **18**, 267.

Fogelholm, R. & Aho, K. (1973) Ischaemic cerebrovascular disease in young adults. 1. Smoking habits, use of oral contraceptives, relative weight, blood pressure and electrocardiographic findings. *Acta Neurologica Scandinavica*, **49**, 415.

Ford, F. R. (1952) Syncope, vertigo and disturbances of vision resulting from intermittent obstruction of the vertebral artery. *Bulletin of Johns Hopkins Hospital*, **91**, 168.

Ford, F. R. & Clark, D. (1956) Thrombosis of the basilar artery with softenings in the cerebellum and brain stem due to manipulation of the neck. *Bulletin of Johns Hopkins Hospital*, **98**, 37.

Ford, R. G. & Siekert, R. G. (1965) Central nervous system manifestations of periarteritis nodosa. *Neurology* (Minneapolis), **15**, 114.

Freedman, P., Moulton, R. & Spencer, A. G. (1958) Hypertension and diabetes mellitus. *Quarterly Journal of Medicine*, **27**, 293.

Frens, D. B., Petrjan, J. H., Anderson, R. & Leblanc, H. J. (1974) Fibromuscular dysplasia of the posterior cerebral artery: report of a case and review of the literature. *Stroke*, **5**, 161.

Friedli, B., Aerichide, N., Grondin, P. & Campeau, L. (1971) Thromboembolic complications of heart valve prostheses. *American Heart Journal*, **81**, 702.

Glaser, G. H. (1952) Lesions of the central nervous system in disseminated lupus erythematosis. *Archives of Neurology and Psychiatry*, **67**, 745.

Gold, A. P. & Yahr, M. D. (1960) Childhood lupus erythematosis; a clinical and pathological study of the neurological manifestations. *Transactions of the American Neurological Association*, **85**, 96.

Goodwin, J. F. (1963) Diagnosis of left atrial myxoma. *Lancet*, i, 464.

Graf, C. J. (1965) Spontaneous carotid-cavernous fistula. *Archives of Neurology*, **13**, 662.

Graveson, G. S. (1949) Retinal arterial occlusion in migraine. *British Medical Journal*, ii, 838.

Greenfield, J. G. (1951) Discussion of some less common cerebrovascular diseases. *Proceedings of the Royal Society of Medicine*, **44**, 855.

Groch, S. N., Sayre, G. P. & Heck, F. J. (1960) Cerebral haemorrhage in leukaemia. *Archives of Neurology*, **2**, 439.

Gunning, A. J., Pickering, G. W., Robb Smith, A. H. T. & Russell, R. W. R. (1964) Mural thrombosis of the subclavian artery and subsequent embolism in cervical rib. *Quarterly Journal of Medicine*, **33**, 133.

Haft, H., Finneson, B. E., Cramer, H. & Fiol, R. (1957) Polyarteritis nodosa as a source of subarachnoid haemorrhage and spinal cord compression. *Journal of Neurosurgery*, **14**, 608.

Hamilton, C. R., Shelley, W. M. & Tumulty, P. A. (1971) Giant cell arteritis including temporal arteritis and polymyalgia rheumatica. *Medicine*, **50**, 1.

Hardin, C. A. (1962) Successful resection of carotid and abdominal aneurysms in two related patients with Marfans syndrome. *New England Journal of Medicine*, **267**, 141.

Harker, L. A., Slichter, S. J., Scott, R. & Ross, R. (1974) Homocystinaemia vascular injury and arterial thrombosis. *New England Journal of Medicine*, **291**, 537.

Harman, J. B. & Leslie, E. M. (1967) Survival of polycythaemia vera patients treated with radioactive phosphorus. *British Medical Journal*, ii, 146.

Hearn, G. W. & Roper-Hall, M. J. (1961) Obstruction of central retinal artery associated with chorea. *British Medical Journal* ii, 684.

Held, K., Jipp, P. & Schreier, A. (1973) Natural history and muscle blood flow of patients with occlusion of the subclavian arteries and aortic arch syndrome. In *Cerebral Vascular Disease: Sixth Salzburg Conference*, ed. Meyer, J. S., Lechner, H., Reivich, M. & Eichhorn, O. Stuttgart: Thieme.

Heyman, A., Nefzger, M. D. & Estes, E. H. (1961) Serum cholesterol in cerebral infarction. *Archives of Neurology*, **5**, 46.

Higashi, K., Hatano, M. & Maza, T. (1974) Disease with abnormal intracranial network complicated with intracerebral haematoma. *Journal of Neurology, Neurosurgery and Psychiatry*, **37**, 365.

Hilal, S. K. (1974) Arterial occlusive disease in infants and children. In *Radiology of the Skull and Brain*, ed. Newton, T. H. & Potts, D. G. Vol. 2, p. 2286–2309. St. Louis: C. V. Mosby.

Hills, J. & Sament, S. (1968) Bilateral agenesis of the internal carotid artery associated with cardiac and other anomalies. *Neurology* (Minneapolis), **18**, 142.

Hockaday, T. D. R. (1959) Traumatic thrombosis of the internal carotid artery. *Journal of Neurology, Neurosurgery and Psychiatry*, **22**, 229.

Holt, J. M. & Lambert, E. H. N. (1964) Heart disease as presenting feature in myotonia atrophica. *British Heart Journal*, **26**, 433.

Houser, O. W. and Baker, H. L. (1968) Fibromuscular dysplasia and other uncommon diseases of the cervical carotid artery: angiographic aspects. *American Journal of Roentgenology*, **104**, 201.

Howie, P. W., Mallinson, A. C., Prentice, C. R. M. & McNicol, G. (1970) Effect of combined oestrogen-progestogen oral contraceptives, oestrogen, and progestogen on antiplasmin and antithrombotic activity. *Lancet*, ii, 1329.

Hughes, J. T. & Brownell, B. (1966) Granulomatous giant-cell arteritis of the central nervous system. *Neurology* (Minneapolis), **16**, 293.

Hutchinson, E. C. & Stock, J. P. P. (1963) Paroxysmal cerebral ischaemia in rheumatic heart disease. *Lancet*, ii, 653.

Illis, L., Kocen, R. S., McDonald, W. I. & Mondkar, V. P. (1965) Oral contraceptives and cerebral arterial occlusion. *British Medical Journal*, ii, 1164.

Inman, W. H. W. & Vessey, M. P. (1968) Investigation of death from pulmonary coronary and cerebral thrombosis and embolism in women of child-bearing age. *British Medical Journal*, ii, 193.

Inman, W. H. W., Vessey, M. P., Westerholm, B. & Engelund, A. (1970) Thromboembolic disease and the steroidal content of oral contraceptives: a report to the Committee on Safety of Drugs. *British Medical Journal*, ii, 203.

Isom, O. W., Williams, C. D., Falk, E. A., Spencer, F. C. & Glassman, E. (1973) Evaluation of anticoagulant therapy in cloth covered prosthetic valves. Supplement III to *Circulation*, **47** and **48**, 48.

Jakobsen, T. (1967) Glucose tolerance and serum lipid levels in patients with cerebrovascular disease. *Acta Medica Scandinavica*, **182**, 233.

Johnson, B. I. (1951) Paradoxical embolism. *Journal of Clinical Pathology*, **4**, 316.

Johnson, R. T. & Richardson, E. P. (1968) The neurological manifestations of systemic lupus erythematosis. *Medicine*, **47**, 337.

Jones, K. S. & Sim, M. (1961) Thrombotic microangiopathy presenting as a psychiatric problem. *British Medical Journal*, i, 1359.

Jörgensen, L. & Torvik, A. (1966) Ischaemic cerebrovascular disease in an autopsy series. *Journal of Neurological Sciences*, **3**, 490.

Kagan, A. R., Bruce, D. W. & Di Chiro, G. (1971) Fatal foam cell arteritis of the brain after irradiation for Hodgkin's disease. Angiography and pathology. *Stroke*, **2**, 232.

Kahn, P. (1973) A histopathological study of three cases of Anderson-Fabry disease. *Journal of Neurology, Neurosurgery and Psychiatry*, **36**, 1053.

Kao, C. C., Messert, B., Winkler, S. S. & Turner, J. H. (1974) Rheumatoid atlanto-axial dislocation: pathogenesis and treatment. *Journal of Neurology, Neurosurgery and Psychiatry*, **37**, 1069.

Kaul, S. N., Du Boulay, G. H., Kendall, B. E. & Russell, R. W. R. (1974) Relationship between visual field defect and arterial occlusion in the posterior cerebral circulation. *Journal of Neurology, Neurosurgery and Psychiatry*, **37**, 1022.

Keen, H., Rose, G., Pyke, D. A., Boyns, D., Chlouverakis, C. & Mistry, S. (1965) Blood sugar and arterial disease. *Lancet*, ii, 505.

Kemball, R. W., Friedman, A. P. & Vallejo, E. (1960) Effect of serotonin in migraine patients. *Neurology* (Minneapolis), **10**, 107.

Kety, S. S. (1950) Circulation and metabolism of the human brain in health and disease. *American Journal of Medicine*, **8**, 205.

Knox, D. L. (1965) Ischaemic ocular inflammation. *American Journal of Ophthalmology*, **60**, 995.

Kudo, T. (1968) Spontaneous occlusion of the Circle of Willis a disease apparently confined to Japanese. *Neurology* (Minneapolis), **18**, 485.

Kurrein, F. (1954) Cerebral mucormycosis. *Journal of Clinical Pathology*, **7**, 141.

Lawrence, J. H., Berlin, N. I. & Huff, R. L. (1953) The nature and treatment of polycythaemia: studies on 263 patients. *Medicine*, **32**, 323.

Lee, J. E. & Haynes, J. M. (1967) Carotid arteritis and cerebral infarction due to scleroderma. *Neurology* (Minneapolis), **17**, 18.

Levesque, M., Lefebvre, J., Bories, J. & Legre, J. (1974) Infantile forms of the syndrome of progressive stenosis of branches of the polygon of Willis. *Journal Neuroradiologique*, **1**, 55.

Lhermitte, F., Gautier, J. C., Derouesne, C. & Buirand, B. (1968) Ischaemic accidents in the middle cerebral artery territory. *Archives of Neurology*, **19**, 248.

Lhermitte, F., Gautier, J. C. & Poirier, J. (1968) Hypoplasia of the internal carotid artery. *Neurology* (Minneapolis), **18**, 439.

Litchfield, H. R. (1938) Carotid artery thrombosis complicating retropharyngeal abscess. *Archives of Paediatrics*, **55**, 36.

Lognelli, G. T. & Buchhert, W. A. (1971) Angiitis in drug abusers. *New England Journal of Medicine*, **284**, 112.

Logothetis, J., Silverstein, P. & Coe, J. (1960) Neurological aspects of Waldenstrom's macroglobulinaemia. *Archives of Neurology*, **3**, 564.

Macmillan, G. C. (1950) Diffuse granulo-arteritis with giant cells. *Archives of Pathology*, **49**, 63.

Mathew, N. T., Abraham, J. & Chandy, J. (1970) Cerebral angiographic features in tuberculous meningitis. *Neurology* (Minneapolis), **20**, 1015.

Mathew, N. T., Abraham, J., Taori, G. M. & Gopalakrishna, V. I. (1971) Internal carotid artery occlusion in cavernous sinus thrombosis. *Archives of Neurology*, **24**, 11.

Matzke, J., Clansen, J. & Guttier, F. (1964) Significance of paraproteinaemia in patients with primary neurologic symptoms. *Acta Neurologica Scandinavica*, **40**, 269.

McCollister, B. D., Bayrd, E. D., Harrison, E. G. & McGuckin, W. F. (1967) Primary macroglobulinaemia. *American Journal of Medicine*, **43**, 394.

McDonald, W. I. & Sanders, M. D. (1971) Migraine complicated by ischaemic papillopathy. *Lancet*, ii, 521.

McKusick, V. (1966) *Heritable Disorders of Connective Tissue*. St. Louis: C. V. Mosby.

Meadows, S. P. (1951) Intracranial aneurysms. In *Modern Trends in Neurology*, Feiling, A. London: Butterworth.

Metz, H., Murray-Leslie, R. M., Bannister, R. G., Bull, J. W. D. & Marshall, J. (1961) Kinking of the internal carotid artery in relation to cerebrovascular disease. *Lancet*, i, 424.

Meyer, J. S., Waltz, A. G., Hess, J. W. & Zak, B. (1959) Serum lipid and cholesterol levels in cerebrovascular disease. *Archives of Neurology* (Chicago), **1**, 303.

Michael, W. F. (1974) Posterior fossa aneurysms simulating tumours. *Journal of Neurology, Neurosurgery and Psychiatry*, **37**, 218.

Miller, H. G. & Daley, R. (1946) Clinical aspects of periarteritis nodosa. *Quarterly Journal of Medicine*, **15**, 255.

Millikan, C. H., Siekert, R. G. & Whisnant, J. P. (1960) Intermittent carotid and vertebrobasilar insufficiency associated with polycythaemia. *Neurology* (Minneapolis), **10**, 188.

Modan, B. (1971) *The polycythaemic disorders*. Thomas, Springfield.

Musoke, L. K. (1966) Neurologic manifestations of malaria in children. *East African Medical Journal*, **43**, 561.

New, P. J. F. (1966) Arterial stationary waves. *American Journal of Roentgenology*, **97**, 488.

Nurick, S., Blackwood, W. & Mair, W. P. G. (1972) Giant cell granulomatous angiitis of the central nervous system. *Brain*, **95**, 133.

Nutter, D. O. & Kramer, N. C. (1965) Macrocryogelglobulinemia. *American Journal of Medicine*, **38**, 462.

Ojemann, R. G., Fisher, C. M. & Roch, J. C. (1972) Spontaneous dissecting aneurysm of the internal carotid artery. *Stroke*, **3**, 434.

Parish, J. G. (1960) Hereditable disorders of connective tissue. *Proceedings of the Royal Society of Medicine*, **53**, 515.

Parker, H. L. & Kernohan, J. W. (1949) Central nervous system in periarteritis nodosa. *Mayo Clinic Proceedings*, **24**, 43.

Peck, F. C. & McGovern, F. R. (1966) Radiation necrosis of the brain in acromegaly. *Journal of Neurosurgery*, **25**, 536.

Picard, L., Andre, J. M., Roland, J., Arnould, G., Lepoire, J., Crouzet, G. & Djindjian, R. (1974) Moya-Moya syndrome of the adult. Transient forms. *Journal Neuroradiologique*, **1**, 69.

Picard, L., Floquet, J., Andre, J. M., Montaut, J. & Salamon, G. (1974) Syndrome Moya-Moya: etude anatomo pathologique. *Journal de Neuroradiologie*, **1**, 113.

Poliak, S. (1957) *The Vertebral Visual System*. University of Chicago Press.

Portnoy, B. A. & Herion, J. C. (1972) Neurologic manifestations in sickle cell disease with review of literature and emphasis on prevalence of hemiplegia. *Annals of Internal Medicine*, **76**, 643.

Poser, C. M. & Taveras, J. M. (1957) Cerebral angiography in encephalotrigeminal angiomatosis. *Radiology*, **68**, 327.

Price, D. L., Harris, J. L., New, P. F. G. & Cantu, R. C. (1970) Cardiac myxoma. *Archives of Neurology*, **23**, 558.

Roach, M. R. & Drake, C. G. (1965) Ruptured cerebral aneurysms caused by microorganisms. *New England Journal of Medicine*, **273**, 240.

Robertson, M. A. & Schroder, J. S. (1959) Pseudoxanthoma elasticum. *American Journal of Medicine*, **27**, 433.

Roger, H., Poursines, Y. & Roger, J. (1955) Les aspects neurologiques de la periarterite nodeuse. *Revue Neurologique*, **92**, 430.

Rose, G. A. & Spencer, H. (1957) Polyarteritis nodosa. *Quarterly Journal of Medicine*, **26**, 43.

Rosen, P. & Armstrong, D. (1973) Non bacterial thrombotic endocarditis in patients with malignant neoplastic diseases. *American Journal of Medicine*, **54**, 23.

Ross, R. S. & McKusick, V. (1953) Aortic arch syndromes. *Archives of Internal Medicine*, **92**, 701.

Rubenstein, M. A. (1959) Unusual remission in a case of thrombotic thrombocytopenic purpura syndrome following fresh blood exchange transfusion. *Annals of Internal Medicine*, **51**, 1409.

Rubenstein, M. K. & Cohen, N. H. (1964) Ehlers Danlos syndrome associated with multiple intracranial aneurysms. *Neurology* (Minneapolis), **14**, 125.

Russell, R. W. R. (1959) Giant cell arteritis: a review of 35 cases. *Quarterly Journal of Medicine*, **28**, 471.

Russell, R. W. R. (1973) The posterior cerebral circulation. *Journal of the Royal College of Physicians*, **7**, 331.

Sarkavi, N. B. S., Holmes, J. M. & Bickerstaff, E. R. (1970) Neurological manifestations associated with internal carotid loops and kinks in children. *Journal of Neurology, Neurosurgery and Psychiatry*, **33**, 194.

'Schimke, R. N., McKusick, V. A., Huang, T. & Pollack, A. D. (1965) Homocystinuria. Studies of 20 families with 38 affected members. *Journal of the American Medical Association*, **193**, 711.

Schneider, R. C. & Crosby, E. C. (1959) Vascular insufficiency of brain stem and spinal cord in spinal trauma. *Neurology* (Minneapolis), **9**, 643.

Schneider, R. C. & Schemm, G. W. (1961) Vertebral artery insufficiency in acute and chronic spinal trauma. Journal of Neurosurgery, **18**, 348.

Schwartz, C. J., Mitchell, J. R. A. & Hughes, J. T. (1962) Transient recurrent cerebral episodes and aneurysm of the carotid sinus. *British Medical Journal*, i, 770.

Segal, J. P., Harvey, W. P. & Gurel, T. (1965) Diagnosis and treatment of primary myocardial disease. *Circulation*, **32**, 837.

Siekert, R. G., Whisnant, J. P. & Millikan, C. H. (1960) Anaemia and intermittent focal cerebral arterial insufficiency. *Archives of Neurology*, **3**, 386.

Siekert, R. G. & Jones, H. R. (1970) Transient ischaemic attacks associated with subacute bacterial endocarditis. *Stroke*, **1**, 178.

Silverstein, A. (1968) Thrombotic thrombocytopenia purpura the initial neurologic manifestations. *Archives of Neurology*, **18**, 358.

Silverstein, A., Gilbert, H. & Wasserman, L. P. (1962) Neurologic complications of polycythaemia. *Annals of Internal Medicine*, **57**, 909.

Sinclair, R. J. G., Kitchin, A. H. & Turner, R. W. D. (1960) The Marfan Syndrome. *Quarterly Journal of Medicine*, **29**, 19.

Skinhøj, E. & Paulson, O. B. (1969) Regional blood flow in internal carotid distribution during migraine attack. *British Medical Journal*, iii, 569.

Smith, K. R., Nelson, J. S. & Dolley, J. M. (1968) Bilateral hypoplasia of the internal carotid arteries. *Neurology* (Minneapolis), **18**, 1149.

Soloman, G. E., Hilal, S. K., Gold, A. P. & Carter, S. (1970) Natural history of acute hemiplegia of childhood. *Brain*, **93**, 107.

Spach, M. S., Howell, D. A. & Harrison, J. S. (1963) Myocardial infarction and multiple thrombosis in a child with primary thrombocytosis. *Pediatrics*, **31**, 268.

Stockman, J. A., Nigro, M. A., Mishkin, M. M. & Oski, F. A. (1972) Occlusion of large cerebral vessels in sickle cell anaemia. *New England Journal of Medicine*, **287**, 846.

Strachan, R. W. (1966) Prepulseless and pulseless Takayasus arteritis. *Postgraduate Medical Journal*, **42**, 464.

Sullivan, J. M., Harken, D. E. & Gorlin, R. (1968) Pharmacologic control of thromboembolic complications of cardiac valve replacement. *New England Journal of Medicine*, **279**, 576.

Susuk, J. & Takaku, A. (1969) Cerebrovascular moya-moya disease. *Archives of Neurology*, **20**, 288.

Swash, M. & Earl, C. J. (1970) Transient visual obscurations in chronic rheumatic heart disease. *Lancet*, ii, 323.

Takayasu, M. A. (1908) A case with peculiar changes of the central retinal vessels. *Acta Societatis Japonicae*, **12**, 554.

Taveras, J. M. (1969) Multiple progressive intracranial arterial occlusions; a syndrome of children and young adults. *American Journal of Roentgenology*, **106**, 235.

Thapedi, I., Ashenhurst, E. & Rozdilsky, B. (1970) Spontaneous dissecting aneurysm of the internal carotid artery in the neck. *Archives of Neurology* (Chicago), **23**, 549.

Tolosa, E. (1954) Periarteritic lesions of the carotid siphon with the clinical features of a carotid infraclinoid aneurysm. *Journal of Neurology, Neurosurgery and Psychiatry*, **17**, 300.

Torvik, A. & Jorgensen, L. (1966) Thrombotic and embolic occlusion of the carotid arteries in autopsy material 2. Cerebral lesions and clinical course. *Journal of the Neurological Sciences*, **3**, 410.

Turnbull, L. (1962) Agenesis of the internal carotid artery. *Neurology* (Minneapolis), **12**, 588.

Vitek, J. V., Halsey, J. H. & McDowell, H. A. (1972) Occlusion of all four extracranial vessels with minimum clinical symptomatology. *Stroke*, **3**, 462.

Walsh, J. P. & O'Doherty, D. S. (1960) A possible explanation of the mechanism of ophthalmoplegic migraine. *Neurology* (Minneapolis), **10**, 1079.

Warren, S., Le Compte, P. M. & Legg, M. A. (1966) *The Pattern of Diabetes Mellitus*. 4th edn. Philadelphia: Lea and Febiger.

Webb, F. W. S., Hickman, J. A. & Brew, D. St. J. (1968) Death from vertebral artery thrombosis in rheumatoid arthritis. *British Medical Journal*, ii, 537.

Weibel, J. & Fields, W. S. (1965) Tortuosity, coiling and kinking of the internal carotid artery. *Neurology* (Minneapolis), **15**, 7.

Weir, R. J., Briggs, E., Mack, A., Taylor, L., Browning, J., Naismith, L. & Wilson, E. (1971) Blood pressure in women after one year of oral contraceptives. *Lancet*, i, 467.

Wells, C. E. (1959) Cerebral emboli the natural history prognostic signs and effects of anticoagulants. *Archives of Neurology and Psychiatry*, **81**, 667.

Wells, C. E. (1961) Premonitory symptoms of emboli. *Archives of Neurology*, **5**, 490.

Whitty, C. W. M. (1953) Familial hemiplegic migraine, *Journal of Neurology, Neurosurgery and Psychiatry*, **16**, 172.

Wilkinson, I. M. S. (1972) The vertebral artery: extracranial and incranial structure. *Archives of Neurology* (Chicago), **27**, 392.

Wilkinson, I. M. S. & Russell, R. W. R. (1972) Arteries of the head and neck in giant cell arteritis. *Archives of Neurology*, **27**, 378.

Winkelman, N. W. & Eckel, J. L. (1932) The brain in acute rheumatic fever nonsuppurative meningoencephalitis rheumatica. *Archives of Neurology and Psychiatry*, **28**, 844.

Wise, D., Wallace, H. J. & Jellinek, E. H. (1962) Angiokeratoma corporis diffusum. *Quarterly Journal of Medicine*, **31**, 177.

Wolman, L. (1959) Cerebral dissecting aneurysms. *Brain*, **82**, 276.

Yaskin, H. E. & Alpers, B. J. (1944) Aneurysm of the vertebral artery. Report of a case in which the aneurysm simulated a tumour of the posterior fossa. *Archives of Neurology and Psychiatry*, **51**, 271.

Zeman, W. (1968) Article in *Pathology of the Nervous System*, ed. Minckler, J. Vol. 1. New York: McGraw-Hill.

Ziment, I. (1969) Nervous system complications in bacterial endocarditis. *American Journal of Medicine*, **47**, 593.

Index

Filmset in Ireland by Doyle Photosetting, Tullamore
Printed by T. & A. Constable Ltd., Edinburgh